P9-CCC-479

This is the eighth volume in the popular Cummings Foundation for Behavioral Health series beginning in 1991 that addresses healthcare utilization and costs. The Nicholas & Dorothy Cummings Foundation, in association with Context Press, is pleased to continue the tradition of distributing complimentary copies to the directors of American Psychological Association approved doctoral programs, to selected leaders in psychology, and to key persons in the field of behavioral healthcare.

It is hoped you will find this series useful in your work. The Cummings Foundation for Behavioral Health requests that after you have finished reading it, you donate it to the library of the institution with which you are affiliated.

Additional copies for individuals only, may be obtained as long as supplies last by sending $5.00 to cover postage and handling to the following address. Regretfully, repeat, multiple, and bulk requests cannot be accommodated.

Janet L. Cummings, Psy.D., President
The Nicholas & Dorothy Cummings Foundation, Inc.
4781 Caughlin Parkway
Reno, NV 89509

Library and Institutional copies may be ordered from CONTEXT PRESS for a charge of $29.95 plus shipping and handling.

Psychological Approaches to Chronic Disease Management

Psychological Approaches to Chronic Disease Management

A Report of the Fifth Reno Conference
on the Integration of
Behavioral Health in Primary Care

Editors:
Nicholas A. Cummings, Ph.D., Sc.D.
William T. O'Donohue, Ph.D.
Elizabeth V. Naylor

Cummings Foundation for Behavioral Health:
Healthcare Utilization and Cost Series,
Volume 8
2005

CONTEXT PRESS
Reno, Nevada

Psychological Aproaches to Chronic Disease Management

Hardback   pp. 270

Library of Congress Cataloging-in-Publication Data

Reno Conference on the Integration of Behavioral Health in Primary Care (5th : 2004 : Reno, Nev.)
   Psychological approaches to chronic disease management : a report of the Fifth Reno Conference on the Integration of Behavioral Health in Primary Care / editors Nicholas A. Cummings, William T. O'Donohue, Elizabeth V. Naylor.
   p. cm. – (Healthcare utilization and cost series ; v. 8)
   Includes bibliographical references.
   ISBN 1-878978-54-3 (hardback)
   1. Chronic diseases–Psychosomatic aspects. 2. Psychotherapy. 3. Medicine, Psychosomatic. 4. Clinical health psychology. I. Cummings, Nicholas A. II. O'Donohue, William T. III. Naylor, Elizabeth V. IV. Title. V. Series.
   RC108.R46 2004
   616'.001'9–dc22

                                                            2005013531

© 2005 Context Press
933 Gear Street, Reno, NV   89503-2729

All rights reserved.

No part of this book may be reproduced, stored in a retrieval system, or transmitted in any form or by any means, electronic, mechanical, photocopying, microfilming, recording, or otherwise, without written permission from the publisher.

Printed in the United States of America

The Healthcare Utilization and Cost Series
of the Cummings Foundation for Behavioral Health

Volume 1 (1991):
Medical Cost Offset: A Reprinting of the Seminal Research Conducted at Kaiser Permanente, 1963-1981
Nicholas A. Cummings, Ph.D. and William T. Follette, M.D.

Volume 2 (1993):
Medicaid, Managed Behavioral Health and Implications for Public Policy: A Report of the HCFA-Hawaii Medicaid Project and Other Readings.
Nicholas A. Cummings, Ph.D., Herbert Dorken, Ph.D., Michael S. Pallak, Ph.D. and Curtis Henke, Ph.D.

Volume 3 (1994):
The Financing and Organization of Universal Healthcare: A Proposal to the National Academies of Practice.
Herbert Dorken, Ph.D. (Forward by Nicholas Cummings, Ph.D.).

Volume 4 (1995):
The Impact of the Biodyne Model on Medical Cost Offset: A Sampling of Research Projects.
Nicholas A. Cummings, Ph.D., Sc.D., Editor.

Volume 5 (2002):
The Impact of Medical Cost Offset on Practice and Research: Making It Work for You. A Report of the Second Reno Conference, May 2002.
Nicholas A. Cummings, Ph.D., Sc.D., William T. O'Donohue, Ph.D., and Kyle E. Ferguson, M.S., Editors.

Volume 6 (2003):
Behavioral Health as Primary Care: Beyond Efficacy to Effectiveness.
A Report of the Third Reno Conference, May 2003.
Nicholas A. Cummings, Ph.D., Sc.D., William T. O'Donohue, Ph.D., and Kyle E. Ferguson, M.S., Editors.

Volume 7 (2004):
Early Detection and Treatment of Substance Abuse within Integrated Primary Care.
A Report of the Fifth Reno Conference, May 2004.
Nicholas a. Cummings, Ph.D., Sc.D., William T. O'Donohue, Ph.D., Melanie Duckworth, Ph.D., and Kyle E. Ferguson, M.A.

The Reno Conferences

Co-sponsored by the University of Nevada, Reno and
The Nicholas & Dorothy Cummings Foundation

The First Reno Conference on Organized Behavioral Healthcare Delivery was convened at the University of Nevada, Reno in January 1999.

The Second Reno Conference on Medical Cost Offset was convened at the University of Nevada, Reno in January 2001.

The Third Reno Conference on Medical Cost Offset and Behavioral Health in Primary Care was convened at the University of Nevada, Reno in May 2002.

The Fourth Reno Conference on Substance Abuse in Primary Care was convened at the University of Nevada, Reno in May 2003.

The Fifth Reno Conference on Psychological Approaches to Disease Management was convened at the University of Nevada, Reno in May 2004.

Preface

This book consists largely of expanded papers that were first presented at the Fifth Reno Conference on Psychological Approaches to Disease Management at the University of Nevada, Reno on May 21-22, 2005. This conference was generously supported by grants from The Nicholas and Dorothy Cummings Foundation and the University of Nevada, Reno.

The primary goal of this conference was to draw together psychologists who have done significant research in the area of chronic disease management so that they could interact publicly in ways that could spur new ideas and collaborations, and in ways that would help define the clinical, research and business agenda for the future. Assembling these experts in chronic disease management provided students, researchers, clinicians, and interested community members from the fields of psychology, medicine, nursing, social work, and health care administration with an opportunity to learn about the latest psychological treatment research addressing some of the leading and most costly chronic conditions in primary care.

A secondary goal of this conference was to illustrate that disease management may be the key to expanding psychology's economic base. This conference elicited discussion around how to actualize this possibility. Given the high costs associated with psychosocial pathways that lead to unnecessary utilization, psychologists have the potential to save billions of health care dollars annually.

The context of this conference is health care has undergone a dramatic change during the past century from tackling acute diseases such as small pox, influenza, and tuberculosis, to a new battle against chronic conditions, including diabetes, asthma, Alzheimer's disease, arthritis, and somatization. The costs associated with these chronic diseases have created a health care crisis in this country. Health care costs are now escalating at triple the rate of general inflation. Chronic disease such as the diabetes, asthma, dementias, arthritis, and coronary problems comprise the largest percentage of these costs. According to claims data compiled from the Oklahoma State Medicaid department for over 244,000 patients, the mean annual health care utilization cost for a patient with one chronic condition is $2,995, while the cost of a patient without a chronic condition is $612, suggesting that individuals with one chronic condition cost almost 5 times more to the health care system than individuals without a chronic condition (Garis and Farmer, 2002). The astronomical costs associated with chronic medical conditions cannot be understated and underscore the imperative for effective treatment and management protocols targeted at these conditions.

Although western medicine has evolved to effectively curb the incidence of acute conditions, it has not had similar success managing chronic conditions. Behavioral and psychological factors have repeatedly been shown to have a profound impact on the onset, progression, and management of chronic diseases. As evidenced by the rising prevalence rates of chronic disease, traditional health care providers lack appropriate tools to tackle the behavioral health issues associated with the current chronic disease epidemic. In addition, the psychological impact of having a chronic medical condition is not well addressed by conventional medical treatments (Friedman, Sobel, Myers, Caudill, & Benson, 1995).

Recently, disease management programs have been created to attempt to supplement the care received by the primary care or specialty care physician. However, these programs have generally been designed by physicians and nurses and do not optimally address the psychosocial drivers and comorbid problems associated with these chronic diseases. Fortunately, some psychologists have been doing important practical work in this area in developing more psychologically sophisticated protocols. Psychologically informed treatment protocols differ from traditional primary-care disease management protocols because they are developed with an understanding of the psychosocial antecedents to medical help seeking; and consequently, can address behavioral health issues associated with chronic conditions. It is imperative that traditional health care providers merge their expertise with behavioral health specialists who have done extensive research in the area of treatment adherence and lifestyle improvement (which are the cornerstones of successful chronic disease management) to create medically-sound, psychologically informed treatment protocols. An integrated approach to disease management in which experts in the fields of physical and behavioral medicine synthesize their knowledge offers a promising alternative to traditional medicine.

This book owes special thanks to Shera Alberti-Annunnzio who provided extensive assistance in organizing this conference. We are exceedingly grateful to our copy editor, Emily Neilan for her dedicated skill and outstanding effort in preparing this manuscript. Finally, we would like to thank all of the chapter authors who participated in the conference and furnished this volume with their excellent work.

References

Garis, R. I., & Farmer, K. (2002). Examining costs of chronic conditions in a medicaid population. *Managed Care, 11,* 43-50.

Friedman, R., Sobel, D., Myers, P., Caudill, M., & Benson, H. (1995). Behavioral medicine, clinical health psychology, and cost offset. *Health Psychology, 14,* 509-518.

Contributing Authors

David O. Antonuccio, Ph.D., ABPP

David O. Antonuccio received his B.A. (1975) in psychology (honors) and economics from Stanford University. He received his M.A. (1979) and Ph.D. (1980) in Clinical Psychology from the University of Oregon. He is currently Professor in the Dept. of Psychiatry and Behavioral Sciences at the University of Nevada School of Medicine and Director of the Stop Smoking Program at the V.A. Medical Center. He served on the Nevada State Board of Psychological Examiners from 1990 to 1998. His clinical and research interests include the behavioral treatment of depression, anxiety, and smoking. He holds a diplomate in Clinical Psychology from the American Board of Professional Psychology and is a Fellow of the American Psychological Association. He was named Outstanding Psychologist in 1993 by the Nevada State Psychological Association (NSPA), received an Award of Achievement from NSPA in 1999 for his work on depression, and was named the 2000 recipient of the McReynolds Foundation Psychological Services Award for outstanding contributions to clinical science. Dr. Antonuccio is internationally known for his work in depression and smoking cessation. His articles on the comparative effects of psychotherapy and pharmacotherapy have received extensive coverage by the national media and are models of careful scholarship.

James A. Blumenthal, Ph.D., ABPP

James A. Blumenthal, Ph.D., is a professor in the Department of Psychiatry and Behavioral Sciences and Professor of Psychology: Social and Health Sciences at Duke University. Dr. Blumenthal received his bachelor of science degree from the University of Pittsburgh and his Ph.D. in clinical psychology from the University of Washington. He completed a predoctoral internship and a postdoctoral fellowship at Duke University Medical Center. Dr. Blumenthal is board certified in clinical psychology from the American Board of Professional Psychology and is a senior fellow at the Duke University Center for the Study of Aging and Human Development. He also received an honorary doctorate in Medicine from the Uppsala University. He is the author of three edited books, 35 book chapters, and more than 200 articles in refereed journals. He is a Fellow in Divisions 12, 20 and 38 of the American Psychological Association, the Society of Behavioral Medicine, the Academy of Behavioral Medicine Research, and the American Association of Cardiopulmonary Rehabilitation. Dr. Blumenthal is past president of both the American Psychosomatic Society and the Division 38 (Health Psychology) of the American Psychological Association. He serves on the editorial board of a number of journals including Health Psychology and Psychosomatic Medicine.

Thomas Creer, Ph.D.

Thomas Creer received his B.A. in 1956 from Brigham Young University, M.S. in psychology from Utah State University in 1963, and his Ph.D. in clinical psychology in 1967 from Florida State University. He has been honored with a National Science Foundation Assistantship, U.S. Public Health Fellowship, and in 2003 and 2004, Who's Who in America. Dr. Creer is currently on the Board of Directors for the American Lung Association of Utah and the Associate Editor for the Journal of Asthma. A referee for over 20 journals, he has been on the Board of Editors for the Annals of Allergy, Asthma, & Immunology, Pediatric Asthma, Journal of Asthma, and Pediatric Asthma, Allergy & Immunology. He has been invited to present papers on asthma in several international conferences including the XII European Conference for Psychosomatic Medicine in Norway, Italian-American Scientific Exchange in Italy, First International Congress of Behavioral Medicine in Sweden, and Second International Congress of Behavioral Medicine in Germany. His consultantships included the Italian-American Scientific Exchange Program, American Academy of Allergy and Immunology Committee, Glaxo Wellcome, Schering, and MURO. He has had numerous committee appointments, and remains an active Committee member of the American Academy of Allergy & Clinical Immunology. He has received over 25 grant awards from agencies including but not limited to the National Institute of Heart, Lung, and Blood, the National Institute of Mental Health, the Academic Challenge Award, Division of Research Resources, Public Health Service, and National Institute of Allergic and Infectious Diseases for his research on asthma. Furthermore, Dr. Creer has published over 160 articles and chapters and 13 books and his most recent writings address asthma management.

Nicholas A. Cummings, Ph.D., Sc.D.

Nicholas A. Cummings, Ph.D., Sc.D. is a Distinguished Professor of Psychology, University of Nevada, Reno; President of the Foundation for Behavioral Health; Chair, Board of Directors for Nicholas and Dorothy Cummings Foundation; Chair, Board of Directors for University Alliance for Behavioral Health, Inc.; and, Member, American Psychological Association

Dr. Cummings is one of the nation's premier experts on the provision of managed behavioral health services. He served as Chief Psychologist and later Senior Psychologist at Kaiser Permanente for over 25 years. In 1985, Dr. Cummings founded American Biodyne, Inc., a practitioner driven national behavioral health service provider that grew to become a major managed behavioral healthcare organization providing services to over 14.5 million enrollees in 39 states by 1992. He led American Biodyne's successful IPO in 1991. Dr. Cummings retired from his position as Chief Executive Officer and Chairman of American Biodyne, Inc. in 1993 following the company's merger with MedCo containment Services and Merck Pharmaceuticals.

Dr. Cummings was the 87th president of the American Psychological Association (1979-1980), and served on two Presidential Mental Health Commissions for Presidents Kennedy and Carter. He was advisor to the U.S. Senate Subcommittee on Health (Senator Ted Kennedy, Chair) for three years, the U.S. Senate Finance Committee for four years, and the Health Economics Branch of what is now the Department of Health and Human Services for six years. He has testified before the U.S. Congress 18 times on behalf of psychology and mental health issues and his research findings have been entered into the Congressional Record 23 times. In 1984, the American Psychological Association conferred upon Dr. Cummings its highest professional award for Distinguished Contributions to Practice.

Furthermore, Dr. Cummings has published 18 books and over 400 journal articles and book chapters on topics including high-utilizers in primary care, somatization in primary-care, substance abuse in primary care and integrated care.

Alan M. Delamater, Ph.D., ABPP

Alan M. Delamater received his Ph.D. from the University of Georgia in 1981. He is currently Professor of pediatrics and Director of clinical psychology at the Mailman Center for Child Development and the Department of Pediatrics at the University of Miami School of Medicine, where he has been since 1991. Prior to that, he was on the psychology faculty at Washington University (1981-1987) and Wayne State University (1987-1991). He has served in a number of leadership roles in professional organizations. With the American Diabetes Association, he served as scientific sessions program chair for the Council of Behavioral Medicine and Health Psychology from 1994-1997, and was a member of the Scientific Sessions Planning Committee from 1995-1997 and the Research Policy Committee from 1998-2000. With the National Institutes of Health, he served on a number of grant review committees since 1992; from 1999-2003 was a member of the Risk, Prevention, Health Behavior (2) Study Section; and from 2003-2004 was a member of the Psychosocial Risk and Disease Prevention Study Section. With the APA Society of Pediatric Psychology, he served as the co-chair for post-doctoral training on the Task Force on Training in Pediatric Psychology, is currently chair of a Task Force on Access to Pediatric Psychology Services, and since 2000 has represented Division 54 on APA's Interdivisional Health Care Committee.

As a researcher, he has consistently received grant funding from NIH and other agencies, and has published widely in the field of pediatric psychology. While most of his research has focused on psychosocial and behavioral aspects of diabetes in children and adolescents, he has also published in a number of other areas, including asthma, cystic fibrosis, and cardiovascular disease, among others. He was awarded the Lifescan Diabetes Research Award on two occasions (1997 and 1999) by the Society of Behavioral Medicine.

As a teacher, he has chaired over 30 dissertations, master's theses, and honor's theses. At the University of Miami, he teaches a graduate seminar in pediatric psychology and provides clinical supervision to interns and post-doctoral fellows;

lectures regularly to interns, post-doctoral fellows, and pediatric residents; and is program director of a training grant from NIH that provides support for pre-doctoral and post-doctoral research training in pediatric psychology. He is active as a clinician, and is board-certified in clinical health psychology.

Joshua Dyer

Joshua Dyer is a graduate student in the Clinical Rehabilitation Psychology program at Indiana University-Purdue University at Indianapolis. His primary area of research is cardiovascular reactivity and recovery in response to psychosocial stressors. With Criterion Health, he has worked on projects related to integrating behavioral medicine into primary care.

Robert Gatchel, Ph.D.

Robert Gatchel, Ph.D. is a professor in Departments of Psychiatry and Rehabilitation Science at the University of Texas Southwestern and the distinguished Elizabeth H. Penn Professor Clinical Psychology. Dr. Gatchel received his B.A. in 1969 from the State University of New York at Stony Brook, and M.S. and Ph.D. in clinical psychology from the University of Wisconsin in 1973. Dr. Gatchel is a diplomate of the American Boards of Professional Psychology, and is on the Board or Directors of the American Board of Health Psychology. He is also the recipient of the consecutive Research Scientist Development Awards from NIH. He is on the editorial boards of numerous journals and is a member or fellow of several professional organizations, including the American Psychological Association, the Academy for Behavioral Medicine Research, and the North American Spine Society. Dr. Gatchel has conducted extensive clinical research, much of it supported by grants from NIH, on the etiology, assessment, and treatment of chronic pain and stress behavior, the comorbidity of psychological and physical health disorders, and the psychophysiology of stress and emotion.

Robert Levy, Ph.D.

Robert Levy, Ph.D. is Director of Research and Evaluation for Criterion Health, Inc. In 2001 he retired, after 33 years, from Indiana State University as Professor Emeritus of Psychology and Coordinator Emeritus of General Education. His areas of specialization within psychology are cognitive processes, research methods, and human-computer interaction. With Criterion he has worked on projects related to the integration of behavioral services into primary care. In addition, he has directed the development of a self-management program for adults with serious and persistent mental illnesses and of a prevention program for youth living in Medicaid recipient families in which there is a member with a serious mental illness or substance abuse. Dr. Levy has served on the board of directors of the Vigo County, Indiana, and National Mental Health Associations; the local community mental health center; the Mental Health Advisory Council and the Addictions Planning Council for the Indiana Department of Mental Health and

Addictions; and chaired the Governor's Advisory Panel for the Grassroots Prevention Coalitions Initiative.

Ronald F. Levant, Ed.D., M.B.A., ABPP

Since earning his doctorate in Clinical Psychology and Public Practice from Harvard in 1973, Ronald F. Levant has been a clinician in solo independent practice, clinical supervisor in hospital settings, clinical and academic administrator, and academic faculty member. He has served on the faculties of Boston, Rutgers, and Harvard Universities. He is currently Dean and Professor, Center for Psychological Studies, Nova Southeastern University. Dr. Levant has authored, co-authored, edited or co-edited over 200 publications, including 13 books and 130 refereed journal articles and book chapters in family and gender psychology and in advancing professional psychology. Dr. Levant has also served as President of the Massachusetts Psychological Association, President of APA Division 43 (Family Psychology), co-founder and the first President of APA Division 51 (the Society for the Psychological Study of Men and Masculinity), two term member and two term Chair of the APA Committee for the Advancement of Professional Practice, two term member of the APA Council of Representatives, Member-At-Large of the APA Board of Directors, and two term Recording Secretary of APA. He is currently serving as President of APA.

Brie Moore, M.A., M.S.

Brie Moore has a Master's degree in Child Development from the University of California at Davis, a Master's degree in Clinical Psychology and is currently a doctoral student in the Clinical Psychology program at the University of Nevada, Reno. Ms. Moore has written practice guidelines for adult weight loss and behavioral pediatric practice, conducted a critical review of empirically-supported treatments of pediatric obesity and has delivered professional trainings and presentations, including at National conferences for the Society for Research in Child Development and the Association for the Advancement of Behavior Therapy on the topics of developmental and behavioral pediatrics. Additionally, Ms. Moore has served as the sole Developmental Specialist for the Children and Families Commission sponsored Integrated Family Support Initiative, a project providing treatment for typically under-served pediatric populations, and is currently the lead behavioral healthcare specialist on an integrated care program evaluation project. Ms. Moore has also recently completed a randomized controlled trial evaluating a primary care behavioral pediatrics intervention she developed (Moore et al., 2004).

Elizabeth V. Naylor

Elizabeth V. Naylor is a doctoral student in the clinical psychology program at the University of Nevada, Reno, Staff Therapist at the University of Nevada, Reno Counseling Services, and former Assistant Director of Research for the Office of Geriatric Medicine at the University of Nevada, Reno. A graduate of Bates College in May 2000, Research Assistant from 2000-2001 at the University of Vermont, and Program Coordinator for the Office of Minority Health, Department of Health and Human Services from 2001-2002, Ms. Naylor is currently working with Dr. Antonuccio and Dr. O'Donohue in a research program that involves the development of behavioral prescriptions as a treatment for depression in the primary care setting.

William T. O'Donohue, Ph.D.

William T. O'Donohue is a professor of Psychology at the University of Nevada, Reno; Nicholas Cumming Professor of Organized Behavioral Healthcare Delivery; and, President and Chief Executive Officer, University Alliance for Behavioral Care, Inc.

Dr. O'Donohue holds academic appointments at the University of Nevada, Reno, in psychology, psychiatry and philosophy and is an Adjunct Professor Psychology at the University of Hawaii Monoa. A licensed psychologist in Nevada, Dr. O'Donohue is widely recognized in the field for his proposed innovations in mental health service delivery, in treatment design and evaluation, and in knowledge of empirically supported cognitive behavioral therapies. Dr. O'Donohue has served as the Director of several psychological clinics, including the Psychological Service Center (1996-1999) and the Victims of Crime Treatment Center (since 1996) at the University of Nevada, Reno. He is a member of the Association for the Advancement for Behavior Therapy and served on the Board of Directors of this organization. Dr. O'Donohue has an exemplary history of successful grant funding. Since 1996, he has received over $1,500,000 in grant monies from sources including the National Institute of Mental Health and the National Institute of Justice. He is currently a standing grant review member for the Substance Abuse Mental Health Service Administration. In addition, Dr. O'Donohue has editted over twenty books, written thirty-five book chapters on various topics, published reviews for seven books, and published greater than seventy-five articles in scholarly journals. Furthermore, he has been a grant reviewer for NIMH, SAMHSA, on the editorial board for four different peer-reviewed journals, and has reviewed manuscripts for 12 different prestigious psychology journals.

Table of Contents

Chapter 1

Disease Management: Current Issues

William O'Donohue
University of Nevada, Reno
Elizabeth V. Naylor
University of Nevada, Reno
Nicholas A. Cummings
University of Nevada, Reno and the Cummings Foundation for Behavioral Health

"Changing the present [health care] system to better treat chronic health conditions is our nation's current health challenge."
(Partnership for Soulutions, 2002, pg. 42)

Chronic Conditions: Genesis of Disease Management

Today, more than 125 million Americans are diagnosed with a chronic medical condition; and, as the population ages, this number is expected to increase to 157 million by 2020 (Wu & Green, 2000). According to the Centers for Disease Control and Prevention, chronic diseases account for over 70% of all deaths in the United States (1999). The four most common causes of death are cardiovascular disease, cancer, cerebrovasular disease, and chronic obstructive pulmonary disease (CDC, 1999). A chronic illness generally lasts a year or longer, limits the activities one can participate in, and requires ongoing medical care (Partnership for Solutions, 2002). Chronic conditions threaten all individuals of our society, transcending every age, race, and socioeconomic category. It is estimated that 24% of Americans have one chronic condition and 21% have two or more (Wu & Green, 2000).

What are the chronic conditions impacting the quality of life of close to half of all Americans? According to the 1998 Medical Expenditure Panel Survey (AHRQ), the most frequent chronic illnesses diagnosed in the nonistitutionalized adult population (which excludes those living in nursing homes or in-patient facilities) in descending order of prevalence include, hypertension (26%), chronic mental health conditions (22%), respiratory diseases (18%), arthritis (13%), heart disease (12%), eye disorders (10%), asthma (10%), cholesterol disorders (9%), and diabetes (9%). Chronic conditions afflicting the noninstitutionalized child population (age 0-17) are respiratory diseases (33%), asthma (28%), emotional/ behavioral disorders (16%), and eye disorders (9%).

Advances in medicine are allowing Americans to live longer than ever before; and as Americans age, they are more likely to develop chronic illnesses. It has been found that of Americans who are 65 and older, 85% have one or more chronic conditions and 62% have two or more chronic conditions (Wu & Green, 2000). A more detailed look at the following data of chronic conditions through ascending age categories further demonstrates that there is a relationship between increasing age and prevalence of chronic conditions: 0-19 years old, 24% one or more and 5% two or more; 20-44 years old, 38% one or more and 13% two or more; and, 45-64 years old, 62% one or more and 35% two or more (Wu & Green, 2000). Considering census data which suggest that the number of older Americans will rise, in 2004 12.7% of the population was 65 or older; however by 2040 this number is projected to increase to 20.5% (U.S. Bureau of the Census, 2000), it is relatively safe to hypothesize that unless our health care system designs effective prevention and early intervention programs to reverse the course of several chronic diseases, chronic conditions are only going to become an increasing problem.

Chronic conditions are gaining significant amounts of attention by various health care systems because they are extremely expensive to treat; and consequently, are draining the resources of the current health care system. In fact, 78% of all health care spending is directed toward people with chronic conditions, while 22% goes towards people without chronic conditions (Medical Expenditure Panel Survey, 1998). When numbers are further analyzed, 57% of health care spending is directed towards individuals with two or more chronic conditions. Not surprisingly, individuals with chronic conditions use the most services; they account for 96% of home health care visits, 88% of prescriptions, 72% physician visits, and 76% inpatient stays. A look at the following average per capita health care spending indicates that as the number of chronic conditions increases, so does health care spending; 0 chronic conditions ($800), 1 chronic condition ($1900), 2 chronic conditions ($3400), 3 chronic conditions ($5600), 4 chronic conditions ($8900), and 5+chronic conditions, ($5000) (1998 Medical Expenditure Panel Survey, AHRQ). It has also been found that health care spending for people with chronic conditions is disproportional to the percent of people with chronic conditions (Partnership for Solutions, 2002). Specifically, 78% of health care spending is attributed to 44% of noninsitutionalized population that has one or more chronic conditions; 68% of private health insurance spending is attributed to the 40% of privately insured people who have chronic conditions; 60% of all health care spending for the uninsured is for care received by the 27% of uninsured people with chronic conditions; and finally, 77% of Medicaid spending is for the almost 40% of nonistiutionalized Medicaid beneficiaries with chronic conditions.

Primary care physicians are generally the first line of defense in the treatment of chronic conditions. In a survey which interviewed over 1200 physicians who have at least 20 hours of weekly patient contact, physicians reported the following on their beliefs regarding treating patients with chronic illness: (1) dissatisfaction with providing care to individuals with chronic conditions (54% very satisfied with care for patients vs. 36% very satisfied with care for patients with chronic conditions); (2) poor outcomes often result from poor care coordination (54% receipt of contradictory information, 49% unattended emotional problems, 44% adverse drug interactions, 36% unnecessary hospitalization, 34% not functioning to potential, 34% experience unnecessary pain, and 24% unnecessary nursing home placement); (3) access to specific services is difficult or very difficult; (84% mental health care, 80% adequate health insurance, 78% respite care for family, 75% patient special education or training, 65% prescription drugs, 56% medical specialists, 55% other health care professionals, and 53% primary care doctors) (Mathmatica Policy Research, Inc., 2001).

In a comprehensive report on the status of chronic disease management in America, *Chronic Care. Making the Case for Ongoing Conditions* Parternship for Solutions (2002) determined that, "changing the present system to better treat chronic health conditions is our nation's current health challenge" (pg. 42). This statement was supported with findings that resulted from an analysis of hard data from a variety of sources. This report made the following conclusions about the current status of managing chronic conditions:

1. The reality of the 21st century is that increasing numbers of individuals with chronic conditions are demanding care that is not appropriately organized to effectively address their needs.
2. Medical technology has rapidly improved; however, the system of financing and delivering care has not changed at a rate necessary to effectively treat chronic disease.
3. The system of health care has begun to embrace disease management programs that target specific chronic conditions; however, has not changed with the times to effectively provide care for people with multiple chronic conditions.
4. A new model of care is needed that provides coordination and quality care for people who suffer from chronic conditions.

The report proposed the following solutions in order to tackle the conclusions drawn above:

1. Financial and reimbursement incentives are needed to encourage early diagnosis with interventions that emphasize a maintenance of health status, and decrease acute episodes and disability associated with conditions. When acute episodes occur, coordinated care (services from a variety of disciplines determined by patient's needs) should aim to bring the individual back to highest functional status that is possible.

2. Financial incentives are needed for coordination of care (vs. splintering of care which is currently the norm).
3. Better connections between supportive and clinical care delivery systems are needed.
4. Training of health care providers need to be examined in order to better prepare them for the changing realities of medical practice and patients' needs associated with providing care to patients with chronic conditions.

Disease Management

Disease management has been proposed as the method for addressing the chronic disease epidemic that most health care systems are ill-equipped to target (as evidenced by prevalence, cost, and physician data previously cited). Disease management has been defined in a variety of ways, an internet search to define the term yields over 20 definitions (Definitions of diseasemanagement on the web, 2004). The lack of consistency in defining disease management may partially explain why success in combating chronic conditions in most health care systems remains minimal at best and expensive without question. For instance, it has been defined generally as, "the process of a physician managing a patient's disease (such as asthma or diabetes) on a long-term, continuing basis, rather than treating it as a single episode" (Sansum-Santa Barbara Medical Foundation Clinic, 2004); to more specifically as, "a system of coordinated health care interventions and communications for populations with conditions in which patient self-care efforts are significant;" (Disease Management Association of America, 2004). The DMAA further identifies a disease management program as one that; (1) supports the physician or practitioner/patient relationship and plan of care, (2) emphasizes prevention of exacerbations and complications utilizing evidence-based practice guidelines and patient empowerment strategies, and, (3) evaluates clinical, humanistic, and economic outcomes on an ongoing basis with the goal of improving overall health. The DMAA specifies the components of disease management programs as: (1) population identification processes, (2) evidence-based practice guidelines, (3) collaborative practice models to include physician and support-service providers, (4) patient self-management education (may include primary prevention, behavior modification programs, and compliance/surveillance), (5) process and outcomes measurement, evaluation, and management, and (6) routine reporting/feedback loop (may include communication with patient, physician, health plan and ancillary providers, and practice profiling).

In the last few decades, disease management has emerged as an important innovation in the manner in which health care is delivered. Traditionally, health care delivery has focused on acute care: a patient problem is assumed to need a delimited episode of care, which results in sufficient recovery or cure so that further care is no longer needed or wanted. This model of service delivery works well for many, but not all, health problems. Simple fractures, strept throat, syphilis, and most gunshot wounds are all well suited for this kind of delivery system. However, many have come to realize that this delivery system fails or at best results in suboptimal care for other chronic medical problems, and particularly those chronic problems that involve both medical and behavioral (e.g., lifestyle) components. This failure is judged to be significant given the high frequencies of these chronic diseases, demographic changes that suggest trends towards even higher frequencies in the future (i.e., longer lifespans), ominous trends in public health (e.g., increased child obesity; see Moore and O'Donohue, this volume) as well as the high costs of failures to manage these diseases. Because of the frequencies of these chronic diseases are both high and predictable, some have regarded disease management programs as requiring a paradigm shift in the way health care services are delivered that involves population management rather than the more traditional individual case management approach.

Another major reason disease management has emerged is because of the spiraling health care costs in the last two decades. Health care has increased at several times the general rate of inflation. It now presents a significant financial burden to employers as well as the government. The trend is particularly worrisome when projected into the future and its impact on the national debt as well as the competitiveness of American companies who have to pay high and constantly increasing premiums are considered. In 1960 health care comprised 4% of the Gross Domestic Product. In 1999 it comprised 11% of GDP and just five years later it consumes approximately 15%. Many regard this as an alarming rate of growth. It is well known that health care utilization is disproportionate: about 20% of patients are responsible for 80% of health care costs. A major percentage of these most costly patients are those with chronic diseases (O'Donohue &Cucciarre, in press). These costs are even higher when one assumes indirect costs such as lower worker productivity. Thus, there has been increasing attention given to chronic diseases as a way to reign in spiraling health care costs. According to the Disease Management Association in 1999, one billion dollars was spent on the implementation of disease management programs (Weingarten et al., 2002). Bodenheimer (2000) suggests that in 1999 there were 200 disease management companies providing these services.

A list of these chronic diseases that need to managed over longer periods of time (including time periods as long as the entire lifetime) include:

1. diabetes
2. asthma
3. COPD
4. heart disease (heart failure, hypertension, angina)
5. arthritis
6. other chronic pain (back pain, migraine)
7. obesity
8. depression
9. Alzheimer's disease and other dementias
10. renal disease
11. peptic ulcer

12. epilepsy
13. osteoporosis
14. AIDs
15. substance abuse

Although some of these programs are associated with demographic variables such as gender or age, another complexity is that sometimes programs need to be designed for certain demographic groups, e.g., pediatric asthma or Spanish speaking diabetics. An increasing important issue pertains to designing optimal disease management programs for patients who have more than one of these chronic diseases. Hoffman, Rice and Song (1996) have data indicating that half of all individuals with one chronic disease have at least one other chronic disease (comprising 39 million Americans in 1987).

Another important way that disease management can be, although not necessarily is, innovative is that it can integrate medical and behavioral care (Cummings, O'Donohue, & Ferguson, 2003). Part of the reason why the traditional acute care model may work better is that it requires less of the patient. The patient may need simply to show up for the appointment and then fairly passively cooperate as medical professionals actively implement the treatment. Often in the traditional acute care system the patient then is simply asked to swallow pills, raise an arm to put on monitors such as blood pressure cuff, lie down, or follow instructions to lie still in bed, etc—all while the medical professional is usually watching or near by to make sure the patient complies. Chronic disease management, on the other hand, requires the patient to engage in long term self management, with behaviors that can be difficult to control (smoking cessation, diet changes) outside the direct monitoring of health professionals.

It is certainly the case that individuals need medical education and support, so, for example, they can monitor their blood sugar levels and administer insulin. This requires an initial medical diagnosis, continued prescriptions, and continued monitoring by medical professionals. But the question becomes, is this all that the patient requires? Will the vast majority of patients provided with just this care successfully manage their chronic disease? Those involved in health care delivery are increasingly realizing that the answer is no. This negative answer appears to be due to several factors. First, many chronic conditions require significant lifestyle changes. Patients will need to learn to eat differently, exercise, identify and avoid certain higher risk situations (asthmatics), and develop new skill sets (e.g., to tolerate pain, arthritics). These behaviors do not emerge automatically nor even once instituted remain over time in most individuals. Patients with a chronic disease may also need to acquire certain psychological skills in order to better accomplish these. Psychological skills such as distress tolerance, self control, urge surfing and acceptance may be key. Finally, because of the chronic and complex nature of these diseases the patient and health care professionals need to form a long term working partnership in order to effectively manage their problem. This may require a new skill set and attitude on the part of both the health care providers and the patients.

For example, Clark and Gong (2000) have suggested that physicians can better form a partnership working with patients in chronic disease and should become competent in the following communication skills:

1. Attend to the patient (signaled by cues such as making eye contact, sitting rather than standing when conversing with the patient, moving closer to the patient, and leaning slightly forward to attend to the discussion).
2. Elicit the patient's underlying concerns about the condition.
3. Construct reassuring messages that alleviate fears (reducing fear as a distraction enables the patient to focus on what you are saying).
4. Address any immediate concerns that the family expresses (enabling patients to refocus their attention toward the information being provided).
5. Engage the patient in interactive conversation through use of open ended questions, simple language, and analogies to teach important concepts (dialogue that is interactive produces richer information).
6. Tailor the treatment regimen by eliciting and addressing potential problems in the timing, dose, or side effects of the drugs recommended.
7. Use appropriate non-verbal encouragement (such as a pat on the shoulder, nodding in agreement) and verbal praise when the patient reports using correct disease management strategies.
8. Elicit the patient's immediate objective related to controlling the disease and reach agreement with the family on a short term goal (that is, a short term objective both provider and patient will strive to reach that is important to the patient).
9. Review the long term plan for the patient's treatment so the patient knows what to expect over time, knows the situations under which the physician will modify treatment, and knows the criteria for judging the success of the treatment plan.
10. Help the patient plan in advance for decision making about the chronic condition (such as using diary information or guidelines for handling potential problems and exploring contingencies in managing the disease).

Those designing and implementing disease management programs have increasingly come to realize that the most effective programs integrate medical care with psychological/behavioral health care to help patients handle problems such as stress, poor social support, depression, treatment adherence, and comorbid psychological problems (e.g., alcoholism) that impact the management of their chronic disease. For example, Lorig and Holman (2000) state:

The role of health care professionals must also change. One of their responsibilities is to act as a partner in care. It is the job of the patient to monitor symptoms, report them accurately, and manage the disease on a day to day basis. It is the job of the health professional to act as a consultant, interpreter of symptoms, and resource person and to offer treatment suggestions (pg.4).

Lorig and Holman view disease management as supporting self management in three areas: (1) medical management of the condition, (2) maintaining, creating or changing meaningful life roles, and (3) emotional regulation. These core areas resulted in a five-prong curriculum covering: (1) problem solving, (2) decision making, (3) resource utilization, (4) forming health care provider/patient collaboration, and (5) taking action. These authors further postulate that Bandura's construct of self efficacy is a key to the success of a self management program.

The Effectiveness of Disease Management

Gordon Paul (1967) has posed a key question regarding understanding and evaluating psychological interventions, namely, "What treatment, by whom is most effective for this individual, with that specific problem, and under what specific set of circumstances?" This question explicates some of the more important dimensions and nuances of the therapeutic enterprise and implies that questions such as, "Does disease management work?", are simply too crude. This is due to both the heterogeneity of disease management programs and the scarcity of careful evaluations of many of these. Some of the major dimensions of this variability will be briefly outlined and discussed below. It is important that patients utilize disease management programs that are evidence based but the variability of these programs and the way they are evaluated make simple judgments regarding their evidential base somewhat difficult.

Disease management programs can differ dramatically. They differ on the modality in which they are delivered. Common modes include:

1. brochures
2. bibliotherapy
3. email
4. websites
5. phone calls
6. one on one face to face encounters
7. group sessions
8. combinations of the above

Disease management programs also differ in terms of the professionals delivering these services. Although no careful surveys have been conducted currently it appears as if nurses are most frequently involved. Health care professionals implementing disease management programs include:

1. physicians (primary care, specialist or subspecialists)
2. psychologists
3. nurses
4. pharmacists
5. social workers
6. master level psychologists
7. health educators
8. nutritionists
9. bachelor level specialty trained professionals
10. some combination of the above (e.g., alternating between a subset of these professionals or being managed by a team of some subset of these professionals)

A very important component of disease management is that it should coordinate the patient's care across diverse health professionals to insure that care is consistent, comprehensive, and nonredundant. Many regard that an optimal way of doing this is that the disease management program involve a multidisciplinary team each with different skill sets that coordinates that patient's care. This may require health professionals who are used to practicing alone to develop skills in functioning as a member of a team.

The content of disease management programs can often differ. Common topics included are:

1. Medical information about the disease
2. Increasing motivation and commitment (e.g., motivational interviewing)
3. Decision support (e.g., regarding treatment options)
4. Training in the requisite medical skills to manage the disease (inhaler use or blood sugar monitoring)
5. General self monitoring/self assessment skills
6. Treatment compliance
7. Skills regarding interacting with the health care system
8. Depression
9. Lifestyle change such as diet and exercise
10. Gaining social support
11. Stress management
12. Lifestyle change
13. Relapse Prevention
14. Reminders
15. Financial incentives

Part of the focus of disease management is prevention. The goal is that by addressing some issues early or even before they occur, problems such as retinopathy in a diabetic due to treatment noncompliance or depression can be prevented. Disease management programs also differ in levels of intensity. Major options include:

1. One or two episodes of interventions
2. Short term (few months of interventions)
3. Longer term interventions (years)

These options also differ in the system used to deliver the disease management program. Major variations are:

1. In the treating physicians office by physician staff
2. By a dedicated external disease management organization external to the treating physician (perhaps hired by the health plan)
3. At the worksite

These can also differ on the kind of patients targeted:

1. All patients with the diagnosis
2. Some subset, such as the most expensive high utilizers with the diagnosis
3. Some subset defined by criteria such as "at risk"

Disease management programs can also vary in whether they also support the health care providers. Some disease management programs provide education, practice guidelines, reminders and even financial incentives to the providers, while others do not. Another complication in making judgments regarding the value of disease management programs is that they also may be evaluated differently. Major options include:

1. No evaluation (this may be all too common)
2. Financial evaluation looking at cost savings or return on investment over
3. Various time periods
4. Clinical evaluation looking at Hemoglobin A1c or depression scores
5. Patient satisfaction
6. Provider satisfaction
7. Quality of life
8. Functional Status

These evaluations can differ in status from ongoing quality improvement to simple research/program evaluations in which outcomes are not used as feedback for real time improvements. The designs of the evaluation can also range from randomly controlled clinical trials (comparing to placebo or treatment as usual) to pre-post studies to case studies. They also vary in whether they are retrospective or prospective, and particularly the length of any follow up evaluations. In addition, their samples can vary from convenience samples to representative samples of some population. They vary on the extent to which a coherent treatment model or theory is guiding the intervention. They can also vary on the quality of the dependent variables (self report of treatment adherence vs. pill counts). They also vary on the range of outcome variables, e.g., medical and behavioral as well as whether these are also measured as process variables. Finally, their analyses differ on the extent to which they control for demographic or severity of illness variables.

Thus, one can see the permutations that are produced just by the variables articulated above. Such variability can be quite good as we should not assume that "one size fits all." One way that this variability can be organized and used to some advantage is through a stepped care approach. In this approach several levels of intervention are organized hierarchically. Patients are then triaged into a level that fits the severity of their problems or is consistent with their choice or ability to pay. Thus, there can be a progression from email, to phone calls, to group intervention, to one on one interventions. This can be consistent with the often ignored ethical dictum of using the least intrusive intervention. Patients who fail at one level can then be placed in a higher level. Stepped care is often recognized as an optimum strategy for population management.

Another important issue is the extent to which other operational and administrative requirements are explicated. Disease management programs are not just clinical entities. They often require information technology (e.g., to identify and track the target population); they require administrative buy in and changes (e.g., who manages and problem solves the implementation; reporting relationships and financial accounting); as well as new skills for support staff (e.g., new record keeping or scheduling). The success or failure of disease management programs can often depend on these kinds of variables which are often give short shrift in descriptions of disease management programs.

Wagner, Davis, Schaefer, Von Korff and Auston (1999) examined 72 disease management programs nominated by experts in the field as being particularly innovative and effective They found that most of the nominated programs were limited in their effectiveness and dissemination by their reliance on traditional patient education rather than modern self-management techniques, poor linkages to primary care, and reliance on referrals rather than proactive population-based approaches. This is an important study as it may show that: (1) the proactive, epidemiologically based population management paradigm is slow to be adopted, even in the disease management field, (2) the clinical pathways to effective disease management are not being implemented, rather more simplistic education models are too often the only modality being tried, and (3) disease management still needs to coordinate health care services better, particularly with the primary chare physician. These are important issues for future researchers to keep in mind.

A Tripartite Stage Model of Disease Management

We believe that disease management needs to be viewed as consisting of three distinct stages. The first stage involves intervention readiness assessments and skills. Prochaska's stages of changes, recent work in acceptance and Miller's motivational interviewing are relevant here. Strategies need to be developed for patients in the precontemplation and contemplation stages rather than just assuming that all patients are ready to change. In addition, good psychological diagnoses is relevant to see if they are comorbid conditions that may need to be treated such as substance abuse or borderline personality disorder. The second stage of disease management involves the processes for change. Lorig has an excellent model as do the authors that follow. Cummings' Biodyne Model which involves a diverse curriculum involving psychoeducation, stress management, treatment adherence, social support, comorbid treatment of depression showed in a randomly controlled trial excellent clinical change as well as decreases in medical utilization of 40% in 18 months (Cummings, 1994). The third stage involves maintenance of change and relapse prevention. The work of Alan Marlatt is key here as well as designing the disease management program in such a way that reentry, continual support, and episodic booster sessions can occur.

The final issue to address is the development of evidence based clinical pathways or practice guidelines. Currently, there is a tremendous amount of variability in what a particular patient may experience across disease management programs. There need to be more data gathered and meta-analysis to reach some consensus regarding what program elements are most associated with what program outcomes. Then, professionals need to participate in effective training programs (another research question) and be monitored to ensure adherence and competence in these evidence based procedures.

Disease Management: Current Research and Contributions

Unfortunately, successful disease management programs are not currently being incorporated into a majority of health care systems. A lack of understanding of what successful disease management programs include and require may explain this expensive and inexcusable phenomenon. More specifically, a lack of integration of treatment targeted at the psychological variables associated with chronic disease frequently account for the inefficient health care system that currently exists to treat chronic conditions. An integrated system of behavioral health care that incorporates a variety of disease management programs offers a promising solution to these concerns raised. Although this approach has already been proven to be both efficacious and cost-effective (as reviewed in this volume by Cummings & Cummings, and; Cummings, Dorken, Pallak & Henke, 1990; Cummings, Cummings & Johnson, 1997), it has not been adopted by a majority of health care systems.

This book, *Psychological Approaches to Chronic Disease Management*, details psychology's role in combating chronic conditions that frequently present in primary care environments. This text was born out of the recognition that psychology may be a significant factor in solving the current health care crisis that is largely attributed to medicine's inability to appropriately treat chronic conditions which has consequently resulted in astronomical health expenditures. A primary objective of this book is to educate leaders in the fields of medicine, psychology, and health care administration on the extensive research that has and continues to be conducted in the realm of behavioral medicine to improve the management of chronic conditions.

Although this book will detail psychological approaches to some of the major chronic conditions plaguing the current health care system, by no means does it represent all of psychology's contributions to the field of chronic disease management. In fact, it only scratches the surface. It is important to recognize that significant work has also been done to develop interventions aimed at improving the management of several other chronic diseases, including but in no means limited to, coronary heart disease, chronic obstructive pulmonary disorder, and end stage renal disease. These conditions will be briefly presented below and will refer readers to literature that give them more deserving attention.

Coronary heart disease (CHD) has and continues to be the leading cause of death in the United States (American Heart Association, 2004). Over 13 million Americans are currently diagnosed with CHD; a chronic condition that costs the nation approximately 133.2 billion dollars (American Heart Association, 2004). CHD has been a focus of behavioral medicine research for the past several decades. Behavioral and psychological factors associated with the prevention and management of the disease are well documented (Smith and Leon, 1992; Rozanski et al., 1999; Swenson and Clinch, 2000). Several disease management programs have been targeted at CHD and an associated condition, congestive heart failure (CHF). Due to the prevalence and cost of CHF, several health care systems have created multidisciplinary disease management programs targeted at preventing heart failure. In an extensive review of the literature from 1983-1998, Rich analyzed sixteen different multidisciplinary disease management programs targeted at CHF and determined that multi-disciplinary heart failure disease management programs are a cost-effective method of reducing morbidity and enhancing quality of life in some patients with heart failure (1999); and, the optimal approach to heart disease management should be the focus of future research. For a detailed review of behavioral medicine's contributions to CHD, see Smith and Ruiz, (2002). For an analysis of CHF disease management programs, the reader is referred to Rich (1999).

Chronic obstructive pulmonary disease (COPD) has been identified as the fourth leading cause of death in the United States (American Lung Association, 2004). In 2004, the annual cost of COPD to the nation was estimated to be 37.2 billion dollars (American Lung Association, 2004). COPD often results in significant disability among older adults and a decreased quality of life (Cugell, 1998). Psychological and behavioral correlates of COPD limiting a patient's quality of life include, decreased social activity, decline in functioning in normal day activities, anxiety, and depression (McSweeny, Grant, Heaton, Adams, & Timms, 1982; Agle

& Baum, 1977). The presence of psychological disorders, like anxiety and depression, in COPD patients significantly affects medical outcome (Singer, Ruchinskas, Riley, Broshek, & Barth, 2001); and often go unrecognized (Gore, Brophy, & Greenstone, 2000). Management of COPD is targeted at early identification, changing smoking habits, the use of bronchiodialaters to improve pulmonary function, quality of life, comorbidities, mortality, symptoms, and acute exacerbation rate (Briggs, 2004); all areas where health psychologists play a crucial role. See Briggs (2004) for a detailed presentation of the research concerning the prevalence, pathogenesis, and treatment of COPD.

End stage renal disease (ESRD) affects over 300,000 Americans. This chronic disease is life threatening, incurable, and requires careful management. In many cases, ESRD is a secondary medical complication that results from an ongoing diagnosis of diabetes or hypertension. Fourty years ago, a diagnosis of ESRD lead to a close death. However, advances in medical technology and an understanding of the psychological correlates of managing ESRD have allowed ESRD patients to live for several years with the disease, if appropriately managed. Treatment options for ESRD include renal transplantation and many different types of renal dialysis (that require adhering to particular diet, fluid-intake, and medication regimens). The modality of treatment for a particular patient is heavily influenced by a variety of nonmedical and psychological variables in both the patient and provider in order to determine which treatment will maximize patient adherence and quality of life (Christensen & Moran, 1998; Davison, 1996). Similar to many other chronic conditions, patient nonadherence and psychological distress have been found to contribute to greater morbidity and earlier mortality of this disease (Christensen & Ehlers, 2002). Thus, effective disease management programs for the management of ESRD must take into account individual patient differences, particularly matching a patient's coping style with the demands of the type of medical intervention (Christensen & Moran, 1998). For a thorough analysis of the current state of affairs regarding psychology's contributions to understanding and managing ESRD, the reader is referred to Christensen and Ehlers (2002).

Several themes are evident in this collection of chapters written by scientist-practitioners who have been active clinicians and researchers in their respective fields of behavioral medicine. The notion that our health care system is outdated and ill-equipped to deal with chronic conditions when psychological services are reserved for mental health problems in a "carve-out" system is consistently supported. The necessity to embrace the biopsychosocial model as the health care model of the future vs. the biomedical model of the outdated past is underscored. Self-management and adherence are presented as crucial treatment components in all interventions designed to target individual or multiple chronic conditions. Decreasing medical expenditures is discussed as an essential component of effective treatment. Reimbursement of behavioral services is presented as an impediment to effective behavioral health care. Additionally, many of the authors highlight the need to remove the stigma associated with mental health care so both patients and physicians can benefit from behavioral health care specialists in an integrated system. Finally, the value of integrated behavioral health care is emphasized again and again as the effective approach to manage chronic conditions.

The first few chapters present research evidence that encourages the integration of behavioral health into the primary care setting. The second chapter, *Psychological Approaches to the Management of Health and Disease: Health Care for the Whole Person*, provides an overview of our current health care system and how it needs and can be changed in order to incorporate behavioral health. The author, Ronald Levant, President 2005 of the American Psychological Association, discusses the magnitude of the Cartesian error, reviews research that underscores the success and impact of psychological interventions on medicine, and emphasizes psychology's changing role from that of a mental health specialty field to a more general behavioral health field. Furthermore, he highlights impediments to change in our health care system and proposes a future vision of health care that integrates behavioral health.

The third chapter, *Behavioral Interventions for Somatizers Within the Primary Care Setting*, presents decades of research conducted by the primary author, Nicholas Cummings, Ph.D, Sc.D, and other notable contributors to the field that support the integration of behavioral health care into primary care. In addition, the two authors provide rationale, a treatment protocol, and research evidence on why and how to treat somatization. They also emphasize the utility of group protocols as a treatment approach for chronic conditions and outline a specific protocol for patients who are diagnosed with borderline personality disorder.

The fourth chapter, *Integrated Model for Changing Patient Behavior in Primary Care*, draws upon research in the field of psychology, health economics, and medicine to propose a model of integrated care where the bottom line is revenue generation. The authors support the utility of their model by discussing the realities of primary care, needs of patients, and components of successful behavior change interventions in the past. They present the logistical and financial issues associated with their proposed integrated model and highlight the need for mental health practitioners, physicians, and other clinicians working in primary care settings to rethink the way behavioral health specialists practice (in terms of the services they provide).

The remaining chapters discuss psychologically-driven interventions for the treatment of specific chronic conditions, including hypertension, diabetes, asthma, pain, depression, and obesity. Although each chapter is unique in its presentation and content, most chapters provide background information on each condition, review relevant research, provide practical advice to clinicians, and discuss evidence-based interventions for specific chronic disease management in the primary care setting.

References

Agency for Healthcare Research and Quality (AHRQ). (n.d.). *1998 Medical Expenditure Panel Survey*. Retrieved November 8, 2004 from http://www.ahrq.gov

Agle, D. P., & Baum, G. L. (1977). Psychological aspects of chronic obstructive pulmonary disease. *The Medical Clinics of North America, 61*(4), 749-758.

American Heart Association. (2004). *2004 Heart and Stoke Statistical Update.* Retrieved on November 20, 2004 from http://www.americanheart.org/downloadable/heart/1079736729696HDSStats2004UpdateREV3-19-04.pdf

American Lung Association. (2004). *Trends in chronic bronchitis and emphysema: Morbidity and mortality.* Epidemiology and statistical unit. Retrieved on November 23, 2004 from http://www.lungusa.org/atf/cf/{7A8D42C2-FCCA-4604-8ADE-7F5D5E762256}/COPD1.PDF

Bodenheimer, T. (2000). Disease management in the American market. *British Journal of Medicine, 320*, 563-566.

Briggs, D. D. (2004). Chronic obstructive pulmonary disease overview: Prevalence, pathogenesis, and treatment. *Journal of Managed Care Pharmacy, 10*(4), S3-S10.

Centers for Disease Control and Prevention. (1999). *Chronic diseases and their risk factors: The nation's leading causes of death.* Washington, DC: U.S. Department of Health and Human Services.

Christensen, A. J., & Ehlers, S. L. (2002). Psychological factors in end-stage renal disease: An emerging context for Behavioral Medicine Research. *Journal of Consulting and Clinical Psychology, 70*(3), 712-724.

Christensen, A. J., & Moran, P. J. (1998). The role of psychosomatic research in the management of end-stage stage renal disease: A framework for matching patient to treatment. *Journal of Psychosomatic Research, 44*, 523-528.

Clark, N. M., & Gong, M. (2000). Management of chronic disease by practitioners and patients: are we teaching the wrong things. *British Medical Journal, 320*, 572-575.

Cugell, D. W. (1988). COPD: A brief introduction for behavioral scientists. In A. J. McSweeny & I. Grant (Eds.), *Chronic obstructive pulmonary disease: A behavioral perspective* (pp. 1-18). New York: Marcel Dekker.

Cummings, N. A. (1994). The successful application of medical offset in program planning and in clinical delivery. *Managed Care Quarterly, 2*, 1-6.

Cummings, N. A., Cummings, J. L., & Johnson, J. N. (Eds.). (1997). *Behavioral health in primary care: A guide for clinical integration.* Madison, CT: Psychosocial Press (an imprint of International Universities Press).

Cummings, N. A., Dorken, H., Pallak, M. S., & Henke, C. J. (1990). *The impact of psychological intervention on health care costs and utilization.* The Hawaii Medicaid Project. HCFA Contract Report # 11-C-983344/9.

Cummings, N. A., O'Donohue, W. T., & Ferguson, K. E. (Eds.). (2003). Behavioral health as primary care: Beyond efifcacy to effectiveness. Reno, NV: Context Press.

Davison, A. M. (1996). Options in renal replacement therapy. In C. Jacobs, C. Kjellstrand, K. Koch, & J. Winchester (Eds.), *Replacement of renal function by dialysis* (4th ed., pp. 1304-1315). Boston: Kluwer Academic.

Definitions of disease management on the web. Retrieved November 23, 2004 from http://www.google.com/search?hl=en&rls=CNDB,CNDB:2004-28,CNDB:en&oi=defmore&q=define:disease+management

Disease Management Association for America. (2004). Retrieved November 2, 2004 from http://www.dmaa.org/

Gore, J. M., Brophy, C. J., & Greenstone, M. A. (2000). How well do we care for patients with end stage chronic obstructive pulmonary disease (COPD)?: A comparison of palliative care and quality of life in COPD and lung cancer. *Thorax, 55,* 1000-06.

Hoffman, C., Rice, D., & Song, H. Y. (1996). Persons with chronic conditions: Their prevalence and costs. *Journal of the American Medical Association, 276* (18), 1473-1479.

Johns Hopkins University, Partnership for Solutions. (2002, December). Chronic conditions: Making the case for ongoing care. Retrieved October 8, 2004 from http://www.partnershipforsolutions.org/DMS/files/chronicbook2002.pdf

Lorig, K., & Holman, H. (2000). *Self management education: Context, definitions, outcomes and mechanisms.* Paper presented at first Chronic Disease Management Conference, Sydney Australia, August, 2000

Mathmatica Policy Research, Inc. (2001). *National Public Engagement Campaign on Chronic Illness Physician Survey, Final Report.* Princeton, NJ: Mathmatica Policy Reserach Inc., 7.

McSweeny, A. J., Grant, I., Heaton, R. K., Adams, K. M., & Timms, R. M. (1982). Life quality of patients with chronic obstructive pulmonary disease. *Archives of Internal Medicine, 142,* 473-478.

O'Donohue, W. T., & Cucciare, M. A. (inpress). The role of psychological factors in medical presentatioins. *Journal of Clinical Psychology in Medical Settings.*

Paul, G. L. (1967). Strategy of outcome research in psychotherapy. *Journal of Consulting Psychology, 31,* 109-118.

Rozanski, A., Bumenthal, J. A., & Kaplan, J. (1999). Impact of psychological factors on the pathogenesis of cardiovascular disease and implications for therapy. *Circulation, 99,* 2192-2217.

Rich, M. W. (1999). Heart failure disease management: A critical review. *Journal of Cardiac Failure, 5*(1), 64-75.

Sansum-Santa Barbara Medical Foundation Clinic. Retreived November 23, 2004 from http://www.sansum.com/site.asp

Singer, H. K., Ruchinskas, R. A., Riley, K. C., Broshek, D.K., & Barth, J. T. (2001). The psychological impact of end-stage lung disease. *Chest, 120,* 1246-52.

Smith, T. W., & Leon, A. S. (1992). *Coronary Heart Disease: A Behavioral Perspective.* Champaign-Urbana, IL: Research Press.

Smith, T. W., & Ruiz, J. M. (2002). Coronary Heart Disease. In A. J. Christensen & M. H. Antoni (Eds.), *Chronic physical disorders: Behavioral medicine's perspective* (pp. 83-111). Oxford: Blackwell Publishers Ltd.

Swenson, J. R., & Clinch, J. J. (2000). Assessment of quality of life in patients with cardiac disease: The role of psychosomatic medicine. *Journal of Psychosomatic Research, 48*, 405-415.

U.S. Bureau of the Census, Population Projections Program. (2000, January). *Projections of the Total Resident Population by 5-Year Age Groups and Sex with Special Age Catagories: Middle Series, 1999 to 2100*. (NP-T3). Retrieved on November 2, 2004 from http://www.census.gov/population/projections/nation/summary/np-t3-b.txt

Wagner, E. H., Davis, C., Schaefer, J., Von Korff, M., & Austin, B. (1999). A survey of leading chronic disease management programs: Are they consistent with the literature? *Managed Care Quarterly, 7*(3), 56-66.

Weingarten, S. R., Henning, J. M. Bardamgarav, E., Knight, K., Hasselbad, V., Gano, A., & Ofman, J. J. (2002). Interventions used in disease management programs for patients with chronic illnesses: Which ones work. *British Journal of Medicine, 325*, 1-8.

Wu, S., & Green, A. (2000, October). *Projection of a Chronic Illness Prevalence and Cost Inflation*. Santa Monica, CA: RAND Project Memorandum.

Chapter 2

Psychological Approaches to the Management of Health and Disease: Health Care for the Whole Person

Ronald F. Levant
Nova Southeastern University
APA President

We are living in truly interesting times, as the ancient Chinese curse goes. The 21st century promises monumental changes in health care. The technology currently available has already provided the tools whereby educated consumers can make critical decisions regarding their own health care, and health care providers can call up databases (such as Epocrates ®) to receive up to date information on pharmaceutical agents. Yet despite these promising technological developments, the status of health care in the U.S. is very troubling.

Health care costs have once again begun to escalate faster than other segments of the economy, and the number of uninsured is now 43.6 million Americans. The Secretary of the Department of Health and Human Services (HHS) met with leaders from the National Academies and challenged them to propose bold new ideas that might change conventional thinking about the most serious problems facing the health care system today. In response, the Institute of Medicine (IOM, 2002, p.1) reported: "The American health care system is confronting a crisis...Tens of thousands die from medical errors each year, and many more are injured. Quality problems, including underuse of beneficial services and overuse of medically unnecessary procedures, are widespread. And disturbing racial and ethnic disparities in access to and use of services call into question our fundamental values of equality and justice for all. *The health care delivery system is incapable of meeting the present, let alone the future needs of the American public.*" (emphasis added; see also IOM 1999, 2001).

These problems are clearly so serious that we need to rethink the U.S. health care system from the ground up. One central assumption that requires re-examination is the idea of the separation of mind from body, the notion pervading our concepts of health and illness that there are some illnesses that are physical and others that are mental, a notion that is enshrined in the current practice in healthcare reimbursement of "carving out," or sub-capitating, mental health benefits. In fact, mind and body are not separate, but rather are inseparable. By maintaining the fiction that mind and body are separate, and, further, assuming that the only role that the mind plays in health and illness is in mental health and illness, we have developed a healthcare system that is hobbled in its ability to deal with the many varied roles that mind and behavior play in so-called physical illness. This system, further, does not even deal with mental health and illness, per se, effectively, as we shall see.

Magnitude of the Cartesian Error

Mind-Body dualism has an enormous negative impact on our health care system. Because of it, our health care system does not systematically attend to the many psychological risk factors for both morbidity and mortality, and it virtually ignores the psychosocial pathways that lead to unnecessary utilization of medical and surgical services. Further, our health care system does not fully utilize appropriate tools to tackle the current chronic disease epidemic, such as the numerous disease management programs aimed at treatment adherence and lifestyle improvement developed and validated by psychologists. Nor does it utilize fully the many well-documented psychological interventions for acute illness and management of stressful medical procedures. In addition, the psychological impact of having a medical illness is not well addressed by the health care system, nor is the fact that many people suffering from a physical illness have comorbid psychological illness, nor is prescription drug abuse. Finally, the lion's share of mental health problems are treated, ineffectively, by primary care providers. Let's take a look at the evidence.

Morbidity and Mortality

1. Seven of the ten leading health and illness indicators identified in *Healthy People 2010* are psychological: Physical inactivity, overweight and obesity, tobacco use, substance abuse, mental illness, irresponsible sexual behavior, and injuries and violence (US DHHS, 2000).
2. Seven of the nine leading causes of death are psychological: Tobacco use, diet and activity patterns, alcohol abuse, firearms, sexual behavior, motor vehicle accidents, and use of illicit drugs. (McGinnis & Foege, 1993). (Recent update in JAMA shows diet and activity patterns are catching up with Tobacco use.)
3. Hence, to reduce morbidity and mortality, we must build in to the nation's health care system the systematic use of psychological health promotion and disease management programs that have been shown capable of addressing these psychological factors.

Unnecessary Utilization and Cost-Offset

1. Approximately 75% of all visits to primary care medical personnel are for problems with a psychological origin (including those who present with frank mental health problems and those who somatize), or for problems with a psychological component (including those with unhealthy lifestyle habits such as smoking, those with chronic

illnesses, and those with medical compliance issues). This leads to unnecessary and ineffective utilization of health care services, which drives up costs (O'Donohue, Ferguson, & Cummings 2002).

2. Stated another way, one study found that less than 16% of somatic complaints had an identifiable organic cause (Kroenke & Mangelsdorff, 1989). The authors concluded that in 74% of the cases with unknown etiology "it was probable that many of the symptoms ...were related to psychosocial factors" (p. 265). The investigators found that the cost of diagnosing an organic complaint was high (e.g., $7,778 for headache). Further, they found that treatment was provided for only 55% of the symptoms and was often ineffective.

3. Furthermore, a large number of studies have demonstrated that providing behavioral health care reduces the utilization of medical and surgical care, and saves money. A recent meta-analysis of 91 studies reported that 90% of the studies showed a decrease in medical utilization following some form of psychological intervention, and that, on the average, psychological intervention reduced the length of hospital stay by over 2.5 days and resulted in per-person savings of $2205. (Chiles, Lambert, & Hatch, 1999; See also Gabbard et al., 1997; Karon, 1995; Mumford et al., 1984).

4. Friedman et al. (1995) pointed out that managed care has reduced costs by focusing on the supply side, i.e., restricting access to care, whereas it has ignored the demand side strategy of managing the psychological factors that influence medical utilization. The authors identified six pathways whereby psychological interventions can both reduce unnecessary utilization and improve care: Providing health information and decision support, reducing psychological stress, changing unhealthy behaviors, providing social support, detecting and treating undiagnosed mental illness, and addressing somatization.

Disease Management

1. There is a growing body of empirical evidence supporting the effectiveness of psychological interventions in ameliorating a wide range of physical health problems, including both acute and chronic disease affecting literally every organ system and encompassing pediatric, adult and geriatric populations. In addition to being clinically effective in improving health outcomes, speeding post-surgical recovery, reducing unnecessary procedures, and improving patient satisfaction, these interventions are dramatically less expensive than alternative somatic interventions across a wide variety of illnesses and disorders, including coronary heart disease, hypertension, diabetes, cancer, arthritis, headaches, chronic pain, asthma, renal disease, peptic ulcer, and inflammatory bowel disease. Groth-Marnat

and Edkins (1996) demonstrated the cost-effectiveness of preparation for anxiety-provoking medical procedures, smoking cessation, rehabilitation of chronic pain patients, and treatment adherence. Sobel (2000) did the same for heart disease, chronic illness, surgical preparation and managing premature infants. A recent special issue on behavioral medicine and clinical health psychology in the *Journal of Consulting and Clinical Psychology* contains 28 articles reviewing the latest empirical evidence for a wide range of behavioral health interventions (Smith, Kendall, and Keefe, 2002).

2. Data regarding the efficacy and cost-effectiveness of psychological interventions for chronic pain are so compelling that the National Institutes of Health (NIH) published a consensus statement calling for wider acceptance and use of behavioral treatments in conjunction with typical medical care (NIH, 1995).

3. Cummings (2003) identified eight criteria for the success of population-based disease management programs: Pervasiveness, system-wide acceptance, co-location of behavior health providers with primary care providers, a program of outreach to the heavy utilizers of medical services, focused, targeted interventions, special training for all providers, and outcome evaluation.

4. Trask et al. (2002) offered the "4T" model for disease management: Target a clinical need where there is sufficient evidence that psychological factors influence outcome, Triage problematic cases, Treat using psychological disease management approaches, and Track patient outcomes.

5. Armed with results from a recent study on cardiovascular disease (Blumenthal et al., 2002), APA convinced the U.S. Congress to direct CMS to conduct a study of the cost saving and quality-of-care benefits from using psychological interventions to treat Medicare beneficiaries with cardiovascular disease (Holloway, 2004). This demonstration project will hopefully help translate the growing body of empirical evidence supporting the effectiveness of psychological interventions in ameliorating a wide range of physical health problems into actual health care practice.

Psychological Effects of Physical Illness, Co-Occuring Mental Illness

1. The psychological impact of having a medical illness is not well addressed by the health care system . It is rarely considered, but should be, given that it could improve outcomes and patient satisfaction.

2. Depression and other mental illnesses often co-occur with medical illnesses, especially heart disease, stroke, diabetes, cancer, and Parkinson's disease, and they can complicate the medical treatment. They are ignored in contemporary heath care. Detecting and treating them would therefore improve medical outcomes. (Trask et al., 2002).

Prescription Drug Abuse

1. An estimated 6.2 million Americans misuse prescription drugs and 4.4 million of them misuse pain medication, yet almost half of all primary care physicians find it very difficult to discuss prescription drug abuse with their patients. (Kelleher & Fins, 2003). Again, here is another area crying out for the integration of behavioral healthcare.

Mental Illness and Substance Abuse Disorders

1. Finally, the vast majority of people receiving mental health treatment are cared for by medical professionals with minimal specific training in mental health (Glied, 1998). This does not augur well for their being able to conduct the first prerequisite for prescribing, namely making an accurate diagnosis. And the data suggests that they don't: One third of primary care patients with major depression remained undetected for up to one year (Rost et al., 1998) and only 20% of primary care patients with major depression were judged as recovered in 8 months as compared to 70% treated by mental health specialists (Schulberg et al.,1996). And it's even worse with the elderly (Heston et al., 1992), and those with substance abuse disorders (Kelleher & Fins, 2003).

Thus, Descarte's 17th century philosophy, which separates mind from body, is, quite simply, bankrupt. We need to transform our *biomedical* health care system to one based on the *biopsychosocial* model, so well articulated by Engel (1977). In this coming transformation, psychology has a tremendous opportunity to evolve into a premier health care profession, serving on the front lines of health care, working collaboratively with physicians and nurses.

Psychological Health Care

What Do Health Psychologists Do?

What do psychologists who function in the physical health care arena actually do? I asked that question of one of my colleagues, Professor Jan Faust of Nova Southeastern University, who is a pediatric psychologist, and here is her response:

- Psychological intervention for adjustment to the diagnosis, treatment, and prognosis of serious illness (pediatric cancer, HIV-AIDS, hemophilia etc.).
- Preparation for anxiety provoking and painful medical procedures including surgery.
- Ameliorating needle and blood phobia and difficulties swallowing pills.
- Reduction of anticipatory nausea and vomiting.
- Pain management for burns, bone marrow aspirations and spinal taps.

- Facilitating medical adherence for diabetes, asthma and other diseases with complex medical regimens.
- Helping adolescents and their families make medical decisions such as terminating life support, choosing experimental chemotherapy protocols, and amputation. Addressing the aftermath of these decisions.
- Preventing pediatric intensive care unit psychosis – altering patterns in living to prevent psychotic symptoms as a response to disrupted circadian rhythms.
- Neuropsychological assessment for accidental injuries (car and bike accidents).
- Emergency room intervention with those patients in crisis.
- End stage counseling and grief work for terminally ill children and their families.
- Developing failure-to-thrive eating protocols.
- Treating obesity, anorexia, and bulimia.
- Therapy for children who have disfiguring, dysmorphic, and debilitating conditions including neurological impairment.
- Treating urinary and fecal incontinence.
- Educating medical personnel on psychosocial issues.
- Enhancing communication between medical personnel, and among medical personnel, patients, and their families.
- Reducing burnout of medical personnel.
- Helping medical personnel with their grief when losing patients.

For another view of psychologists' roles in primary care, see O'Donohue, Cummings and Ferguson (2003, pp 20-22), which reports a typical day in the work life of a behavioral healthcare provider, Dr. Aaron Kaplan.

"The Times They Are A'Changing"

The foregoing suggests tremendous opportunities for psychology to play a major role in resolving some of this nation's health care problems with regard to cost, quality, and access. In order to do this psychology must define itself as a health profession rather than as a mental health profession. An APA Board of Professional Affairs Work Group recognized this when it called for a "figure-ground reversal" in professional psychology. The Work Group advocated that, rather than viewing psychology as a mental health profession with health psychology representing a subset of its expertise, psychology should be viewed as a health profession, with mental health as a subset of its expertise.

This change in perspective, to viewing psychology as health discipline operating from a biopsychosocial perspective, would, of course, require a dramatic change in our training programs. If psychology truly wishes to rise to the challenge presented by the failures of the US health care system and respond effectively to the tremendous opportunities in health care, we would have to deliberately and with dispatch adopt a biopsychosocial model, and change not only the doctoral curriculum but also the undergraduate pre-requisites. Both are long on the "psycho" and "social" parts, but short on biology and the related areas of mathematics, physics, and chemistry. So too, training programs are highly variable in the degree to which students gain experience working in interdisciplinary collaboration in the broader health care arena, whether it be primary care, general hospitals, academic medical centers and the like, and this would have to change to ensure at least a modicum of training in psychological health care.

We would also need to redefine some parts of the profession[1] from specialty mental health care to primary health care. As a specialty profession of mental health care, we have dealt primarily with people who self-identify as having psychological problems and who have access to a mental health specialist. This is just a fraction of those who need psychological services. As a primary health care profession, working in the broader health care arena, we would be able to serve the much larger group of people who do not have access to mental health care or who do not identify their problem as psychological.

This would also require a change in practitioners' behavior. A 1995 study by the American Psychological Association (APA) Practice Directorate of 16,000 practicing psychologists found that psychologists' patterns of practice appeared to have changed little in response to the negative effects of managed care on their practices (Phelps, Eisman, & Kohout, 1998). The majority of respondents devoted three-quarters of their time to providing traditional mental health assessment and psychotherapy services in independent practice settings. Only a small number of them were working outside mental health and in the broader delivery system. Only about 13% of respondents reported a medical setting as their primary work site. There were some generational differences, however, with recent graduates more likely than previous generations to work outside traditional mental health settings. For example, about 20% of psychologists licensed in the 1990s were practicing in medical settings. Nevertheless, private practice was still the most likely setting for these young psychologists, with 40% in independent practice. The question that needs to get addressed is: In the face of a changing healthcare environment, will clinging too tenaciously to old patterns of practice place the profession at risk?

The American Psychological Association took a major stride, when, in 2001, under the leadership of then-President Norine Johnson, the mission statement was amended to include health as part of its mission, which now reads: "to advance psychology as a science and a profession, and as means of promoting health, education, and human welfare." This bylaw change was approved by one of the largest pluralities ever.

Health and Behavior Codes

In fairness, we have to point out that a serious limitation on psychologists' ability to participate in the broader health care arena has been the absence of payment mechanisms to reimburse psychological services within general health care settings. Psychologists have not been permitted to bill under procedure codes such as evaluation and management of medical disorders, patient education, and preventative services. As a consequence, they were forced to bill under mental health codes, which are often inappropriate, or to make arrangements with care systems to bundle their services. Moreover, psychologists did not have easy access to reimbursement for services provided to patients related to non-psychiatric diagnoses, even when these services are well accepted clinically and are strongly supported by the empirical literature. However, the recent approval the Center for Medicaid and Medicare Services of the Health and Behavior codes for psychologists may well be the vehicle to address these problems. This allows psychologists to see patients for medical diagnoses in their private offices and bill for assessment and intervention (Foxhall, 2000).

Impediments to Change

Psychology thus offers a key to saving billions of dollars annually and dramatically improving the U.S. health care system. It is therefore imperative that psychologists be more centrally involved in the healthcare system. An integrated biopsychosocial approach to health promotion and disease management in which experts in the fields of medicine and psychology synthesize their knowledge offers a most promising alternative to the current biomedical health care system, and could become an increasingly significant component of psychology's future. Undertaking a change of this scope will, of course, not be easy. However, to put this in perspective, consider that psychology now has before it a rare transformational opportunity, on the scale of what took place more than 50 years ago at the end of World War II. Prior to World War II professional psychologists had very limited roles as psychodiagnosticians working under the direction of psychiatrists. The war and its aftermath brought with it a tremendous demand for mental health services, including treatment, which helped wrest control of psychotherapy from psychiatry and opened this field up to psychology. This, in turn, led to a tremendous expansion of the scope of practice for professional psychology (Humphries, 1996).

How are we going to get there? It is not going to be easy. Trask et al. (2002, p. 76) point out that, despite the overwhelming evidence, "numerous practical, social, and economic barriers for integrating clinical behavioral science into mainstream healthcare have yet to be overcome." Let's briefly review some of them: weakness in the evidentiary base, and resistance from medicine, government and industry.

Do Psychological Health Interventions Reduce Mortality?

Some of these impediments have to do with weaknesses in the evidentiary base, particularly with regard to reducing mortality. Two recent clinical trials found that psychological treatments improved emotional and social functioning in patients suffering from cancer and cardiovascular disease, but had no effect on physical morbidity and mortality (Goodwin et al., 2001; National Heart, Lung and Blood Institute, 2001).

Commitment to the Biomedical Model

Some of the impediments are due to the resistance of the medical community to the adoption of a biopsychosocial model. Friedman et al. (1995, p. 515) comment that "even when hard data on cost and health outcomes are reported for soft psychological interventions, medical professionals too often dismiss or ignore such studies…[because] prevailing attitudes toward the origin of disease has emphasized biological explanations." Even in the area of the treatment of depression in primary care, Coyne et al. (2002) note that there is "a profound medicalization" (p. 803), and that it is "unrealistic to expect…a wholesale integration into primary care of psychologists providing conventional psychotherapy" (p. 805). I would also note in passing that, in the tradition of double-blind medical research, psychological effects were viewed as in the same category as placebo and thus devalued.

This is not new. Medicine has long been committed to the biomedical model. Pickren (2004) noted that an important effort to integrate psychology as one of the basic sciences of medicine around the turn of the twentieth century failed, largely because psychologists were unable to gain as allies the leaders of the medical reform movement. Interestingly, in the same paper, Pickren also noted that one of the areas of successful collaboration between psychology and medicine was psychosomatic medicine, where psychology offered scientific and organizational expertise that brought a new interdisciplinary field into being.

Resistance of Government and Industry

Resistance to change also comes from government and industry. A striking example is the failure of the federal government to enact Mental Health Parity legislation, which would extirpate the mind body dualism and outright discrimination against mental illness that pervades our national laws governing health care insurance. Newman (1999) described the resistance of the businesses who pay a large share of their employees' health insurance tab. One important factor is the short term perspective of employers, who might not be willing to make investments in improving the health of their employees for a cost-offset that they might not realize for years, for fear that the employee might leave the company and a competitor would reap the benefits.

Onward to the Future

The Patient as Primary Care Provider

The medical community has traditionally placed patients in a very passive dependent role. This is an outmoded practice. Patients are not only educated consumers today, but they are also the primary decision maker with regard other own health care. The definition of evidence-based practice recently adopted by the Institute of Medicine (2001, p. 147) recognizes the important role of the patient:

> *Evidence-based practice* is the integration of best research evidence with clinical expertise and patient values… *Patient values* refers to the unique

preferences, concerns and expectations that each patient brings to a clinical encounter and that must be integrated into clinical decisions if they are to serve the patient.

Friedman et al. (1995, p. 510) go even further and sagely observe: "With over 80% of all illness episodes self-diagnosed and self-treated without professional consultation, patients are in fact the true primary care providers in the health care system." Most patients, are, it would seem, *resilient*, when it comes to illness. This certainly fits with what we have learned about individual's resilience in response to disasters, war, and terrorism (Levant, Barbanel, & DeLeon, 2003).

Presidential Initiative: Health Care for the Whole Person

Given the important role of consumers, I believe that in order to reform the U.S. health care system we must appeal directly to the public, not alone, but in collaboration with other like-minded physician and provider groups. We need to articulate the public's dissatisfaction with the biomedical health care system that results in their care provider not having time to listen to all of their concerns or offering ineffective care. We need to put forth a vision of integrated care, a care system that offers Health Care for the Whole Person. This will in fact be one of my initiatives as President of the American Psychological Association in 2005.

References

Blumenthal, J. A., Babyak, M., Wei, J., O'Connor, C., Waugh, R., Eisenstein, E., et al. (2002). Usefulness of psychosocial treatment of mental stress induced myocardial ischemia in men. *The American Journal of Cardiology, 89,* 164-168.

Chiles, J. A., Lambert, M. J., & Hatch, A. L. (1999). The impact of psychological interventions on medical cost offset: A meta-analytic review. *Clinical Psychology: Science and Practice, 6,* 204-220.

Coyne, J. C., Thompson, R., Klinkman, M. S., & Nease, D. E., Jr. (2002). Emotional disorders in primary care. *Journal of Consulting and Clinical Psychology, 70,* 798-809.

Cummings, N. A. (2003). Advantages and limitations of disease management: A practical guide. In N. A. Cummings, W. T. O'Donohue, & K. E. Ferguson (Eds.), *The impact of medical cost offset on practice and research: Making it work for you.* Reno, NV: Context Press.

Engel, G. (1977). The need for a new medical model: A challenge for biomedicine. *Science, 196,* 129-136.

Foxhall, K. (2000). New CPT codes will recognize psychologist's work with physical health problems. *Monitor on Psychology, 31,* 46-47.

Friedman, R., Sobel, D., Myers, P., Caudill, M., & Benson, H. (1995). Behavioral medicine, clinical health psychology, and cost offset. *Health Psychology, 14,* 509-518.

Gabbard, G. O., Lazar, S. G., Hornberger, J., Spiegel, D. (1997). The economic impact of psychotherapy: A review. *The American Journal of Psychiatry, 154,*147-155.

Glied, S. (1998). Too little time: The recognition and treatment of mental health problems in primary care. *Health Services Research, 33,* 891-910.

Goodwin, P. J., Leszcz, M., Ennis, M., Koopmans, J., Vincent, L., Guther, H., et al. (2001). The effect of group psychosocial support on survival in metastatic breast cancer. *The New England Journal of Medicine, 345,* 1719-1726.

Groth-Marnat, G., & Edkins, G. (1996). Professional psychologists in general health care settings: A review of the financial efficacy of direct treatment interventions. *Professional Psychology: Research and Practice, 27,*161-174.

Heston, L. L., Garrard, J., Makris, L., Lane, R. L., Cooper, S., Dunham, T., et al. (1992). Inadequate treatment of depressed nursing home elderly. *Journal of the American Geriatrics Society, 40,* 1117-1122.

Holloway, J. D. (2004, March). A federal boost to psychological care for cardiac patients. *Monitor on Psychology ,35*(3), 32.

Humphries, K. (1996). Clinical psychologists as psychotherapists: History, future, and alternatives. *American Psychologist, 51,* 190-197.

Institute of Medicine. (1999). *To err is human: Building a safer health system.* Washington, DC: National Academy Press.

Institute of Medicine. (2001). Crossing *the quality chasm: A new health system for the 21ˢᵗ century.* Washington, DC: National Academy Press.

Institute of Medicine. (2002). *Fostering rapid advances in healthcare: learning from system demonstrations.* Washington, DC: National Academy Press.

Karon, W. (1995). Collaborative care: Patient satisfaction, outcomes, and medical cost-offset. *Family Systems Medicine, 13,* 351-365.

Kelleher, W. J., & Fins, A. I. (2003). *Integration of behavioral healthcare services and primary care.* Paper presented at the Florida Coalition for Optimal Health and Aging Conference, Ft. Lauderdale, FL.

Kroenke, K., & Mangelsdorff, D. (1989). Common symptoms in ambulatory care: Incidence, evaluations, therapy, and outcome. *The American Journal of Medicine, 86,* 262-26.

Levant, R. F., Barbanel, L. H., & DeLeon, P. H. (2003). Psychology's response to terrorism. In F. Moghaddam & A. J. Marsella (Eds.), *Understanding terrorism: Psychological roots, consequences, and interventions* (pp. 265-282). Washington, DC: American Psychological Association.

McGinnis, J. M., & Foege, W. H. (1993). Actual causes of death in the United States. *Journal of the American Medical Association, 270,* 2207-2212.

Mumford, E., Schlesinger, H. J., Glass, G. V., Patrick, C., & Cuerdon, T. (1984). *The American Journal of Psychiatry, 141,* 1145-1158.

National Heart, Lung, and Blood Institute. (2001). *Study finds no reduction in deaths or heart attacks in heart disease patients treated for depression and low social support.*

Retrieved October 28, 2001 from http://www.hlbi.nih.gov/new/press/01.11-13.htm

National Institutes of Health (NIH). (1995, October). *Integration of behavioral & relaxation approaches into the treatment of chronic pain & insomnia (NIH Technology Assessment statement)*. Washington, DC: National Institutes of Health Publications.

Newman, R. (1999). Comment on Chiles et al. *Clinical Psychology-Science & Practice*, *6*(2), 225-227.

O'Donohue, W. T., Ferguson, K. E., & Cummings, N. A. (2002). Introduction: reflections on the medical cost offset effect. In N. A. Cummings, W. T. O'Donohue, & K. E. Ferguson (Eds.), *The impact of medical cost offset on practice and research: Making it work for you*. Reno, NV: Context Press.

Phelps, R., Eisman, E. J., & Kohout, J. (1998). Psychological practice and managed care: Results of the CAPP practitioner survey. *Professional Psychology: Research and Practice*, *29*, 31-36.

Pickren, W. (2004). *Psychology and health care: A historical foundation for future collaboration*. Unpublished manuscript, American Psychological Association.

Rost, K., Zhang, M., Fortney, J., Smith, J., Coyne, J., & Smith, G.R. (1998). Persistently poor outcomes of undetected major depression in primary care. *General Hospital Psychiatry*, *20*, 12-20

Schulberg, H. C., Block, M. R., Madonia. M. J., Scott, C. P., Rodriquez, E., Imber, S. C., et al. (1996). Treating major depression in primary care practice. *Archives of General Psychiatry*, *53*, 913-919.

Smith, T. W., Kendall, P. C., & Keefe, F.J. (2002, Eds.). Special issue: Behavioral medicine and clinical health psychology. *Journal of Consulting and Clinical Psychology*, *70*, 459-851.

Sobel, D. S. (2000). Mind matters, money matters: The cost effectiveness of mind/body medicine. *Journal of the American Medical Association*, *282*, 1705.

Trask, P. C., Schwartz, S. M., Deaner, S. L., Peterson, A. G., Johnson, T., Rubenfire, M., et al. (2002). Behavioral medicine: The challenge of integrating psychological and behavioral approaches in primary care. *Effective Clinical Practice*, *5*, 75-83.

U.S. Department of Health and Human Services. (2000, November). *Healthy people 2010: Understanding and improving health*. Washington, DC: U.S.G.P.O.

Footnotes

1. Some professional areas would clearly remain specialty care, e.g., neuropsychology

Chapter 3

Behavioral Interventions for Somatizers within the Primary Care Setting

Nicholas A. Cummings
Janet L. Cummings
University of Nevada, Reno and the
Cummings Foundation for Behavioral Health

> *"The nice thing about hypochondriacs is that they never complain about other people's problems."*
> An anonymous but weary
> primary care physician

Healthcare costs are once again on a steep rise, premiums are increasing by double digits, health plans are avoiding or attempting to abandon coverage for problematic sectors of our population, the "baby boomer" generation is aging, and over 40 million Americans remain uninsured. The debate over healthcare has become a political issue, but no one has an immediate answer to escalating costs other than to pass on some of these costs to the insured through higher co-pays and shifting a greater portion of the premium from the employer to the employee. Some health economists remain more optimistic, and we agree with Gilmartin (2004) and others who maintain that those healthcare providers that develop cost-effective, innovative delivery systems that demonstrably improve the health and well-being of patients will prosper.

Most healthcare plans strive to become price competitive by operational efficiencies, shifting claims processing to Ireland, outsourcing case management and patient telephonic contact to India, and developing computer algorithms that can be monitored by employees with minimal education. As important as these efficiencies are, there is a point of diminishing returns, and they leave dangling the reservoir of costs that can only be addressed by a clinically driven system. This is especially true of the managed behavioral health organizations (MBHOs). Having long ago lost their hands-on clinical acumen, they are dependent more and more on bean-counter approaches to cost savings. But their lack of clinical knowledge can leave holes in what might appear to be a tight monitoring system. As just one example, recently a large MBHO was startled when one of the few remaining clinicians in their employ informed them that practitioners in their network were consistently billing, and the company was paying for patients who missed their appointments. Top management, having no appreciation for the fact that for decades psychotherapists have billed their "no shows," asked incredulously, "Why would they ever submit such a claim?" This hole was quickly plugged up, but how many other and more expensive gaps continue?

There are five major wasteful health expenditures, all of which have direct solutions:

1. Frivolous/exorbitant malpractice costs.
   Solution: Tort reform, such as the California plan in effect for decades.
2. Defensive medicine, resulting in billions of unnecessary expenditures.
   Solution: Again, tort reform.
3. Medical mistakes, the third largest cause of death after heart attacks and cancer.
   Solution: Electronic records and medical informatics.
4. Non-compliance to medical regimen.
   Solution: Behavioral interventions.
5. Somatization.
   Solution: Behavioral interventions.

Although behavioral care can do little to impact on the first three, the last two are essentially our province. Non-compliance results from a set of attitudes and behaviors for which psychology has developed interventions. Somatization as used in this chapter has nothing to do with the diagnostic nomenclature of somatiform disorder and as defined here, is impacted only by behavioral interventions:

Somatization is the translation of stress and distress into physical symptoms in the absence of physical illness, or the exacerbation of physical disease by psychological factors (Follette & Cummings, 1967; Cummings & Follette, 1968).

The term somatization was introduced in the late 1950s by the senior author as an alternative to the usual diagnostic parlance of the time. Following exhaustive tests that elicited no physical illness, physicians were prone to enter a diagnosis of hypochondria, a term that had unfortunate pejorative connotations. A number of alternatives were proffered to the Kaiser Permanente Health Plan, all of which were rejected until the terms somatization and somatizer were coined and came into standard usage in San Francisco and eventually to most of the national medical community.

In our society, persons in psychological difficulty will reflect this in physical symptoms, for which they seek medical attention for relief. Somatization then, is only the physical reflection of a broad spectrum of psychological diagnoses, and addressing somatization is an effective way to triage most, if not all psychogical conditions.

Effectively Delivering Behavioral Interventions

Somatization accounts for 10% to 15% of the $1.4 trillion healthcare budget, or $140 billion to $210 billion per year. Research (to be described below) has consistently demonstrated that behavioral interventions could save 5% to 10% of the healthcare budget. Taking the lowest, conservative figure of 5% savings yields $70 billion, equivalent to the entire annual mental health and substance abuse budget of the United States, and a sum that could provide health insurance for the 40 million Americans who have no coverage.

Creating a delivery system in which behavioral health is totally integrated into primary care is a formidable task, requiring considerable effort and expertise. The Kaiser Permanente Health Plan in Northern California spent two years and expended millions of dollars retooling their delivery system to reflect full integration. A less formidable task, but remarkably effective is a delivery system that provides extensive, but targeted behavioral interventions for the somatizers. It impacts sufficiently on healthcare so that overall medical costs can be reduced by 5% to 10%. The key is an aggressive but sensitive outreach program that assures a steady, high volume flow of somatizers into the system to which a broad array of effective, targeted interventions are provided. This is a significant undertaking, but the rewards in patient and physician satisfaction, coupled with equally significant cost savings, makes the effort worthwhile. Merely parachuting one or two disease management programs into an otherwise conventional healthcare system has limits. Even if each individual program is shown to be effective, the savings are not sufficient to effect the over-all budget. Somatization has varied causes and reflects many psychological conditions, with high medical utilization being the common denominator. A comprehensive outreach program will tap almost all of the diagnoses reflected in the mental health nomenclature.

A Viable Outreach Program

The successful treatment of somatization is not so much about money as it is about bringing the appropriate treatment and subsequent relief to patients who have been suffering, often for years. Measuring the medical cost offset (the savings in medical dollars after subtracting the cost of the behavioral interventions) is a convenient way to measure treatment outcome. Convinced that he has a medical condition and that eventually this will be established, the patient demands more and more tests and procedures. The physician, trained to elicit disease, complies, creating an inordinately large medical record. Somatizers have been known to seek emergency attention in the morning, be reassured, only to return for another non-appointment visit in the afternoon. A medical record revealing two to three hundred physician visits per year is not rare. When behavioral interventions result in resolution of the underlying stress and emotional distress, the patient ceases her incessant medical visits and the resultant cost-savings is a good measure of treatment success. The question remains: how can somatizers get into a behavioral care system?

The following sequence is classic: The physician works diligently to find the physical cause of the patient's symptoms. Scores, sometimes hundreds of tests are performed and repeated, and the reassurance they elicit may satisfy the patient for as much as a few days, or only a few hours. The reassurance is short lived because repeating medical examinations and tests actually is reinforcing the belief in a physical illness that ultimately just the right test will discover. Eventually, the physician becomes exasperated, tells the patient "it is all in your head," and makes a referral for psychotherapy. The patient remains convinced she has a physical disease and feels hurt, betrayed and angry. Most often the referral is rejected, but even if the patient keeps an initial appointment, he quickly sabotages attempts to engage him in psychotherapy. He seeks out a new and hopefully more sympathetic physician, and the process is repeated again. It is not unusual to see a patient who over a number of years had repeated this sequence with several physicians.

The answer to the dilemma is a carefully constructed outreach program that does not challenge the patient's belief in the physical nature of her symptoms. The target of this outreach is the 15% of highest utilizers of healthcare by *frequency of physician visits,* not dollar amount. The latter reflects the high ticket items such as terminal cancer and massive heart attacks, while the somatizer is characterized by repeated visits to the physician in an attempt to establish a medical diagnosis. In constructing the outreach program it is important to adhere to the following proven principles:

1. Awaiting a physician referral is problematic as it is slow at best, and often not forthcoming at all. Many physicians are intent on eliciting the implied physical illness, while others who suspect somatization do not refer because they have had unfortunate experiences with irate patients after making a referral to a psychotherapist.
2. A direct outreach to the 15% of the highest utilizers by frequency of physician visits nonetheless requires physician buy-in. A patient sensitive and a physician respectful system that is meticulously followed, keeps physicians informed, and results in no patient complaints is readily accepted.
3. The behavior healthcare providers must be a part of the medical system so as not to be in violation of HIPPA laws and regulations. In other words, when computer records of the targeted population are accessed, this outreach must qualify as a referral method from physician to behavioral care provider (psychologist, social worker) within the same medical system.
4. Mailings are of little success in bringing in the somatizers. Direct telephone contact has been shown to be highly effective, but it is important for the caller to identify oneself as calling from the patient's physician's office and thus differentiating the call from telemarketing.
5. It is equally important not to challenge the patient's conception of her "illness."

An approach that accompanies a sympathetic understanding with the invitation to come in for an appointment is surprisingly successful because a somatizer welcomes another service, especially if it is not threatening. We have found particularly successful the statement, "Anyone that is having as much illness as you are having must be upset and depressed about it. Perhaps we can help you with that." If the patient questions the utility of this, and complains about the lack of understanding from the physician, it frequently is helpful to add, "Perhaps we might be able to find you a more sympathetic physician."

6. Most patients called will make an appointment on the spot. Others need to be called a second or even third time. This will bring in approximately 85% of the somatizers called, with about 10% flatly refusing to participate, and a remaining 5% not saying no, but resisting making an appointment. In what we have termed extreme outreach, a house call will result in the cooperation and participation of most of the latter. A caveat is necessary here: a house caller dressed in street or office clothes is seldom admitted, but a nurse dressed in full regalia and carrying a black bag has never been refused entry. The interview often takes place around the dining room table with other members of the family present.

In a program where behavioral care providers (BCPs) are co-located in the primary care setting with primary care physicians (PCPs), a substantial portion of the outreach is eliminated because a PCP can walk the somatizer down the hall and directly to the BCP's office. This process, termed the "hallway handoff," essentially eliminates refusals, and when the telephone outreach is added, the result is as many as 95% of the somatizers will participate in at least one session, but most frequently in the full program. The strength of the program, therefore, is dependent upon first getting the somatizers in, and second having them participate in meaningful, effective treatment programs that will cut across almost all of the mental health diagnostic nomenclature.

The Research Evidence

At a personal meeting in February 2004 with a member of the President's New Freedom Commission on Mental Health, the Commission member expressed to the senior author how startled he was to recently become acquainted with the massive empirical evidence on both medical cost offset and the integration of behavioral health into primary care. He confessed that before being appointed to the President's Commission he had been so busy as a health plan executive that he had remained unaware of the research findings that would have been so useful to him in his work. Indeed, the research is so extensive that only landmark studies will be highlighted. For the reader wishing more information, there is an overview by Cummings, Cummings, and Johnson (1997) as well as a number of books for those who wish more detailed information (Blount, 1998; Cummings, O'Donohue,

Hayes, & Follette, 2001; Cummings, O'Donohue, & Ferguson, 2002; Cummings, O'Donohue, & Ferguson, 2003).

Principal finding: Traditional psychotherapy delivered in a conventional manner increases medical costs. Following the seminal research on somatizers and medical cost offset at Kaiser Permanente (Follette and Cummings, 1967; Cummings and Follette, 1968), the National Institute for Mental Health sponsored over twenty replications (summarized in Jones and Vischi, 1979) in the hope that research would demonstrate the universality of medical cost offset. Although most studies revealed medical cost offset, there was wide variation in the amount, and some studies showed little or no savings and even cost increases. To look into this disparity the government convened the Bethesda Consensus Conference (Jones & Vischi, 1980) in which all the medical cost offset researchers were present. The conclusion was that the more traditional the delivery system and the behavioral health interventions, the less likely will be the potential cost savings in medical care.

Principal finding: Targeted, focused behavioral interventions in an innovative delivery system renders significant medical cost offset (i.e., beyond the cost of providing the behavioral services). The Health Care Financing Administration, through its Medicaid and Medicare programs, and as part of their Hawaii Project I, co-sponsored with the State of Hawaii, the establishing of a new delivery system on Oahu (Honolulu). Named Hawaii Biodyne, the cost of recruiting and training the providers, and creating a number of centers was recovered within eighteen months, and the next three years accrued millions of dollars in savings in medical care. The populations served were the 36,000 Medicaid recipients and 92,000 federal employees on Oahu, all randomly assigned by intact family to control and experimental groups. Those in the control group were eligible for psychological and psychiatric services with any licensed practitioner in the community, and coverage included 52 sessions a year renewable every January. The experimental group received services at the Biodyne Centers, by self-referral, physician referral, or through the outreach. Both control and experimental subjects were classified as whether they manifested (1) psychological stress with no medical co-morbidity; (2) had co-morbidity with one of six chronic medical conditions: asthma, diabetes, emphysema and other airways blockages, hypertension, ischemia, and rheumatoid arthritis (including fibromyalgia); and (3) patients whose primary problem was addiction and substance abuse.

Results consistently revealed that the new delivery system saved medical dollars, while traditional care in the private practice community increased medical costs. (Health Care Financing Administration, 1991; Cummings, Dorken, Pallak, & Henke, 1993). As Figure 1 reveals, those in the non-chronic disease (psychological distress only group) demonstrated a savings of over $200 annually per patient seen, while patients in the control group revealed an almost $200 annual increase in medical costs, or a $400 spread. The results in Figure 2, the chronic disease group, are even more remarkable. The experimental group (Biodyne patients) showed a saving of almost $550 a year per patient, while those in the control group raised medical costs by over $500 per patient annually, resulting in a differential of over

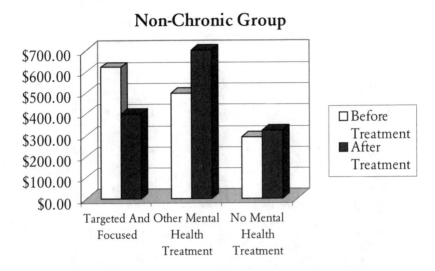

Figure 1. Non-chronic Group. Average medical utilization in constant dollars for the Hawaii Project Non-Chronic Group for the year before (white column) for those receiving targeted and focused treatment, or other mental health treatment in the private practice community, and no mental health treatment, and for the year after (black columns) for each treatment condition (Cummings, Dorken, Pallack, & Henke, 1993).

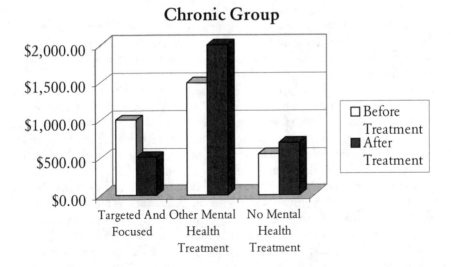

Figure 2. Chronic Group. Average medical utilization in constant dollars for the Hawaii Project chronically ill group for the year before (white columns) for those receiving targeted and focused treatment, other mental health treatment in the private practice community, and no mental health treatment, and for the year after (black columns) for each treatment condition (Cummings, Dorken, Pallak, & Henke, 1993).

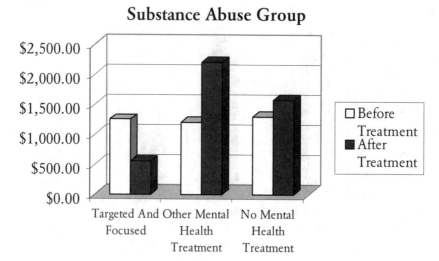

Figure 3. Substance Abuse Group. Average medical utilization in constant dollars for the Hawaii Project substance abuse group for the year before (white columns) for those receiving targeted and focused treatment, other mental health treatment in the private practice community, and no mental health treatment, and for the year after (black columns) for each treatment condition (Cummings, Dorken, Pallak, & Henke, 1993).

$1,000). The treatment of the substance abusers demonstrated the most savings and the greatest differential (Figure 3). Whereas the patients seen at Biodyne elicited a $700 saving, those seen in the private practice community raised their costs by almost $900, yielding a $1,600 differential per patient.

The Hawaii Project II (Laygo, et al., 2003) was conducted in three well established community health centers on Oahu. The model went beyond the collaborative model of the Hawaii Project I into the full integration of behavioral health in primary care that included co-location of behavioral care providers working side-by-side with primary care physicians. Preliminary findings reflect medical cost offset similar to that of Hawaii Project I.

Be careful what you wish for. Convinced that these studies are flawed and unlimited access and services in the psychological/psychiatric private sector would vindicate traditionally delivered psychotherapy, the American Psychological Association (APA) prevailed upon the government to fund such a study with the Champus population at Fort Bragg, North Carolina (Bickman, 1996). The population was the civilian dependents of military personnel, primarily children, and the degree of negative results surprised everyone. Instead of saving healthcare costs, there was an astounding ten-fold increase in costs from $8 million to $80 million annually (Figure 4). The APA reported and embalmed the study in the *American Psychologist,*

The Fort Bragg Champus Study

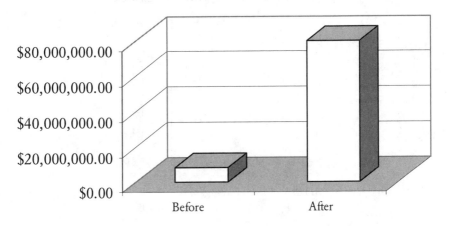

Figure 4. the annual Fort Bragg Champus expenditure the year before the study was $8 million dollars (first column) and $80 million the year after the study (Bickman, 1996).

never again to refer to it. It remains, however, well-known to actuaries and managed care executives.

The Behavioral Intervention Program

The implications for public policy are that if somatizers are effectively outreached and treated, conservatively there could be a 5% savings ($70 billion) annually that would pay the premium for the 40 million uninsured Americans. Projecting a plausible 10% annual savings ($140 billion), this amount would double the nation's mental health and substance abuse (MH/SA) treatment budget, while all the enacted parity laws have resulted in a decrease rather than an increase in the amount of money the nation spends on MH/SA. The relationship among our current MH/SA budget, the potential 10% savings in medical care, and the total current $1.4 trillion dollar healthcare budget are graphically seen in Figure 5.

Mindful that the range of patients the somatizer outreach has bought into the system will encompass the mental health diagnostic gamut, it is imperative that the subsequent behavioral interventions are targeted and focused, relying upon empirically derived treatments that have been further field tested for appropriate adaptation and modification, completing the journey from the laboratory to the real world of healthcare delivery. Effectively implemented, the treatment program will incorporate a host of individual disease and population management protocols, supplant others, and add a markedly increased behavioral dimension to disease management that is typically lacking in adequate behavioral emphasis. In short,

A 10% savings in medical costs can exceed twice the total MH/SA budget for the United States

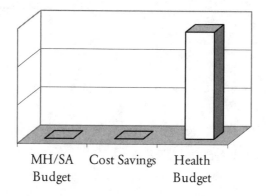

MH/SA   Cost Savings   Health
Budget   Budget

Figure 5. The annual mental health and substance abuse treatment budget (MH/SA) of the United States is $70 billion dollars (first column). A 10% reduction in mental health costs through behavioral interventions would result in a $140 billion savings, or twice the MH/ SA budget (second column). The total healthcare budget of the United States is $1.4 trillion (third column). All dollar amounts are for the fiscal year 2003.

outreaching somatizers is a rapid method of triaging a broad spectrum of patients into a full-fledge disease and population management program. This has direct impact on the cost-therapeutic effectiveness of the entire delivery system, whereas one or two disease and population programs, no matter how efficacious, can not make a noticeable difference on the bottom line.

The Delivery System

The outreach would be of little consequence if the patients flowing into the program were not treated in a seamless system with immediate access to appropriate treatment. In highly collaborative or fully integrate primary care settings, the patient is in programs that are perceived as part of healthcare and are absent the stigma of *mental* healthcare. In addition, the patient's belief in the *physical* nature of his or her illness is not challenged, thus removing an anticipated threat that would cause the somatizer to bolt and run. The patients get into the treatment program by physician referral (hallway hand-off in co-located systems), the outreach, or self-referral. In primary care in which physician referral and outreach are aggressive and effective, self-referral becomes relatively unnecessary and is usually under 5% of those treated. The effectiveness of outreach to augment physician referral results in as many as 90% of those needing behavioral interventions actually receiving it, a 900% increase over the traditional system in which only 10% of those referred for behavioral interventions ever enter treatment.

The hallway handoff sequence. In the integrated primary care system in which BCPs are co-located with PCPs, the hallway handoff results in a 15 to 20 minute session with the BCP. Most patients will return for one or two additional full (45-50 minute sessions) and find sufficient resolution to their problems as demonstrated by patient satisfaction and their subsequent participation in the healthcare system. This will be as high as 40% of the patients entering the system through the hallway handoff. About 50% of the others will go into the appropriate treatment program, and 10%

Patient Flow in Hallway Handoff and Somatizer Outreach

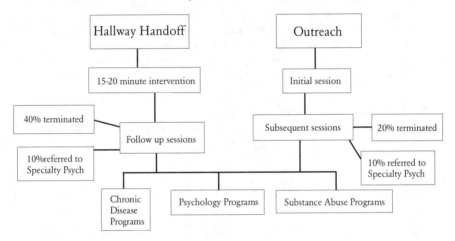

Figure 6. In the integrated primary care setting hallway handoffs and somatizer outreach compliment each other, resulting in 90% of the patients being seen in the primary care setting.

will be chronically mentally ill persons who are referred to specialty care. This sequence is shown graphically in Figure 6.

The outreach program sequence. In a successful outreach program, 90% of those outreached will be seen within six months in an individual session, with most of these within one or two months. Following an initial individual session or two, about 20% of the patients will have resolved the underlying cause of their somatization and opt out of further treatment. The majority will enter one of the appropriate behavioral programs, as shown in Figure 6.

The Biodyne model of individual and group behavioral interventions is extensively described in a number of books (Cummings & Cummings, 2000a; Cummings, Runyon, et al., In Press; Cummings & Sayama, 1995) and can only be alluded here. In this model the BCP's time will be apportioned as follows: 25% in individual sessions, including the initial 15-20 minute session; 50% in group disease and population programs; and 25% in group psychotherapy. There are six chronic disease group programs: asthma, diabetes, emphysema and chronic obstructive pulmonary disease (COPD), hypertension, ischemia, and rheumatoid arthritis, including fibromyalgia (see Cummings & Cummings, 1997). There are eight group programs for psychological conditions: bereavement (Hartmann-Stein, 2000), agoraphobia and multiple phobias, borderline personality disorder, depression (see note below), independent living for schizophrenics, panic and anxiety; perfectionistic personality, including obsessive-compulsive disorder (Cummings & Cummings, 2000a; Cummings, Cummings & Johnson, 1997; Cummings & Sayama, 1995); and child and adolescent attention deficit/hyperactivity disorder, or AD/HD (Cummings & Wiggins, 2001). Finally, there are four addictive and substance abuse group programs: pre-addictive program for those not convinced they are addicted (and following which most go into an addictive program that includes compulsive gambling and sexual addiction as well as chemical addiction, all with a goal of abstinence), adult children of alcoholics (ACOA), and, obesity (Cummings & Cummings, 2000b; Cummings, Duckworth, O'Donohue, & Ferguson, 2004). These are summarized in Table 1.

Group Protocols		
Chronic Diseases	**Psych Conditions**	**ADDICTIVE**
Asthma	Agoraphobia and	Pre-addictive
Diabetes	multiple phobias	Addiction
Emphysema (COPD)	Bereavement	ACOA
Hypertension	Borderline Personality*	Obesity
Ischemia	Depression**	
Rheumatoid Arthritis	Indep. Living: Schizophrenic	
(and fibromyalgia)	Panic/Anxiety	
	Perfectionist/OCD	

*BPD patients are treated in their own programs for all co-morbidities.
**Depression that accompanies other conditions is treated within those programs.
  Separate depression programs: bipolar, chronic and reactive depressions.

Table 1. The six chronic diseases, eight psychological conditions, and four addictive programs of the Biodyne model, using eighteen group protocols (from Cummings, Cummings, & Johnson, 1997).

In most disease and population management systems depression is regarded as a unitary condition, where actually there are several different types of depression, all of which should be treated in separate programs. For example, depressions accompanying a chronic illness, stemming from a severe loss, or reflecting a generalized unhappiness with life have little in common with bipolar depression that follows its own internal and probably biological cycle. Further, a patient depressed over years of pain with rheumatoid arthritis is not likely to understand or fully appreciate the depression that might accompany diabetes. The depressions that invariably accompany every chronic illness are best treated separately within the group program for each chronic medical condition. Furthermore, bereavement is not a variant of depression, but nature's own method of healing a severe loss, and requires its own program that will allow the patient to grieve and thus promote recovery from the loss. The Biodyne model does have, however, a program for the depression that results when bereavement is derailed or otherwise unsuccessful, usually because of lingering hostility toward the deceased. Inappropriately prescribed antidepressants will also interfere with the mourning process. Another depression program is geared toward the reactive depressions resulting from loss of job, a divorce, flunking out of college, and so forth, and a still separate program addresses those chronically depressed persons who reflect a lifelong depression stemming from the loss of a parent(s) or other severe loss at the critical developmental stages in infancy and childhood.

There is an important caveat regarding borderline personality disorder (BPD). These patients can wreck any program while they compete with their fellow patients for attention, impulsively reacting with jealousy and hostility, and trampling the boundaries of the program. In the Biodyne model, BPD patients with co-morbidity, whether this be depression, diabetes, addiction, or whatever, are treated in their own separate group programs within each co-morbidity. Years of experience has demonstrated that where this caveat is ignored, not only is the BPD patient not helped, but the other patients are deprived of treatment.

The Group Protocols

A half a century of experience with the Biodyne model in such complex delivery systems as Kaiser Permanente, both Hawaii Projects, and American Biodyne indicates that most conditions can be treated efficiently and effectively in a combination of initial individual sessions and subsequent group programs, with the main emphasis on the latter. The group culture that derives from these programs greatly facilitate treatment and propel the patient toward recovery. Furthermore, each group program has three aspects: *treatment* of the medical psychological components of each condition, *management* of the chronic aspects, and *prevention* of relapse or serious untoward developments. Some protocols will have a greater or lesser emphasis on each depending on the condition. For example, management with compliance to medical regimen are primary in diabetes, whereas treatment and ultimate recovery are the goals in panic attacks.

Group protocols, whether for substance abuse, psychological conditions, or chronic illness all share certain characteristics and facilitate mixing and matching.

1. There is an *educational component* for each condition. Information describing these conditions and their psychological components will be found in

usable forms in such books as *Mind Body Medicine* (Goleman & Gurin, a 1993 *Consumer Reports Book*), but care must be exercised to update the medical information by readily available booklets from the various charitable organizations pertaining to each (e.g., American Heart Association, American Diabetes Association). There is evidence that gaining a better understanding of one's condition in itself is therapeutic. Practitioners are admonished to include frank information about their disorder to the patients in the borderline personality program. If sensitively and candidly presented, this enhances the group's ability to anticipate and comprehend the impulsiveness that accompanies this disorder.

2. *Pain management* is a part of program that addresses painful chronic illnesses.

3. *Relaxation techniques,* including guided imagery, can be helpful in all of the conditions addressed.

4. *Stress management* is an important component of all programs, but especially for those who anticipate sudden panic and anxiety attacks, and for recovering addicts who are taking it one day at a time.

5. Group programs provide a *support system,* important to all patients. This feature is especially important to those social isolates who lack family and friends. Learning from others with the same condition that "I am not the only one feeling like this" results in a group spirit that facilitates the program. The protocols also pair patients in a buddy system, encouraging each patient to call one's buddy when the going gets tough between group meetings. The borderline personality disordered patients are required to call one's buddy and are restricted from calling the therapist.

6. A *self-evaluation component* addresses physical monitoring (e.g., blood pres sure and blood sugar), as well as psychological monitoring (e.g., stress levels, exercise regimen). Training patients to monitor blood pressure and blood sugar is relatively easy with current home apparatus' but they can also be trained to evaluate psychological progress. For example, training them on a five-point scale of compliance to their own medical or exercise regimen markedly improves compliance, especially since the patients share the results of all self-monitoring in the group.

7. *Homework* is given to each patient after each session. There is no cookbook of homework assignments, and homework is tailored to help the patient (and the group) attain the next level of understanding and mastery.

8. The *treatment of depression* that accompanies most of the conditions reflects the context in which depression is occurring. The Biodyne model does not subscribe to the notion that depression is primarily a medical condition without psychological etiology and behavioral components.

9. *Self-efficacy* (after Bandura, 1977) refers to the belief that one can perform a specific action or complete a task. Although this involves self-confidence in general, it is the confidence to perform a specific task. Positive changes

can be traced to an increase in self-efficacy brought about by a carefully designed protocol that will advance the sense of self-efficacy.

10. *Learned helplessness* (after Seligman, 1975) is a concept that holds helplessness is learned and can be unlearned. Some patients with chronic illnesses fall into a state of feeling helpless in the face of their disease. A well-designed protocol will enable a patient to confront and unlearn helplessness.

11. A *sense of coherence* (after Antonovsky, 1987) is required for a person to make sense out of adversity. Patients with chronic physical or mental illness feel not only that their circumstances do not make sense, but neither does their life. The ability to cope often depends on the presence or absence of this sense of coherence, and the protocol should be designed to enhance it.

12. *Exercise* is an essential component of every protocol, and is the feature most neglected by patients and not enforced by therapists. Exercise ameliorates depression, raises the sense of self-efficacy, and promotes coping behavior. The patient should be encouraged to plan and implement his or her own exercise regimen, and then stick to it.

13. *Modular formatting* enables a protocol to serve different but similar populations and conditions by inserting or substituting condition-specific modules. There is utility in deriving protocols that facilitate mixing and matching.

The Borderline Personality in the Healthcare System

To date several hundred group protocols have been identified, some with an impressive empirical base (as those in Beck, Steer, and Garbin, 1988), while others reflect extensive clinical experience and judgment and no empirical base (for example Beckfield, 1994). Recently there has been a wave of proprietary protocols for sale, while others are published and remain in the public domain. Chapters in this volume discuss programs with chronic medical conditions (see, for example, Delamater), so we have selected a group protocol for a pervasive behavioral problem: borderline personality disorder (BPD). This is a condition that no one else treats in its own group, allowing it to insidiously impact negatively on all other programs. This condition has been shown to be more responsive to group than to individual psychotherapy (Cummings & Sayama, 1995).

The thought of having more than one borderline patient in the office at the same time strikes terror in the hearts of most psychotherapists. Yet the group method is less volatile as these patients can not manipulate each other as they do the physician, psychotherapist, and the healthcare system. They immediately identify manipulative behavior in each other and do not hesitate to confront their fellow patients with a bluntness not possible for the psychotherapist. They are antiauthoritarian and quick to condemn the psychotherapist, but their peer orientation renders them susceptible to the criticism of fellow patients.

This protocol was selected because more than any other of our patients, BPDs raise havoc with the medical system. PCPs are manipulated into being overly sympathetic toward these initially charming and seemingly needy patients, but the more attention and services they provide, the more the patient demands. The first time the physician does not live up to the patient's ever-increasing expectations a rampage of hostility is unleashed, complaints are filed, and there are even more demands for attention from the now beleaguered physician. They overly use the emergency room and non-appointment (emergent) care, while they telephone at all hours of the day and night, ostensibly with a medical crises. A similar fate can befall the unwary psychotherapist, and many if not most malpractice suits toward psychologists are initiated by borderline patients (Welch, 2000).

There have been recent attempts to normalize BPD by extending the bipolar diagnosis to include the borderline patient. This is unfortunate, as it has the potential to deprive both the borderline and bipolar of the appropriate, but different treatment. The BPD group protocol (from Cummings & Sayama, 1995, pp. 241-248) is detailed below.

The BPD Group Protocol

The borderline group protocol implies all of the attributes of group process, and assuming the psychotherapist is skilled in these, they will not be repeated here. What will be stressed are the unique aspects, as there are features that differ from usual group therapy procedure. The approach is contrary to the prevalent professional belief that BPDs require long term, and even continuous psychotherapy. The BPD individual naturally slows down the acting out about the age of forty, and this is often misinterpreted that long term psychotherapy has been effective. The five month program leverages the group milieu into a powerful learning experience, resulting in changed attitudes that continue far into the future, requiring only occasional contact with the therapist.

The subjects. The group is composed of as many as ten patients, with eight as the ideal number. In smaller systems with less critical mass the group can be conducted with as few as four. All the patients are women. There are just as many male borderline personalities as there are female. Yet, most of the borderlines we see are women. This is because BPD men are usually remanded to the criminal justice system, while women borderlines invariably find themselves in the mental health system. We have had rare male groups when sufficient numbers presented themselves, but it is important not to assign the one or two males who appear to the women's group. The flirtation, seductiveness, and grandstanding that occurs across genders will wreck the group. Overwhelmingly, the protocol is intended for women's groups, with either a male or female therapist equally effective.

The buddy system. Early in the first session the therapist circulates a sheet of paper upon which each group member writes her first name and telephone number. This is photocopied so that each group member receives a copy, with instruction that when personal crisis occurs the patient is to call the patient just below her name. The person at the bottom calls the first name on the list. Each patient is allowed one phone call to the therapist per week, which must take place during business hours and is subject to a majority of the group voting that the call to the therapist was justified. If the group votes that it was not justified, the patient forfeits her entitlement to call the therapist the following week. If the patient calls the therapist more than once in a week's time, it isunderstood that the therapist will not return the call.

Boundaries. It is explained in the first session that the group is closed and time-limited to 20 sessions at one per week. Once the group has begun no one else can join, but a group member can be expelled by majority vote of the group if that group member refuses to abide by the rules. Each group member signs an agreement which embodies all of these and the following provisions.

It is further explained that each group member is entitled to one psychiatric emergency room visit during the 20 weeks, with the group voting at the next session whether or not this was necessary. If the group finds it was not, the patient forfeits two weeks worth of entitlements to call the therapist. More than one emergency room visit during the 20 weeks is considered a refusal to abide by the rules.

Each group member is entitled to one, and only one psychiatric hospitalization during the 20 weeks, providing the majority of the group votes *in advance* that it is necessary, and the hospitalization does not result in the individual missing more than one group session. This is an interesting twist on the managed care concept of prior authorization that is generally resented by providers and patients alike. In this case the authorization is rendered by one's peers, a decision that is quickly accepted and acknowledged by the borderline who is seeking hospitalization. In all matters subject to vote, the therapist conducts the vote but does not vote. This is to deflect the hostility from the therapist to the group. A tie vote goes in favor of the respective patient.

Attendance at all group sessions is mandatory. If a group member is ill or otherwise detained, at the next session the patient explains the reason and a vote is taken as to whether or not the absence was avoidable. If the majority of the group finds it was avoidable, it is recorded as an unauthorized absence. Two unauthorized absences require a vote to consider expulsion.

In the beginning, the patients tend to be lenient with each other, but soon they realize they have been had, and the therapist's task now becomes a matter of helping them to not be overly harsh.

Psychoeducation. It is imperative that the therapist sensitively but thoroughly explain the characteristics of the borderline personality, making understandable the behaviors known as *splitting* and *projective identification.* BPD is the product of a dysfunctional environment but the the patient has adopted the role of a victim and uses it to excuse untoward behavior and manipulate a sympathetic environment. Understanding by the therapist is warranted, but this should not lead to sugar-coating the characteristics of borderline behaviors. Frank explanation will prove helpful, enabling fellow patients to see through each others behaviors and to suggest better alternatives.

Role of the therapist. Patients never cease to direct questions to the therapist. It is imperative that the therapist *never* get sucked in and that she or he always defer the question to the group. It often behooves the therapist to be a bit clever and redirect the question to a group member who has already caught on to that particular patient's brand of manipulation. The therapist is most successful when she imparts knowledge and guides the group process toward a patient self-monitoring system.

It is critical that the therapist never become angry (especially unconsciously) with the patient. One way of preventing this is to be straightforward (yet not punitive) when annoyed. The patient will set out to make the therapist angry, and will triumph when the well-meaning therapist not only becomes angry, but feels compelled to deny it. These are annoying patients, and it is best to acknowledge it when it happens. To say to a patient, "You're usually hard to take, but today you are behaving downright obnoxiously. What's up?" may be the most assuring and therapeutic thing the therapist can do.

Dwelling on the past. The patients are not allowed to dwell on their sordid pasts. Once they have told their story, that's it. Borderlines are enamored of retelling the abuse they have suffered, embellishing the story with each retelling to the point of outright exaggeration and fabrication. Even worse, dwelling on the past fosters a decompensation rather than a corrective emotional experience. When a patient falls into rehashing the past, the therapist calls this to the attention of the group and asks what should be done. The group will invariably curtail the behavior, if for no other reason than "If I can't, you can't."

The group is encouraged to look at today's work, school, social and other relationships, offering realistic ways of handling the problem or crisis without "flipping out." When the therapist is tempted to offer suggested solutions, she should bite her tongue. Remember, we are creating a peer system for patients who (1) are incapable of *really* bonding, and (2) who would not tolerate therapist (parental) authority.

Termination. At the end of the 20 weeks, the group disbands as a group. Some of the patients will want to continue when the next group is formed, and this is welcomed. It is part of the therapeutic plan that in each succeeding group there will be a "veteran" who though still a patient, is more identified with stability and the avoidance of acting out than are the new group members. If a group member is expelled by the group, that patient may enter a subsequent group, but only after the group from which she was expelled has concluded the last of its 20 sessions.

Splitting. Two procedures must be noted to avoid splitting of the therapist. First, if there are two co-therapists conducting the group, extra care must be taken to be ever alert to the patients' unrelenting attempts to split the co-therapists. Second, these patients will demonstrate sheer genius in attempting to manipulate an individual contact with the therapist. This should be seen as an example of splitting and avoided. If the patient makes it impossible to avoid, such as waiting for the therapist in the parking lot, the therapist should end the encounter and bring it up in the group at the next session. The group's reaction is what will effectively curtail any further such acting out. Invariably some group members will attempt to split the group into two camps, and in such cases the therapist must take the lead to identify the behavior.

Borderline games. Borderline patients delight in well-meaning games. They are so adept at game playing that they are positively amused when the therapist suggests some poignant paradoxes, such as conferring the Yours-Is-the-Saddest-Story-I-Have-Ever-Heard Award. And, as is not unusual under this kind of peer process, if one group member becomes seemingly prudish, the Holier-Than-Thou Award may be in order. The therapist is encouraged to innovate awards as might be helpful. The recipient may protest, but the therapist can always tell when the patient is positively engaged, even in the face of a negative tirade. There will be a momentary, split-second sparkle of amusement in the eyes, or an involuntary, almost imperceptible grin before the patient launches into the tirade. Though therapeutic decisions are usually vigorously protested, the proof of effectiveness is the patient's change in behavior.

Projective identification. The repetition compulsion propels the patient to prove that no one (including the therapist) is any better than her dysfunctional parents. When this is accomplished, she "wins" the game that says, "It is not I who is bad, but my parents and the entire world are bad." But alongside this aggressiveness exists the terror of a perpetual five-year-old, who fears. "If I can manipulate everyone, who is strong enough to be there for me?" This part of the patient wants the therapist to "win," and is most enraged when the therapist allows himself to be manipulated. In one patient's words, "The person who can be there for me has to be someone I can't deceive or manipulate." The BPD reserves a special hell for the therapist whose attempts to be nice allow him to be manipulated. This is perceived as weakness and betrayal. This group protocol gives the therapist the tools to be, on behalf of the patient, that strong person who is not manipulated.

BPD and suicide. Borderlines are prone to threaten suicide, and the crescendo is loudest in direct proportion to how successful it is in intimidating the therapist. These patients are survivors, having survived abuse that would destroy most of us. They seldom kill themselves, but the therapist is always faced with the dilemma that this suicide attempt may be the one in a thousand that is lethal. If it is, not to hospitalize the patient may result in a suicide. If it is not, to hospitalize the patient is to be manipulated and thus, in the patient's eyes, disqualified to be the strong, effective therapist. Unnecessary hospitalization only encourages suicidal gestures, as the patient has learned these intimidate the therapist. The therapist in such a quandary can rely on the accuracy of the group when it votes whether to hospitalize. Remember, they are world class experts on manipulative behavior.

Concluding note. Therapists, even those with considerable experience, who have not conducted borderline groups will be skeptical. Why would the patient not just quit or get expelled by refusing to abide by the rules? Those who have conducted these groups are amazed that seldom does a patient quit or get expelled. The reason is two-fold.

First, the patient wants to stick around and defeat the therapist and the group; and second, the terrified child within the patient is hoping that finally this will be the person for her. One psychologist who was trained in the method and became exceptionally successful in conducting these groups put it this way: "I always wondered why Nick would say borderlines who do not succeed in manipulating the therapist will not quit, commit suicide, or get expelled from the group. It's because they want to see the end of the movie and if they get kicked out of the theater they'll never know how the movie ends. Part of them wants everyone dead, while the other part is hoping for a happy ending."

Summary

Outreaching the somatizer will elicit a broad spectrum of psychological distress, encompassing almost the entire psychiatric diagnostic nomenclature. In addition, it will elicit those with chronic diseases for whom psychological distress is exacerbating their physical illness. This provides a constant flow of patients to be addressed by a well-designed behavioral care delivery system in which there is strong collaboration between primary care physicians and behavioral care providers, and ideally one in which behavioral health is integrated in primary care with BCPs co-located with PCPs.

References

Antonovsky, A. (1987). *Unraveling the mystery of health: How people manage stress and stay well.* San Francisco: Jossey-Bass.

Bandura, A. (1977). Self-efficacy: Toward a unifying theory of behavioral change. *Psychological Review, 84,* 191-215.

Beck, A. T., Steer, R. A., & Garbin, M. G. (1988). Psychometric properties of the Beck Depression Inventory: Twenty-five years of evaluation. *Clinical Psychology Review, 8,* 77-100.

Beckfield, D. F. (1994). *Master your panic and take back your life! Twelve treatment sessions to overcome high anxiety.* San Luis Obispo, CA: Impact.

Bickman, L. (1996). A continuum of care: More is not always better. *American Psychologist, 51,* 689-701.

Blount, A. (1998). *Integrated primary care: The future of medical and mental health collaboration.* New York: W.W. Norton.

Cummings, J. L., Runyon, C., Cucciare, M., Cummings, N. A., & O'Donohue, W. T. (Eds.) (In Press). *Primer of integrated care.*

Cummings, N. A., & Cummings, J. L. (2000a). *The essence of psychotherapy: Reinventing the art in the new era of data.* San Diego: Academic Press.

Cummings, N. A., & Cummings, J. L. (2000b). *The first session with substance abusers: A step-by-step guide.* San Francisco: Jossey-Bass (Wiley).

Cummings, N. A., Cummings, J. L., & Johnson, J. N. (Eds.). (1997). *Behavioral health in primary care: A guide for clinical integration.* Madison, CT: Psychosocial Press.

Cummings, N. A., Dorken, H., Pallak, M. S., & Henke, C. J. (1993). The impact of psychological interventions on health care costs and utilization: The Hawaii

Medicaid Project. In N. A. Cummings & M. S. Pallak (Eds.), *Medicaid, managed behavioral health and implications for public policy*. Vol. 2: *Healthcare and utilization cost series* (pp. 3-23). South San Francisco, CA: Foundation for Behavioral Health.

Cummings, N.A., Duckworth, M. P., O'Donohue, W. T., & Ferguson, K E. (Eds.). (2004). *Early detection and treatment of substance abuse within the primary care setting*. Vol. 7: Healthcare utilization and cost series. Reno, NV: Context Press.

Cummings, N.A., & Follette, W. T. (1968). Psychiatric services and medical utilization in a prepaid health plan setting: Part 2. *Medical Care, 6,* 31-41.

Cummings, N. A., O'Donohue, W. T., & Ferguson, K. E. (Eds.). (2002). *The impact of Medical cost offset on practice and research: Making it work for you*. Vol. 5: Healthcare and Utilization Cost Series. Reno, NV: Context Press.

Cummings, N. A., O'Donohue, W. T., & Ferguson, K. E. (Eds.). (2003). *Behavioral health as primary care: Beyond efficacy to effectiveness*. Vol. 6: Healthcare Utilization and Cost Series. Reno, NV: Context Press.

Cummings, N. A., O'Donohue, W. T., Hayes, S. C., & Follette, V. (Eds.). (2001). *Integrated behavioral healthcare: Positioning mental health practice with medical/surgical practice*. San Diego: Academic Press.

Cumming, N. A., & Sayama, M. (1995). *Focused psychotherapy: A casebook of brief intermittent psychotherapy throughout the life cycle*. Madison, CT: Psychosocial Press.

Cummings, N. A., & Wiggins, J. G. (2001). A collaborative primary care/ behavioral health model for the use of psychotropic medication with children and adolescents: The report of a national retrospective study. *Issues in Interdisciplinary Care, 3*(2), 121-128.

Follette, W. T., & Cummings, N.A. (1967). Psychiatric services and medical utilization in a prepaid health plan setting. *Medical Care, 5,* 25-35.

Gilmartin, R. V. (2004). *Annual report, Merck and Company*. Whitehouse Station, NJ: Merck Press.

Goleman, D., & Gurin, J. (Eds.). (1993). *Mind body medicine: How to use your mind for better health*. Yonkers, NY: Consumer Reports Books.

Hartman-Stein, P. E. (Ed.). (1998). *Innovative behavioral healthcare for older adults*. San Francisco, CA: Jossey-Bass.

Health Care Financing Administration (1991). The impact of psychological intervention on health care costs and utilization. The Hawaii Medicaid project. Washington, DC: *HCFA Contract report #11-C-983344/9.*

Jones, K.R., & Vischi, T.R. (1979). The impact of alcohol, drug abuse, and medical care utilization: A review. *Medical Care, 17* (suppl.), 43-131.

Jones. K. R., & Vischi, T. R. (1980). *The Bethesda Consensus Conference on medical cost offset: Alcohol, drug abuse and mental health administration report*. Rockville, MD: Alcohol, Drug Abuse, and Mental Health Administration (ADAMHA).

Laygo, R., O'Donohue, W., Hall, S., Kaplan, A., Wood, R., Cummings, J., et al. (2003). Preliminary report from the Hawaii Integrated Healthcare Project II. In

N. A. Cummings, W. T. O'Donohue, & K. E. Ferguson, *Behavioral health as primary care: Beyond efficacy to effectiveness,* (pp. 111-144). Reno, NV: Context Press.

Seligman, M.E.P. (1975). *Helplessness: On depression, development, and death.* San Francisco: W.H. Freeman.

Welch, B. (2000). *If you treat borderline patients, you will be sued: Get ready.* Private mailing to psychologists insured by the APA Insurance Trust.

Chapter 4

An Integrated Model for Changing Patient Behavior in Primary Care[1]

Joshua R. Dyer
IUPUI, Clinical Rehabilitation Psychology, Indianapolis, IN
Robert M. Levy
Criterion Health, Inc., Terre Haute, IN
Robert L. Dyer
Criterion Health, Inc., Bellevue, WA

Typical primary care patients enter the doctor's office expecting the expert to give them a pill or diagnose something significant and send them to a specialist in order to be cured. This system has been in place with largely unchanged expectations by either patients or medical staff since WWII. In spite of demographic changes in our society and advances in the behavioral sciences, it is still the norm. Fortunately, there is a growing movement of researchers and healthcare providers that now recognize the need to change not only the method of service delivery but also the very notion of the patients' activity on their own behalf. Patients, especially those with chronic conditions, are increasingly being seen as active partners in their care. Treatment and rehabilitation for these patients do not happen passively in the doctor's office; rather, both the patient and the health care staff create a treatment plan and share in the patient's implementation of it.

Patients with chronic conditions have unique needs that are difficult to meet in the typical 12-minute primary care physician (PCP)-patient interaction. Successful treatment often requires that patients make permanent lifestyle changes, such as changes in diet, smoking cessation, medication compliance, and implementing exercise regimens. These patients must also learn new skills such as self-monitoring and communicating with healthcare professionals. Likewise, patients with behavioral problems or mood disorders such as sleep disorders, depression, or anxiety can benefit from short behavioral interventions that are beyond the scope of the PCP's practice but do not necessarily demand referral to outside specialists.

[1] *The helpful and supportive comments of Capt. Nicholas Lind, Shaw Air Force Base, are greatly appreciated.*

One way to better serve these patients is to integrate a behavioral health practitioner, Behavioral Health Specialist (BHS) into the primary care practice. This will improve patient care and outcomes and also ease the burden for the PCP. The BHS will have two functions. First, he/she will be available as a mental health professional at all times to the PCP. For example, if the PCP treats a depressed patient in crisis, he/she can immediately take the patient to the BHS who is trained to deal with this situation. The PCP and BHS can then work together to create a treatment plan. The second function is to serve high service utilizing patients in the practice. People with chronic conditions as well as many of those with behavioral problems often need to make lifestyle changes that a structured psychoeducational program can facilitate. The BHS will assess their readiness to change and, if necessary, use focused, brief interventions to help the patient become ready to change. Once it is determined that the patient is ready, he/she will enter a self-efficacy based group self-management program. The Figure below depicts the essential components of this model, which is called Prime Behavioral Health

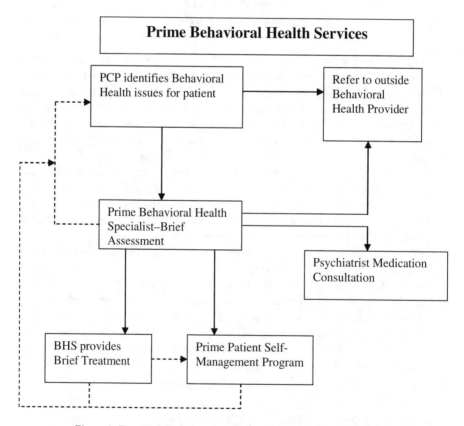

Figure 1. Essential Components of Prime Behavioral health Services.

Services. It is based on a review and analysis of systems issues, recognition of the different needs of individual patients as a function of their readiness for change, and recognition of the importance of group self-management.

If the psychiatrist or behavioral health provider are outside of the practice, the PCP very rarely gets feedback (this probably varies greatly from community to community). One option may be to refer all potential mental health patients to the BHS for him or her to act as a gatekeeper. If the BHS has a working relationship with the local mental health providers, he or she can request monthly written updates on each of the patients. The BHS could then brief the PCP.

A successful behavioral health program working in a primary care setting must: (1) help extend the primary care physician, (2) help patients in a way they recognize, (3) be founded in science, and (4) make money for the practice.

Realities of Primary Care

One of the most noticeable characteristics of the primary care setting is the speed of service delivery. The average patient-physician contact is 12 minutes. PCPs see 130 patients and bill over 50 hours per week totaling a financial productivity of gross billings exceeding $400,000 per year. (In contrast, the average productivity of a master's level psychiatric social worker includes billing 26 hours per week and annual gross billings equaling $87,000- a significantly different standard). From this, each PCP supports an average of 4.6 full time employees (Medical Group Management Association 2003 Annual Survey). So, what happens in the 12 minutes upon which this business is built? The physician and patient address an average of six symptoms. Over half of the total visits are for chronic conditions (see Table 1).

- Diabetes (5%)
- Anxiety (33% of acute chest pain visits are anxiety or panic)
- Hypertension/ coronary disease (17% Americans)
- GI problems (>75% have no physiological basis)
- Chronic obstructive pulmonary disorder (10% health costs; pediatric asthma is epidemic)
- Pain (50% physician visits; arthritis 12% office visits of elderly)
- Insomnia (when asked 69% primary care patients acknowledged)
- Depression for grief/ loss (6-10% PCP patients; 80% report physical symptoms of chronic medical illness first)
- Substance abuse (5%, complicating physical factor)
- Somatization-high users of primary care- with little physiological basis

---

Table 1. Disposition of primary care patients (American Academy of Family Physicians, 2004).

While behavioral health issues are diagnosed in less than 10% of encounters, "psychological issues" are suspected in over 30% of encounters. This discrepancy may be due to many issues including that physicians focus primarily on physical symptoms and acute problems; they may have inadequate training to deal with "psychological issues"; they may be afraid of alienating their patients by giving them a diagnosis associated with potential stigma; it may be because of the time consuming nature of "psychological issues" or because of a lack of financial incentives.

Primary care physicians do not have much incentive to refer patients out to a behavioral health specialist. In the US Surgeon General's Report on Mental Health (2003) it was reported that 72% of patient encounters end in a prescription, *29% are referred for in house "counseling"* (diet, medication taking, activity planning, etc.), 5% are referred to another physician specialist, and *only 2% are referred out to a behavioral health specialist.* This said, physicians care about the well-being of their patients. As long as it will work financially and with minimal disruption to their patient flow, physicians are interested in adding services that target lifestyle management issues to increase the breadth of care they offer. The following are the results of a survey of 120 primary care physicians in the North West (Yurdin, *Northwest Physician,* 1997):

71% of office visits were follow up to chronic conditions
70% to 89% of PCPs prefered treating diabetes, hypertension, pain, asthma
    with lifestyle management, yet 71% of patients with these disorders
    only saw PCPs
74% of PCP practices did not offer lifestyle management
86% of PCPs would be interested in adding revenue by offering lifestyle
    management
60% of PCPs reported revenue generation would increase utilization
80% of PCPs interested in adding a "qualified health educator and care
    coordinator" to their practice

What Patients Need

Not surprisingly, one reason physicians do not refer patients out for counseling is that the patients send a fairly clear message they are not interested in "extra" help. They do not want the stigma or the inconvenience of another set of appointments. What they do want is a noticeable decrease in their symptoms and to achieve some insight into their pattern of symptom escalation. Patients want this to occur within the context of their "normal" health care service. What they get is 12 minutes with the doctor to cover six symptoms and receive a medication prescription; this is not necessarily conducive to achieving insight into symptom escalation. As a result, over half of the medications prescribed are not taken as directed (Haynes, McKibbon, & Kanani, 1996). Additionally, in spite of strong evidence of the effectiveness of diet and exercise for multiple populations, patients are not receiving the advice and skills necessary to start and maintain regimens (Brunner et al., 1997; Dubbert, 2002; U.S. Preventive Services Task Force, 2003; McInnis, 2003)

The treatment given in this traditional model is not matching the needs of patients. The current system of primary care evolved from a time when most patients were treated infrequently and most often only for acute diseases. Demographics, medical science, and an increasingly health conscious America have conspired to change the role of the family doctor. As is evident in Table 2 below, there are key differences in the nature and treatment of acute versus chronic diseases. The end result of this is that the role of the healthcare professional shifts from solely selecting and conducting therapy to include the additional roles of teacher and motivator. Similarly, the patient no longer just follows orders for a limited duration of time, but now is responsible for his or her own daily management. The responsibilities of each have changed, yet the 12 minute interview ending with a prescription remains the standard of care.

	Acute Disease	**Chronic Disease**
Beginning	Rapid	Gradual
Cause	Unually one	Many
Duration	Short	Indefinite
Diagnosis	Symptoms align with diagnosis	Often uncertain, especially early
Diagnostic Tests	Often decisive	Often of limited value
Treatment	Cure common	Cure rare
Role of Professional	Select and conduct therapy	Teacher, partner, and motivator
Role of Patient	Follow orders	Responsible for daily management, partner of health professional

Table 2. Acute versus chronic disease (adapted from Lorig, Holman, Sobel, et al., 2000).

Being responsible for the daily management of (a) chronic disease(s) demands that patients make and sustain a number of changes. Nearly all of them have to learn to become adherent to medications. Often, dietary changes and exercise routines are necessary. They need to learn what to do during symptom flare-ups; this is especially relevant for patients suffering from chronic pain. They need to learn how to find and use relevant information. In addition, they need to learn how to elicit proper support from family and peers during difficult times. These are all issues well suited to behavioral medicine interventions.

Readiness to Change

Given this laundry list of changes that patients need to make, it is critical that we ensure they are ready and committed to change. In the *Stages of Change Model*, Prochaska et al identify five stages through which people progress in order to successfully change health related behaviors (Prochaska, DiClemente,& Norcross, 1992). Table 3 below describes these stages and the types of interventions that help patients progress through each.

Stage of Change	Description	Interventions
Precontemplation	Denial- no thoughts about change	Consciousness raising Dramatic relief Environmental reevaluation
Contemplation	Identify that there is a problem and consider change in the near future	Self-reevaluation
Preparation	Gathering resources, information, and support to begin behavior change	Self-liberation
Action	Beginning and continuing change	Reinforcement management Helping relationships Counterconditioning Stimulus control
Maintenance	Incorporating lifestyle changes into core behaviors; adoption of behaviors into value system	

Table 3. Stage appropriate intervention strategies.

Interventions that utilize the *Stages of Change* model have been successfully applied to smoking-cessation, exercise, mammography, safe sex behaviors, medical compliance, and stress management programs (Prochaska, Redding, & Evers, 1997). For a review, see Burkholder & Evers, 2002. The findings of these programs are that the vast majority of people in need of change are not in the action stage. For example, aggregating across studies and populations 10-15% of smokers are prepared for action, 30-40% are in the contemplation stage, and 50-60% are in the precontemplation stage (Prochaska, DiClemente,& Norcross, 1992). Similar percentages have been found for weight loss, diet, and exercise (Campbell et al., 2000; Natarajan, Clyburn, & Brown, 2002). Additionally, the amount of progress individuals make following interventions tends to be a function of the pretreatment stage of change; and, having patients progress from any one stage to the next within two weeks is a strong predictor of later success (Miller, 2002; Prochaska, DiClemente, & Norcross, 1992; Steptoe, Kerry, Rink, & Hilton, 2001).

One approach that can effectively help patients progress toward the action stage is *Motivational Interviewing* (Miller, 2002). *Motivational Interviewing* is an evidence-based practice based on the *Stages of Change* model. It uses brief, focused sessions to bring about behavior change and has been demonstrated to be effective for problems involving alcohol, drugs, diet, and exercise (Burke, 2003).

The real value of the *Stages of Change* model is as a heuristic to address patients' readiness to change. That is, in precontemplation and contemplation stages, brief motivational interviewing sessions or even phone calls may be an effective way to help patients progress towards the action stage. Once in the action phase, group programs provide the most efficient and effective format to accomplish sustained lifestyle changes.

The Effectiveness of Groups

The efficiency of groups is obvious. One provider can bill and treat multiple patients at the same time. However, the effectiveness of the therapeutic benefits may be surprising to readers.

A group treatment modality offers several unique benefits including a shared sense of "normalcy" and decreased feelings of isolation; the experience of acceptance within the group that combats the sense of demoralization; and the opportunity to help others, thus rebuilding self-esteem and problem solving skills. Group treatment has been found to be superior to individual treatment for chronic pain, substance abuse, weight control, parenting problems, vocational problems, and when treatment lasted for ten or fewer total sessions (McRoberts, Burlingame, & Hoag, 1998). Group psychotherapy was found to be equally as efficacious as individual therapy regardless of patient demographic variables, diagnoses, amount of time spent in therapy, theoretical orientation approach of provider to group, and training level of provider (McRoberts et al., 1998). The finding that a group format is more effective for ten or fewer sessions when compared to individual treatment is both clinically and practically significant given that in addition to optimal patient care, time and cost-efficiency are driving forces in today's health care industry. The efficiency and effectiveness of group modality makes it an appropriate format with which to foster self-management skills in a primary care environment.

Self-Management Group Model

A self-managing patient is one who is informed, compliant to medications, adherent to necessary lifestyle changes, and, most importantly, is an active partner in his or her care. Successful programs rely on a collaborative process to define problems, set priorities, establish goals, identify barriers, create treatment plans, and solve problems (Glasgow et al., 1999).

An example of an established program of self-management is Stanford's Chronic Disease Self Management Program (CDSMP). The CDSMP is a community-based intervention built on Bandura's self-efficacy theory. "Perceived self-efficacy refers to beliefs in one's capabilities to organize and execute the courses of action required to produce given attainments" (Bandura, 1997, p. 3). The CDSMP is a six-week small group intervention taught by two lay leaders from a highly structured manual. The CDSMP emphasizes skill building, modeling, problem-solving strategies, and social persuasion to achieve behavior change in patients with a physician-confirmed diagnosis of heart disease, lung disease, stroke, or arthritis. Lorig and colleagues found that after one year of participation in CDSMP, patients experienced statistically significant improvements in cognitive symptom management, communication with the physician, self-efficacy, depression, and health distress. Results also demonstrated savings in health expenditures (Lorig, Sobel, et al., 1999).

There are several important lessons to be learned from the CDSMP.

1. A self-management program based on self-efficacy is effective; and, the benefits gained from achieving self-efficacy are still evident up to four years later (K. R. Lorig, Mazonson, & Holman, 1993).
2. Patients with different chronic diseases have similar symptom management problems that are addressed with a self-efficacy based program. In other words, heterogeneous groups shift the focus off the disease per se and onto symptom self-management. In terms of the reality of primary care practices, it will be easier to constitute heterogeneous groups than homogeneous groups for a program. Furthermore, for the facilitators the focus is on the group process and does not assume specialized knowledge about the diseases.
3. Not only can more people be served within one program model, a single program will, by definition, be able to be more inclusive than one targeting only a single condition.
4. Lay leaders who complete a four-day training session can implement such a program effectively. No significant differences were found between groups led by two peer leaders, two professionals, or one of each (Lorig, Sobe, Ritter, Laurent, & Hobbs, 2001).
5. As effective as this program may be, it is not reaching its full potential. As a recent NIH report on treatment approaches to osteoarthritis

stated, "Until sociobehavioral interventions are incorporated into medical care, their benefits may go largely unrealized" (Felson et al., 2000, p. 732).

The Stanford work on self-management provides a framework for building self-management programs. Lorig and Holman recently defined three essential self-management tasks - medical management, role management, and emotional management and six skills - problem solving, decision making, resource utilization, the formation of a patient-provider partnership, action planning, and self-tailoring (Lorig, & Holman, 2003).

An Issue to Address for Effective Integration

An essential step when considering changing patient care is to define a model that will ensure that the program has a chance to be effective and will fit within the current healthcare system. Wagner and colleagues developed a heuristic model, called the Chronic Care Model (CCM), that identifies changes needed in the healthcare system, the provider, and the patient in order to improve patient outcomes (Wagner, Austin, & Von Korff, 1996; Wagner, Glasgow, et al., 2001). They developed the CCM by reviewing and synthesizing successful interventions used across multiple settings and multiple diseases. Their findings provide a framework for tailoring a chronic disease program to fit the specific needs of the provider and patient population.

In a review of the CCM, 32 of 39 studies found that interventions based on CCM components improved at least one process or outcome measure for diabetic patients. Additionally, 18 of 27 studies across conditions (congestive heart failure, asthma, and diabetes) found reduced health care costs or lowered use of health care services (Bodenheimer, Wagner, & Grumbach, 2002). The following are the six key elements identified by the CCM.

1. External healthcare organization - Make chronic illness care a key goal of the organization and insure that leadership is committed and visibly involved.
2. Community linkages - Provide linkages with community resources.
3. Patient self-management support - Collaborative process to define problems, set priorities, establish goals, identify barriers, create treatment plans and solve problems.
4. Provider decision support - Use evidence-based practice guidelines.
5. Care delivery design - Use specialists such as nurse case managers, pharmacists, or health educators to provide programs and follow-up.
6. Clinical information management - Establish a registry.

While disease management programs have had success, in a survey of 72 chronic disease management programs, Wagner et al. found that only one addressed all six key elements (1999). While the majority claimed to offer self-management support, only 18% emphasized patient activation/empowerment, collaborative goal setting, and problem solving. These have been shown to be more effective than traditional information-oriented programs (Wagner, Davis, Schaefer, Von Korff, Austin, 1999). The good news is that Health Resources and Services Administration (HRSA) has adapted the CCM model and we can anticipate increased initiatives emphasizing these organized components in publicly funded disease management programs.

Logistics/Financial Issues

As is implied by these six elements, traditional mental healthcare providers must change their practice patterns in order to succeed in primary care. The 50 minute individual session is not practical in an environment where speed and accessibility are essential. Individual sessions should be brief, well under 30 minutes (15-20 minutes being ideal), and appropriate for the patient's stage of change. If more intense, longer duration therapy is needed, the behavioral health specialist should refer the patient to a traditional setting. When appropriate, patients utilizing behavioral interventions should be spending the majority of their time in structured groups focused on self-management.

A major impediment in adapting these new modes of service delivery is the historic payment system and the historic separation of bureaucratic systems. Services are often reported differently for behavioral health and physical health. Physical healthcare providers use the Classification of Procedures Terminology (CPT) codes and behavioral healthcare providers use the American Psychiatric Associations Diagnostic and Statistical Manual of Mental Disorders (DSM-IV) terms. Behavioral health providers delivering services without a primary or secondary psychiatric diagnosis typically have their invoices denied. Perverse incentives exist that make services delivered by mid-level primary care extenders (nurse practitioners or physician assistants) eligible for payment while those same services if delivered by behavioral health professionals are denied. In 2002, Medicare demanded that all program administrators adopt a new set of codes that allowed behavioral health practitioners to help in physical health even when a DSM-IV diagnosis is not primary or secondary (the 96150-155 codes). Commercial plans are adopting these guidelines. Previously, we have observed that the use of physician extenders in providing education and support has been addressed in most plans through the guidelines for billing services that are "incident to" the care of the physician. Several of the key management issues in billing are summarized in the Table 4 as a function of whether behavioral services are provided in the context of integrated care in a primary practice or as separate psychiatric services.

Another historic problem in incorporating behavioral health into a primary care setting has been the need to achieve "relevance." Too often the Behavioral Health Specialist comes into the primary care setting but is quickly viewed as relevant to see only depressed adults, acting out children, and domestic disturbances. This encourages the traditional 50-minute therapy hour, it means that the BHS is going

	In PCP Practice as Primary Health	As Psychiatric Practitioner Services
Diagnosis	Physical	Psychiatric*
Authority	PCP prescribes	BH Practitioner
Billing under	PCP bundled services (incident to) 99201-5, 11-15 series 99242-5 office consultations 99078 educational services- group 99401-4, 11-12 prevention interventions 0108 & 0109 for diabetes	MH benefit* 90804-29 series, individual 90853,57 group 90849-49 family 99150-5 codes as come on line
Documentation	In medical chart	BH Practitioner records
Liability	PCP practice (& BHP as provider)	BH Practitioner

Table 4. Billing overview.

to see only twenty five people a week, and it also means that the BHS is not readily accessible to the medical staff. In order to reach the scope of relevance in a practice, experience has shown the BHS must offer services that touch a significant percent of the practice patients–demanding brief, group oriented interventions. If the behaviorist offerings to the medical staff aren't relevant to over 30% of patients in the practice, they probably are not going to have much impact on the practice.

Examples of Successful Programs

By way of example, the following three presentations from 2004 conferences address different components necessary for the successful integration of behavioral health into primary care.

The SAMHSA Prime-E Study, Primary Care Research in Substance Abuse and Mental Health for the Elderly (Quijano, 2004), is a large multi-site (10) and year (now in its 6th year) study that examines the elderly's use of mental health and substance abuse services in primary care. They compare the effectiveness of two service delivery models: one incorporates enhanced referral to access behavioral health care in specialty settings and the other collocates the behavioral health services within the primary care settings. Preliminary results are encouraging in that they show significantly in-creased engagement. Engagement is defined as getting a person into necessary services and is the crucial first step for an effective intervention. This study showed a 72% rate of engagement in the collocated services vs.

48% for specialty care. The differences are even greater for alcohol related abuse: 72% vs. 29%, respectively.

Swope Health Services in Kansas City, Missouri is in the process of implementing a major integration project (Wilson, 2004). Two important lessons learned from their work thus far include the following: a need to provide the behavior health specialist with additional training in behavioral medicine and psychotropic medicine, working in medical settings, and delivering brief interventions; and, the need to provide primary care physicians and staff with training and scripts in how to make effective referrals to behavioral health specialists that prevent them from using stigmatized phrases, like "refer you to the shrink."

The Air Force has had a large integration project under way for several years that follows a behavioral health consultant model (referral) using clinical psychologists and social workers (Oordt, 2004). They are members of the primary care team and are trained in brief assessments and interventions. Initial evaluations show superior levels of both patient and primary care physician satisfaction. They have found that less than 10% are referred to specialty care. Patients average about 1.5 visits with the behavioral health consultant with most of these being for depression (36.6%) and anxiety (15.7%). The study found that for 2003 there was an estimated value of $369,040 for the 5272 non-active duty visits with no incremental overhead cost. They reported that they will be doing more group work and addressing lifestyle issues.

Summary

From a physician's perspective, the ideal patient is one who can adequately inform the physician of his or her symptoms and coping strategies and who is willing and able to carry out the physician's advice. Unfortunately, this patient is rare, especially when significant lifestyle changes need to be made. Behavioral medicine technologies can help patients approach this ideal by focusing on empowerment and change. As previously shown, they can greatly improve patient outcomes, patient satisfaction, and cost-effectiveness. Additionally, since Behavioral Health Specialists are mental health professionals, they will increase the number and quality of services provided by the PCP's office. It has been estimated that medically unexplained symptoms account for 25%-50% of primary care visits; psychosocial concerns appear to play a prominent role in these visits (Barsky & Borus, 1995). Also, up to 70% of depressed patients seek treatment solely from PCPs (Hoffman, Rice, & Sung, 1996). These patients take more time, are less compliant, and have more health problems than other patients. They are inadequately treated because they do not fit into the current healthcare system and they are not seeking mental health treatment because of stigma, lack of awareness as to the nature of the problem, or simply because it is inconvenient. By including a mental health professional in the treatment team, stigma is minimized and behavioral issues can be addressed in a non-threatening, convenient manner.

Adding a mental health provider to the Primary Care team, however, requires a coherent model that addresses both the primary care practice's management needs as well as the patient's needs.

Putting it All Together: The Prime Behavioral Health Services Model

At the beginning of this chapter we introduced the Prime Behavioral Health Services model, which we now present again below and detail. The logic steps are straightforward. The PCP identifies potential behavioral health issues for a patient and, using protocols, makes a decision to either refer the patient to an outside behavioral health provider (BHP) or to the in-practice Behavioral Health Specialist, (BHS).

Another option is to do both. It may take a while for the patient to be seen by an outside provider and we know from the literature that the majority of those referred don't make it. It may be appropriate to see the patient for three sessions of case management to make sure that the person is, in fact, hooked up with their provider, to make sure the patient is satisfied with the provider, and to provide the PCP assurance that the patient is being well attended.

The BHS is an independent practitioner level mental health provider, for example, clinical psychologist, MSW, or nurse equivalent who will have received specialized training on brief interventions and assessment as well as on working in a primary care setting. This person will be available to the PCP as much as possible. The BHS will conduct a brief assessment using standardized protocols and either provide a brief intervention, or, if appropriate, refer the patient to a more traditional service model outside behavioral provider. The other option is that the BHS can refer the patient to the Prime Self-Management program either on its own or in conjunction with the brief treatment they would provide. In addition, the BHS would use motivational interviewing techniques to address the patient's readiness to change. Either the BHS or a trained "behaviorist," who would work with the BHP, delivers the Prime Self-Management group program. The behaviorist also would provide the patients with prompting on their medication compliance as well as other lifestyle programs.

Prime Self-Management Program

The Prime Self-Management Program addresses the three essential self-management tasks (medical management, role management, and emotional management) and six skills (problem solving, decision making, resource utilization, the formation of a patient-provider partnership, action planning, and self-tailoring) defined by Lorig and Holman (K. R. Lorig, Holman, H.R., 2003). Importantly, Prime Health Program utilizes professional Behavioral Health Specialists in the primary care practice. The Behavioral Health Specialists are accountable and available to the physicians and patients at all times. They perform the following duties:

Provide assessments and brief interventions for such behavioral/emotional
   problems as depression and anxiety
Help the physician make decisions about referrals to behavioral health
   practitioners if longer term interventions are needed
Help move patients toward an appropriate level of readiness to make the
   lifestyle changes needed to more effectively become a partner in their
   care
Conduct self-management groups

Providing these services within and as a part of the primary care practice also
means that they are billable.

Impact

The decision to extend the services offered in a primary care setting is not new.
Primary care groups have long included education and support. What we have
learned is that organized, structured activities can significantly impact emotional
well-being and adherence to the steps necessary to minimize adverse symptoms in
patients' lives. In staff model health maintenance organizations, organized disease
management programs are routine for chronic illnesses. What is still novel is finding
a way to offer cost-effective programs in small commercial settings. Building a
program that incorporates the following criteria:

Quick, brief assessments,
Prompt appropriate referral to specialized behavioral health services,
In-practice brief interventions to emotionally unstable patients,
In-practice brief interventions to patients needing assistance in making
   lifestyle adjustments to medication, diet, or activity, and,
In-practice interventions to high service utilizing patients

can make a difference in peoples' lives and the bottom line of a medical practice.

References

American Academy of Family Physicians. (2004). *Mental health care services by family
   physicians. Position paper.* Retreived November 7, 2004, from http://www.aafp.org/
   x6928.xml
Bandura, A. (1997). *Self-efficacy: The exercise of control.* New York: W. H. Freeman and
   Company.
Barsky, A. J., & Borus, J. F. (1995). Somatization and medicalization in the era of
   managed care.[see comment]. *Journal of the American Medical Association, 274*(24),
   1931-1934.
Bodenheimer, T., Wagner, E. H., & Grumbach, K. (2002). Improving primary care
   for patients with chronic illness: The chronic care model, part 2. *Journal of the
   American Medical Association, 288*(15), 1909-1914.

Brunner, E., White, I., Thorogood, M., Bristow, A., Curle, D., & Marmot, M. (1997). Can dietary interventions change diet and cardiovascular risk factors? A meta-analysis of randomized controlled trials. *American Journal of Public Health, 87*(9), 1415-1422.

Burke, B. L., Arkowitz, H., & Menchola, M. (2003). The efficacy of motivational interviewing: A meta-analysis of controlled clinical trials. *Journal of Consulting & Clinical Psychology, 71*(5), 843-861.

Burkholder, G. J., & Evers, K. A. (2002). Application of the Transtheoretical Model to several problem behaviors. In P. M. Burbank & D. Riebe (Eds.), *Promoting exercise and behavior change in older adults: Interventions with the transtheoretical model* (Vol. xxii, pp. 317). New York: Springer Publishing Co.

Campbell, M. K., Tessaro, I., DeVellis, B., Benedict, S., Kelsey, K., Belton, L., et al. (2000). Tailoring and targeting a worksite health promotion program to address multiple health behaviors among blue-collar women. *American Journal of Health Promotion, 14*(5), 306-313.

Dubbert, P. M. (2002). Physical activity and exercise: Recent advances and current challenges. *Journal of Consulting & Clinical Psychology: Special Behavioral Medicine and Clinical Health Psychology, 70*(3), 526-536.

Felson, D. T., Lawrence, R. C., Hochberg, M. C., McAlindon, T., Dieppe, P. A., Minor, M. A., et al. (2000). Osteoarthritis: new insights. Part 2: treatment approaches.[see comment]. *Annals of Internal Medicine, 133*(9), 726-737.

Force, U. S. P. S. T. (2003). Behavioral counseling in primary care to promote a healthy diet: recommendations and rationale. *American Journal of Nursing, 103*(8), 81-92.

Glasgow, R. E., Wagner, E. H., Kaplan, R. M., Vinicor, F., Smith, L., & Norman, J. (1999). If diabetes is a public health problem, why not treat it as one?: A population based approach to chronic illness. *Annals of Behavioral Medicine, 21*(2), 159-170.

Haynes, R. B., McKibbon, K. A., & Kanani, R. (1996). Systematic review of randomised trials of interventions to assist patients to follow prescriptions for medications.[erratum appears in Lancet 1997 Apr 19;349(9059):1180]. *Lancet, 348*(9024), 383-386.

Hoffman, C., Rice, D., & Sung, H. Y. (1996). Persons with chronic conditions: Their prevalence and costs. *Journal of the American Medical Association, 276*(18), 1473-1479.

Lorig, K., Sobe, L. D., Ritter, P., Laurent, D., & Hobbs, M. (2001). Effect of a self-management program on patients with chronic disease. *Effective Clinical Practice, 4*, 256-262.

Lorig, K. R., & Holman, H.R. (2003). Self-management education: History, definition, outcomes, and mechanisms. *Annals of Behavioral Medicine, 26*(1), 1-7.

Lorig, K. R., Mazonson, P. D., & Holman, H. R. (1993). Evidence suggesting that health education for self-management in patients with chronic arthritis has sustained health benefits while reducing health care costs. *Arthritis and Rheumatism, 36*(4), 439-446.

Lorig, K. R., Sobel, D.S., Stewart, A.L., Brown, B.W., Bandura, A., Ritter, P., et al. (1999). Evidence suggesting that a chronic disease self-management program can improve health status while reducing hospitalization. *Medical Care, 37*(1), 5-14.

McInnis, K. J. (2003). Diet, exercise, and the challenge of combating obesity in primary care. *Journal of Cardiovascular Nursing, 18*(2), 93-100.

McRoberts, C., Burlingame, G. M., & Hoag, M. (1998). Comparative efficacy of individual and group psychotherapy: A meta-analytic perspective. *Group Dynamics: Theory, Research, and Practice, 2,* 101-117.

Miller, W. R., & Rollnick, S. (2002). *Motivational interviewing: Preparing people for change* (2 ed.). New York: Guilford Press.

Natarajan, S., Clyburn, E. B., & Brown, R. T. (2002). Association of exercise stages of change with glycemic control in individuals with type 2 diabetes. *American Journal of Health Promotion, 17*(1), 72-75.

Prochaska, J. O., DiClemente, C. C., & Norcross, J. C. (1992). In search of how people change: Applications to addictive behaviors. *American Psychologist, 47*(9), 1102-1114.

Prochaska, J. O., Redding, C. A., & Evers, K. E. (1997). The transtheoretical model and stages of change. In L. F. Glanz & B. K. Rimer (Eds.), *Health Behavior and Health Education* (2 ed., pp. 60-84). San Francisco: Jossey-Bass.

Steptoe, A., Kerry, S., Rink, E., & Hilton, S. (2001). The impact of behavioral counseling on stage of change in fat intake, physical activity, and cigarette smoking in adults at increased risk of coronary heart disease. *American Journal of Public Health, 91*(2), 265-269.

Wagner, E. H., Austin, B.T., & Von Korff, M. (1996). Improving outcomes in chronic illness. *Managed Care Quarterly, 4*(2), 12-25.

Wagner, E. H., Davis, C., Schaefer, J., Von Korff, M., & Austin, B. (1999). A survey of leading chronic disease management programs: Are they consistent with the literature? *Managed Care Quarterly, 7*(3), 56-66.

Wagner, E. H., Glasgow, R. E., Davis, C., Bonomi, A. E., Provost, L., McCulloch, D., et al. (2001). Quality improvement in chronic illness care: A collaborative approach. *The Joint Commission Journal on Quality Improvement, 27*(2), 63-80.

Wilson, S. B. (2004). Mind and body: Integrating approaches to reduce health disparities. *National Council for Community Behavioral Healthcare.* Retrieved November 4, 2004, from http://www.nccbh.org.html/learn/PCI/04CONF/A1/A1-Wilson.pdf

Chapter 5

Lifestyle Approaches to the Treatment of Hypertension

James A. Blumenthal, Andrew Sherwood, Lara J. LaCaille,
Anastasia Georgiades, & Tanya Goyal
Duke University Medical Center

Hypertension (HTN) is a major health problem, affecting more than 50 million people in the United States and 1 billion worldwide (Joint National Committee, 2003). One out of every four adult Americans currently has HTN, and this number is projected to increase over the next decade. Given the known risks associated with HTN (e.g., stroke, myocardial infarction [MI], congestive heart failure [CHF], kidney failure), reducing blood pressure (BP) is of great importance. In fact, HTN is the most common primary diagnosis in the United States and is responsible for 35 million office visits with HTN as the primary diagnosis (Joint National Committee, 2003). Despite the prevalence of HTN, BP management and control is often inadequate (Berlowitz et al., 1998). Although anti-hypertensive medications can lower BP in many hypertensive individuals (Joint National Committee, 2003; Systolic Hypertension in the Elderly Program Cooperative Research Group, 1991), they are not effective for everyone, and prohibitive costs and unwanted side effects may impair quality of life and reduce adherence (Breckenridge, 1991; Israili & Hall, 1992; Pahor, Guralnik, Furberg, Carbonin, & Havlik, 1996; Suissa, Bourgault, Barkun, Sheehy, & Ernst, 1998). Additionally, some antihypertensive medications may exacerbate abnormalities associated with HTN, such as insulin resistance and hyperlipidemia (Grimm et al., 1996; Weingerger, 1985; Pollare, Lithell, & Berne, 1989; Lithell, Pollare, & Vessby, 1992). Consequently, there has been increasing interest in the development and application of lifestyle modifications for assisting in the management of HTN.

Hypertension is defined as chronically elevated BP, with systolic blood pressure (SBP) of 140 mm Hg or greater, diastolic blood pressure (DBP) of 90 mm Hg or greater, or taking anti-HTN medication (Joint National Committee, 2003). The 2003 report of the Joint National Committee on Prevention, Detection, Evaluation and Treatment of High Blood Pressure (JNC 7) recently provided a new classification system for HTN as well as guidelines for the prevention and management of HTN (See Table 1). One of the most notable changes in the new report is the inclusion of a "prehypertension" category, defined as BPs of 120-130/80-89 mm Hg,

BP Classification	Systolic BP, mm Hg*		Diastolic BP, mm Hg*	Lifestyle modification	Management*	
					Initial drug therapy	
					Without compelling indication	With compelling indications
Normal	<120	and	<80	Encourage		
Prehypertension	120-139	or	80-89	Yes	No antihypertensive drug indicated	Drug(s) for the compelling indications
Stage 1 hypertension	140-159	or	90-99	Yes	Thiazide-type diuretics for most; may consider ACE inhibitor, ARD, B-blocker, CCB, or combination	Drug(s) for the compelling indications. Other antihypertensive drugs (diuretics, ACE inhibitor, ARB, B-blocker, CCB) as needed
Stage 2 hypertension	≥ 160	or	≥ 100	Yes	2-drug combination for most (usually thiazide-type diuretic and ACE inhibitor or ARB or b-Blocker, or CCB)	Drug(s) for the compelling indications. Other antihypertensive drugs (diuretics, ACE inhibitor, ARB, B-blocker, CCB) as needed

Abbreviations: ACE, angiotensin-convertin enzyme; ARB, angiotensin-receptor blocker; BP, blood pressure; CCB, calcium channel blocker. *Treatment determined by highest BP category.

Table 1. JNC 7 Guidelines for the Classification and Management of Blood Pressure. Table adapted from JNC 7 report (Joint National Commission, 2003). Source: Journal of the American Medical Association (2003), 289, 2561. Reprinted with permission.

which in the previous guidelines (Joint National Committee, 1997) identified "high normal" (130-139/85-89 mm Hg) and "normal' (<130/<85 mm Hg) BPs. The "prehypertension" category underscores evidence that cardiovascular risk increases continuously with rising BP and that individuals with prehypertensive BPs are at significant risk for developing HTN and its complications (see Figure 1).

The prevalence of HTN is related to age, gender, and ethnicity. In both men and women, prevalence generally increases markedly across the lifespan. However, in young adults prevalence is much greater in men than women, but this difference progressively diminishes with age, ultimately reversing at around 50 years to a greater prevalence in women than men (Burt et al., 1995). For women, the more dramatic rise in BP associated with age is linked to the occurrence of menopause (Staessen, Bulpitt, Fagard, Lijnen, & Amery, 1989). HTN is also more prevalent among African Americans than Americans of European heritage, especially in the southeastern United States (Hall et al., 1997).

HTN is associated with significant adverse health consequences (Kochanek, Smith, & Anderson, 2001). For instance, a 5-6 mm Hg DBP elevation has been shown to predict a 35-40% increased risk of stroke and a 20-25% increased risk of ischemic heart disease (IHD) and MI (Collins et al., 1990; MacMahon et al., 1990). MI and stroke are not directly due to HTN, however, but rather to the resulting structural changes in the heart and blood vessels. For example, left ventricular hypertrophy (LVH), a structural consequence of HTN, is one of the strongest known predictors, other than advancing age, of IHD and fatal and non-fatal MI. In fact, enlarged LV mass, independent of other conventional risk factors, is associated with increased morbidity and mortality in individuals with HTN (Casale et al., 1986) as well as healthy individuals (Levy, Garrison, Savage, Kannel, & Castelli, 1990).

Although the rate of stroke-related mortality can be reduced considerably with anti-HTN medications, the expected reduction in IHD-related deaths has not been as consistently demonstrated in treatment trials (Collins et al., 1990; MacMahon et al., 1990). The relatively modest reduction in IHD-related death following anti-HTN medication intervention underscores the need for implementing alternative treatments such as lifestyle changes of diet, exercise, weight loss and stress management. Notably, such lifestyle interventions have been found to improve other risk factors, such as hyperinsulinemia and dyslipidemia (Dengel, Galecki, Hagberg, & Pratley, 1988; Pratley et al., 2000; Smutok et al., 1993; Wallace, Mills, & Browning, 1997).

There exists a great need to identify effective interventions to reduce HTN and to retard/ reverse the structural changes associated with elevated BP. Stress reduction interventions, such as biofeedback, relaxation, meditation, and cognitive-behavioral therapies (CBT), do not appear to be as effective as mono therapies as once thought. However, there is now good reason to believe that exercise and diet interventions represent two of the best lifestyle approaches to treat persons with HTN and prevent people with high BP from developing HTN. In fact, the 2003 report of the Joint National Committee on Prevention, Detection, Evaluation and Treatment of High

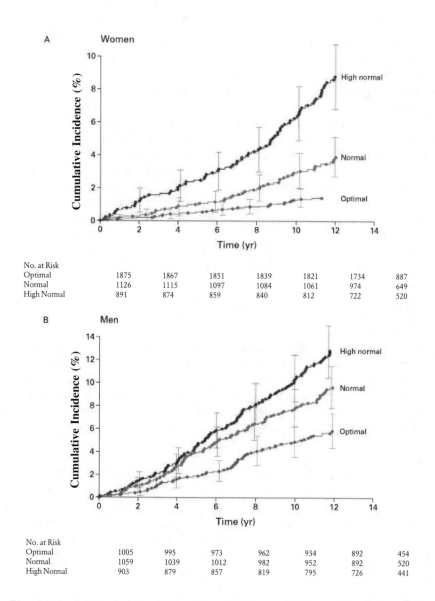

A   Women

No. at Risk

Optimal	1875	1867	1851	1839	1821	1734	887
Normal	1126	1115	1097	1084	1061	974	649
High Normal	891	874	859	840	812	722	520

B   Men

No. at Risk

Optimal	1005	995	973	962	934	892	454
Normal	1059	1039	1012	982	952	892	520
High Normal	903	879	857	819	795	726	441

Figure 1. Cumulative Incidence of Cardiovascular Events in Women (Panel A) and Men (Panel B) without Hypertension, According to Blood-Pressure Category at the Base-Line Examination. Vertical bars indicate 95 percent confidence intervals. Optimal blood pressure is a systolic pressure of less than 120 mm Hg and a diastolic pressure of less than 80 mm Hg. Normal blood pressure is a systolic pressure of 120 to 129 mm Hg or a diastolic pressure of 80 to 84 mm Hg. High-normal blood pressure is a systolic pressure of 130 to 139 mm Hg or a diastolic pressure of 85 to 89 mm Hg. If the systolic and diastolic pressure readings for a subject were in different categories, the higher of the two categories was used. Source: New England Journal of Medicine (2001), 345, 1295. Reprinted with permission.

Blood Pressure (2003) recommends that lifestyle modifications be the initial treatment strategy for lowering HTN. Figure 2 displays a clinical algorithm for the stepped care approach to treating HTN, beginning initially with lifestyle modification and progressing to more aggressive medical management. Among the lifestyle factors that have been studied, exercise and dietary modification are generally regarded as being most promising. This is an area where psychologists are especially likely to make significant contributions to the development, delivery, and assessment of lifestyle behavior change programs.

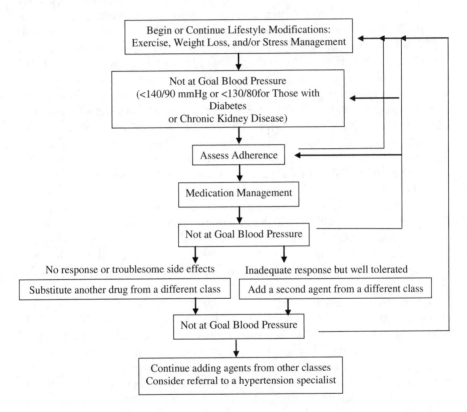

Figure 2. Algorithm for the Treatment of Hypertension. A stepped care approach is suggested beginning with lifestyle modification (e.g., diet, exercise and stress management) and progressing to include different pharmacologic regimens as needed. The minimum goal is to achieve BP levels <140/90 mm Hg, but optimal BP is <120/80 mm Hg. Adapted from JNC 7 (2003). Source: Journal of the American Medical Association (2003), 289, 2564. Adapted with permission.

Efficacy of Exercise Training in the Treatment of HTN

Numerous reviews (American College of Sports Medicine, 1994; Arroll & Beaglehole, 1992; Blumenthal, Sherwood, Gullette, Georgiades, & Tweedy, 2002; Halbert et al., 1997; Kelley, 1999; Kelley & McClellan, 1994; Linden & Chambers, 1994; Siegel & Blumenthal, 1991; Tipton, 1991) have supported the value of physical activity and aerobic exercise. Most cross sectional studies have consistently demonstrated an association between higher levels of fitness and lower BP. The strengths of these studies lie in the diversity of patient populations included, their large sample sizes, and consistency of results despite widely differing methodologies. Additionally, these findings have been replicated with several large longitudinal studies (Paffenbarger, Thorbe, & Wing, 1968; Lee, Hsieh, & Paffenbarger, 1995; Paffenbarger Wing, Hyde, & Jung, 1983). One particular longitudinal study (Blair, Goodyear, Gibbons, & Cooper, 1984), that investigated 6,039 men and women who were normotensive at the time of self-referral to a preventive medicine clinic, found that the relative risk of HTN in the low fitness individuals, relative to those considered high fitness, was 1.52 (confidence interval 1.08-2.15). This association remained after controlling for age, body mass index (BMI), baseline BP, and follow-up interval.

We have previously reviewed the major randomized trials of exercise in patients with HTN (Blumenthal et al., 2002; Siegel & Blumenthal, 1991). Most exercise interventions typically involve aerobic exercise such as walking, jogging or biking. A typical exercise prescription involves 3 dimensions: frequency (e.g., 3-5 times per week), intensity (e.g., 70-85% of a person's age-predicted maximum heart rate [estimated as 220-age]), and duration (e.g., 30-45 minutes). Typically, cardiovascular "training effects" are induced in 8-12 weeks, although it has been noted that BP changes may occur as early as 2 weeks from the initiation of an exercise program. Despite claims by organizations such as the American College of Sports Medicine (1994) that exercise will produce a 10 mm Hg reduction in both SBP and DBP, results from well-controlled studies offer more conservative estimates. Moreover, most studies have been limited because of high dropout rates, unplanned crossover, imprecise measurement of BP or aerobic fitness, or failure to precisely measure other potential confounders (e.g., body weight), and few studies included adequate numbers of women. Better designed studies with greater methodological rigor generally demonstrate smaller exercise-related BP reductions than studies with less rigorous controls. Interestingly, recent meta-analyses (Kelley, 1999; Whelton, Chin, Xin, & He, 2002) demonstrated more modest reductions in BP due to exercise, suggesting that only a 2% reduction in resting SBP and a 1% reduction in DBP, with an average BP reduction of 3.8/2.5 mm Hg is more likely to be achieved. Thus, moderate exercise alone, without weight loss or dietary modification generally appears to produce only modest BP reductions.

Efficacy of Diet and Weight Loss in the Treatment of HTN

Weight Management

The relationship between obesity and BP is well-established (Jeffery, 1991). Given that the prevalence of overweight and obesity is rapidly increasing (Flegal at al., 2002), the burden of HTN and cardiovascular-related mortality also can be anticipated to increase. In fact, the prevalence of overweight and obesity in US adults in the year 2000 was 64.5% and 30.9%, respectively. Numerous intervention studies have examined the effect of weight loss on BP, but few have specifically targeted hypertensive patients. Additionally, few studies compared weight loss alone to a usual diet/exercise control condition. Consequently, these studies leave unanswered the specific effect of weight loss on BP. Several interventions have included multiple dietary/lifestyle components, compared weight loss to exercise, or included a dietary intervention for all groups (e.g., Blumenthal et al., 2000; Dengel et al., 1998; Gordon, Scott, & Levine, 1997; Perez-Stable et al., 1995). Reviews of these interventional studies (e.g., Mulrow et al., 2002; Staessen, Fagard, & Amery, 1988) have shown significant reductions in BP resulting from weight loss, as well as a magnitude of change that is considered clinically meaningful. MacMahon and colleagues (1987), pooled the results from a number of interventional studies, and found that a weight loss of 9.2 kg was associated with a reduction of 6.3 mm Hg SBP and 3.1 mm Hg DBP. Similarly, in a recent meta-analysis of 25 randomized controlled trials of weight reduction and BP, a net weight loss of 5.1 kg reduced SBP by 4.44 mm Hg and DBP by 3.57 mm Hg (Neter, Stam, Kok, Grobbee, & Geleijnse, 2003). Larger BP reductions were found in populations that lost more weight. Examining the longer-term of effects of weight loss on BP, Avenell et al. (2004) conducted a meta-analysis of randomized controlled trials of weight loss with follow ups of at least a year, and calculated that a 10% weight loss was associated with a fall in SBP of 6.1 mm Hg. These results support the conclusion that weight loss interventions are efficacious in reducing BP in both normotensive and hypertensive overweight individuals.

In general, group behavioral weight loss interventions for obesity are the standard of care, and have not changed substantially over the past decade (Wadden, Foster & Brownell, 2002). On average, participants in a 20-week program lose 8.5 kg, but without continued treatment or a maintenance program, one third of that weight is typically regained within one year. Consequently, there have been increased efforts to incorporate maintenance programs into well-established, empirically-validated manualized behavioral weight loss programs, such as the LEARN Program (Brownell, 2004) and Cooper, Fairburn and Hawker's (2003) cognitive behavioral treatment manual.

Although exercise is often emphasized in many weight management programs, it is not usually associated with significant weight loss unless accompanied by caloric restriction. For instance, studies examining exercise alone (without diet modifications) have found decreases of < 2 kg body weight and < 1-2% body fat

(Wilfley & Brownell, 1994; Wilmore, 1983). Furthermore, exercise is associated with minimal changes in hip-to-waist circumference ratio, which suggests that adipose distribution is not significantly altered (Bouchard, Bray, & Hubbard, 1990). However, exercise appears to be associated with increased maintenance of weight loss (Craighead & Blum, 1989; Bahlkoetter, Callahon, & Linton, 1979; Blair & Holder, 2002; Wing & Klem, 2002), which appears central to sustaining BP changes associated with weight loss. There is also some evidence that exercise and diet modification may act synergistically to improve aerobic capacity and reduce body weight (Hagan, Upton, Wong, & Whittam, 1986). Moreover, it has been shown that exercise enhances adherence as well as weight loss compared to instructions to increase exercise on one's own (Craighead & Blum, 1989). Thus, it appears that behavioral weight loss programs that include supervised exercise are likely to be the most effective intervention to promote and maintain weight loss.

Dietary Components

Several specific dietary nutrients have been implicated in affecting BP, which has resulted in numerous interventions targeting these specific dietary factors. Reduction of alcohol use and sodium intake, as well as supplementation of potassium, magnesium, and calcium have all been found to lower BP, particularly in those populations with HTN (e.g., Cutler, Follmann, & Allender, 1997; Whelton et al., 1997).

Alcohol. Epidemiological studies have generally shown that alcohol consumption is associated with elevated BP (see Beilin, Puddey, & Burke, 1996), and a direct relationship between change in alcohol consumption and change in BP has been observed (Gordon & Doyle, 1986; Gordon & Kannel, 1983; Kromhout, Bosschieter, & Coulander, 1985). These findings have prompted the Joint National Committee (2003) to recommend limiting alcohol intake to no more than 1 oz of ethanol per day. However, much of the research on alcohol restriction and BP has focused on alcoholics during and after detoxification (Aguilera et al., 1999; Saunders, Beevers, & Paton, 1981), and fewer studies have examined the relationship in light to moderate drinkers. Despite these limitations, the overall findings in studies of alcohol restriction and BP do indicate that reducing alcohol intake can lower BP, particularly in heavy drinkers. In a review of the literature on alcohol and BP over the past 30 years, Keil and colleagues (Keil, Liese, Filipiak, Swales, & Grobbee, 1998) concluded that a direct and causal relationship exists between chronic intake of $\geq$ 30-60 g of alcohol per day and elevated BP, and that reducing alcohol intake is effective in lowering BP. Thus, recommending moderate alcohol consumption appears warranted, but complete abstinence in non-problem drinkers does not appear necessary, especially in light of the beneficial effects of moderate alcohol consumption on CAD risk (Joint National Committee, 2003).

Sodium. Dietary sodium intake is thought to be related to the development of HTN, in large part based on observations of increased BP in cultures with higher intake of dietary salt (Midgley, Matthew, Greenwood, & Logan, 1996). However, individuals vary greatly in their BP response to sodium (Joint National Committee,

2003) and results of within-population studies of the relationship between sodium and BP have been mixed (Midgley et al., 1996). Additionally, there is some evidence that overly restrictive sodium intake may actually have detrimental effects on other variables, such as lipids (e.g., Egan, Weder, Petrin, & Hoffman, 1991) and may even promote increased cardiovascular morbidity and mortality (e.g., Alderman, Madhavan, Cohen, Sealey, & Laragh, 1995). Recent reviews of both epidemiological studies and randomized controlled trials of sodium reduction and HTN (Cutler et al., 1997; He & Whelton, 1997; Midgley et al., 1996) have supported the benefits of sodium restriction on BP. In a review of 32 studies with outcome data for 2635 subjects, Cutler et al. (1997) observed a dose-response relationship in which a 100 mmol 24-hr sodium reduction was associated with a decrease of 5.8 mm Hg SBP and 2.5 mm Hg DBP for hypertensives and 2.3 mm Hg SBP and 1.4 mm Hg DBP for normotensives. Similarly, a meta-analysis of 83 studies examining the effects of reduced sodium on BP determined a similar relationship, with a reduction of 3.9 mm Hg SBP and 1.9 mm Hg DBP among those with HTN, but only 1.2 mm Hg SBP and 0.23 mm Hg DBP in non-HTN patients (Graudal, Galloe, & Garred, 1998). Collectively, these reviews indicate that sodium restriction interventions have a moderately beneficial effect on BP, particularly for SBP and in individuals with HTN, with the greatest benefit seen in those who are salt-sensitive.

Other minerals. A variety of other minerals have been implicated in affecting BP including potassium, magnesium, and calcium. Of these, potassium supplementation has been found to have the most robust effect on reducing BP and perhaps protecting against the development of HTN. Whelton et al. (1997) performed a meta-analysis of 33 randomized controlled trials, and found that potassium supplementation was significantly associated with reductions of 3 mm Hg SBP and 2 mm Hg DBP. Furthermore, there was a relationship between the effect of potassium and sodium intake, highlighting the importance of the sodium-potassium ratio.

Early studies of environmental factors related to BP that suggested a relationship between hard water and HTN prompted interest in the contribution of minerals, including calcium and magnesium, to elevated BP. A meta-analysis of epidemiological studies of the association between dietary calcium intake and BP (Cappuccio et al., 1995) evaluated 23 population studies and found an inverse relationship between dietary calcium intake and BP. However, a secondary meta-analysis of data from 22 randomized clinical trials of the effects of dietary calcium supplementation on BP (Allender et al., 1996), reported a drop in BP of slightly less than 1 mm Hg SBP and 0.2 mm Hg DBP, with larger decreases in SBP among hypertensives than among normotensives. Studies that have examined the relationship between magnesium supplementation and BP generally have been small, but results often have suggested a beneficial effect of magnesium supplementation on BP (Dyckner & Wester, 1983; Motoyama, Sano, & Fukuzaki, 1989; Widman, Wester, Stegmayr, & Wirell, 1993). Larger randomized trials of magnesium supplementation on BP have found mixed effects (Kawano, Matsuoka, Takishita, & Omae, 1998; Yamamoto et al., 1995), and thus it remains unclear whether magnesium supplementation alone is beneficial, and therefore cannot be recommended as a preventive measure or treatment for HTN at the current time.

A recent review of dietary interventions in the treatment of HTN including studies of sodium restriction, alcohol restriction, and potassium, magnesium, and calcium supplementation, concluded that a balanced approach to eating was the optimal dietary approach to BP reduction (Blumenthal, et al., 2002).

Combination Dietary Interventions

A series of recent studies have begun examining the effects of combining a number of dietary nutrients into whole diet approaches to reducing BP. The initial DASH (Dietary Approaches to Stop Hypertension) study was a NHLBI-sponsored multi-center, randomized feeding trial developed to examine the effects of three dietary patterns on BP among unmedicated persons with higher than optimal DBP or with stage 1 HTN (Appel et al., 1997; Windhauser et al., 1999; Conlin et al., 2000). All meals were provided to participants over an 8-week treatment period. The three dietary patterns included: a "control" diet reflecting a typical American diet; a fruits and vegetables diet that was high in these foods, but otherwise similar to the control diet, and a "combination" diet (i.e., the DASH diet) that was high in fruits, vegetables, and low-fat dairy products as well as low in total fat, saturated fat, and cholesterol. More specifically, the DASH diet was rich in magnesium, calcium, and potassium, minerals which have all been individually identified as being associated with reduced BP. Sodium content and body weight were kept constant through the entire study. The DASH diet, compared to the control diet, reduced both SBP and DBP by 5.5 and 3.0 mm Hg, respectively. Patients with HTN experienced the greatest reduction in BP (11.4/5.5 mm Hg) whereas non-HTN participants had more modest reductions (3.5/2.1 mm Hg) (Appel et al., 1997). Figure 3 displays the primary results. Interestingly, African Americans experienced the greatest effects of the DASH diet (Appel et al., 1997).

A second DASH study (Sacks et al., 2001) compared the effects of three levels of sodium intake and two dietary patterns on BP among unmedicated participants with stage I HTN. In this controlled feeding study, participants were randomly assigned to the DASH diet or to a control diet representing a typical American diet. Using a crossover design, participants were assigned 3 different sodium levels (150, 100, 50 mmol/d for a 2100 kcal diet) for 30 days each. SBP reduction was superior with the DASH diet across all sodium levels, while reductions in sodium intake were associated with further decreases in SBP for both the DASH and control diets.

Thus, it appears that the DASH diet is effective in all segments of the population and it is particularly effective in African Americans, a group dispropor-tionately affected by HTN and its consequences (Svetkey et al., 1999). Not surprisingly, the DASH diet has now become part of the current JNC 7 (Joint National Commission, 2003) recommendations for the prevention and treatment of HTN. It should be emphasized, however, that the initial DASH studies were "feeding studies," which provided participants with prepared food for the treatment

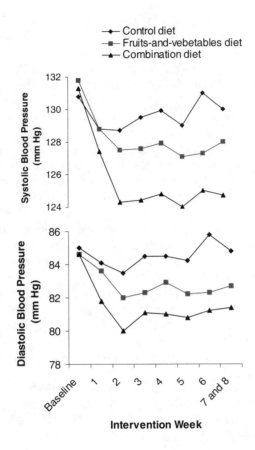

Figure 3. Results from the DASH Study. Mean Systolic and Diastolic Blood Pressures at Base Line and during Each Intervention Week, According to Diet, for 379 Subjects with Complete Sets of Weekly Blood-Pressure Measurements. Source: New England Journal of Medicine, 1997, 336, 1122. Reprinted with permission.

period. Moreover, the study was designed to assess the impact of diet, independent of weight loss. Consequently, caloric consumption was adjusted to maintain body weight and thus, the effects of weight loss were not studied (Appel et al., 1997).

Combination Dietary and Weight Loss Interventions

Recently, a few randomized controlled trials have begun to explore the added benefits of weight loss when combined with making specific dietary changes, such as reducing sodium or eating the DASH diet. The TONE study (Whelton et al., 1998) included 975 participants who were receiving a single anti-HTN medication.

The 585 obese participants were randomized to one of 4 conditions: (a) low-sodium diet, (b) weight loss, (c) low-sodium + weight loss, or (d) usual care. BP reductions were greatest in the combined intervention (-5.3 mm Hg SBP, -3.4 mm Hg DBP), but slightly smaller reductions were also found in the weight loss group (-4.0 mm Hg SBP, -1.1 mm Hg DBP) and the low-sodium group (-3.4 mm Hg SBP, -1.9 mm Hg DBP). Relative to usual care, hazard ratios among the participants were 0.60 for low-sodium intake alone, 0.64 for weight loss alone, and 0.47 for weight loss plus low-sodium diet, indicating decreased morbidity and mortality.

The DEW-IT (Diet, Exercise, and Weight Loss Intervention Trial) study was the first randomized controlled trial that assessed the efficacy of a multi-dimensional intervention involving the DASH diet in combination with weight loss, aerobic exercise, and sodium reduction (Miller et al., 2002). Forty-four participants who had "pre-HTN" or HTN, were overweight, and were taking one anti-HTN medication were randomized to either (a) a 9-week comprehensive lifestyle intervention, in which they received all of their meals (DASH-diet, low-sodium, and reduced calorie) and participated in 3 supervised exercise sessions per week; or (b) a no-intervention control group. No instruction in diet or weight loss was provided to the intervention group, other than asking participants to eat all of their meals and nothing additional. The lifestyle group mean net reductions in 24-hour ambulatory BP were 9.5 mm Hg SBP and 5.3 mm Hg DBP (See Figure 4). Although the sample size was small, these results indicate that individuals who are taking anti-HTN medications can further reduce their BP when provided with a highly structured diet and exercise intervention.

In another extension of the DASH studies, PREMIER (PREMIER Collaborative Research Group, 2003) assessed the added effects of the DASH diet when paired with a multi-component lifestyle intervention. PREMIER was an 18-month, multicenter trial examining the effect of different levels of lifestyle intervention on BP in prehypertensive or hypertensive patients who were not taking anti-HTN medications. Across sites, 810 individuals were randomly assigned to one of three groups: (a) advice-only, which involved a 30-min educational lesson on ways to reduce BP; (b) "established intervention," involving a 6-month behavioral intervention for weight loss (if indicated), reduction in sodium intake, increased physical activity, and limited alcohol intake; or (c) the established intervention plus instruction in the DASH diet. At the completion of the 6-month intervention, SBP was reduced in all three groups, though both groups receiving the behavioral interventions experienced the most significant reductions. Specifically, SBP was reduced 6.6 mm Hg, 10.5 mm Hg, and 11.1 mm Hg for the above three groups, respectively (see Figure 5). Although this study clearly supports the efficacy of nonpharmacologic interventions, PREMIER did not assess the impact of the DASH diet alone nor did it control for weight loss, making it difficult to determine the relative impact of different components of behavioral interventions.

Currently, the ENCORE Study at Duke University Medical Center is examining the independent contributions of the DASH diet alone and the DASH diet

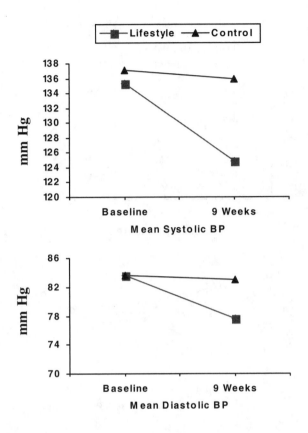

Figure 4. Results from DEW-IT (Miller et al., 2002). Mean systolic and diastolic BP over time by randomized group. Source: Hypertension (2002), 40, 612-618. Printed with permission.

combined with a behavioral weight loss program compared to usual care in healthy persons with pre-HTN and HTN, delivered in "free-living" setting over a 4 month treatment period. Key endpoints include not only clinic and ambulatory BPs, but also vascular markers of disease, including arterial stiffness and endothelial dysfunction.

Biofeedback, Relaxation Therapies, and Stress Management

Numerous intervention studies designed to reduce psychological stress have been conducted over the past three decades and their effectiveness has been evaluated in several meta-analytic reports (Jacob, Chesney, Williams, Ding, & Shapiro, 1991; Eisenberg et al., 1993; Linden, & Chambers, 1994). The most commonly used techniques applied in stress reduction interventions can be divided into 3 major areas: biofeedback, relaxation techniques and cognitive behavioral therapy.

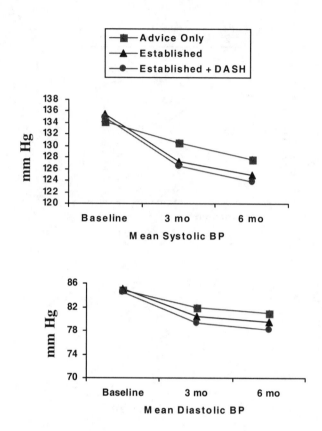

Figure 5. Results from PREMIER Study in which patients received the DASH diet plus lifestyle modification (JNC 7), diet (JNC 6) or usual care (Adapted from PREMIER, 2003). Mean systolic and diastolic BP over time by randomized group. Source: Journal of the American Medical Association (2003), 289, 2090. Reprinted with permission.

Biofeedback has been investigated as a potential treatment method in the behavioral management of hypertension in a number of studies. Biofeedback is a treatment technique designed to teach patients self-regulation of somatic processes. A variety of biofeedback methods have been used, including electromyographic (EMG) feedback, heart rate feedback, and blood pressure (BP) feedback. EMG biofeedback has been most widely used, principally as an adjunct to relaxation training. BP biofeedback is more difficult to perform; standard sphygmomanometry is too cumbersome, automated devices are too slow and distracting, and direct BP measurement using arterial catheterization are too invasive. Shapiro (Shapiro et al., 1969) developed a non-invasive procedure using a constant cuff technique in which BP is measured with each heart beat. In this approach, a microphone is placed near the elbow to detect Korotkoff (K) sounds and an EKG record permits detection of a K-sound with each heartbeat. To train patients to lower BP, the cuff is inflated so that the K-sounds are detected half of the time. Patients are reinforced using operant conditioning for those heart beats that are no followed by a K-sound. Once this is achieved, a process of shaping is introduced in which the cuff is deflated by 2 mm Hg and the entire process is repeated until a new median SBP is reached. Although Sharpiro et al. demonstrated that it is possible to lower BP with this method, the technique is not easily adapted for clinical practice and is seldom used. Agras and Jacob (1979) noted that BP biofeedback "has no greater clinical effect than relaxation therapy, thus the extra investment in blood pressure feedback equipment would seem unwarranted" (p 225). Indeed, any modality of biofeedback as a single method treatment has only showed limited effectiveness in reducing BP (Jacob et al., 1991; Eisenberg et al., 1993). In addition, in the studies where an effect was evident it was usually not significantly different from that of a placebo or sham biofeedback interventions (e.g., Blanchard et al., 1996; Henderson, Hart, Lal, & Hunyor, 1998; Hunyor et al., 1997).

Relaxation techniques, such as progressive muscle relaxation, meditation, and yoga have also been utilized as interventions for HTN. In the Hypertension Intervention Pooling Project, Kaufmann et al. (1988) reviewed 12 randomized controlled trials of relaxation therapies in the treatment of HTN. The studies involved the use of relaxation therapy alone, relaxation in combination with biofeedback, or relaxation in combination with other treatments such as dietary counseling or cognitive restructuring. The meta-analysis showed a significant, although modest, decrease in DBP for patients who were not pharmacologically treated, but no significant improvement for medicated patients; the effect on SBP was not significant. It also was evident that patients with higher pretreatment BP levels showed the greatest change. In one of the more definitive meta-analyses, Jacob et al. (1991) concluded that relaxation therapy had no significant effects on BP levels.

It has been reported that cognitive behavioral stress management therapy can reduce excessive stress arousal by changing cognitive and emotional responses to events, include cognitive restructuring, adaptive emotional learning strategies, imagery, and psychosocial or mental relaxation. Work by Patel (1991) has consistently been the most promising. She has reported significant reductions in BP and medication use using a combination of meditation, breathing techniques, stress management, and biofeedback. In one study she reported BP reductions from 168/100 to 141/84 mm Hg in the treated group compared to 169/101 to 160/96 mm Hg in controls (Patel & North, 1975). Other studies have been far less impressive. In a study by Batey et al. (2000), stress management was one of seven non-pharmacologic approaches evaluated in Phase I Trials of Hypertension Prevention (TOHP-I) for efficacy in lowering DBP in healthy men and women aged 30 to 54 years with DBP 80-89 mm Hg. The only significant effect was a 1.36 mm Hg reduction in DBP relative to controls at the end of the trial for stress management participants who completed at least 61% or more of the intervention sessions. It was concluded that stress management is an unlikely candidate for primary prevention of HTN in a general population sample similar to study participants.

After the somewhat discouraging results from single treatment trials, it was suggested that the use of multi-component stress reducing therapies may prove to be more beneficial than using a single approach alone. Some meta-analytic reviews consequently attempted to compare single component interventions to combination therapies. In Jacob et al.'s (1991) meta-analysis of 75 treatment groups and 41 control groups, it was concluded that single component interventions, such as meditation or relaxation therapy, showed small effects or no reduction in BP levels (-5.7 to +3.5 mm Hg for SBP and -3.1 to +2.3 mm Hg for DBP). In a subsequent meta-analysis of more than 80 studies, Eisenberg et al. (1993) concluded that there were no significant effects on BP from single component interventions (SBP effects between –1.5 mm Hg and +2.9 mm Hg; DBP effects between –0.8 mm Hg and +1.2 mmHg), whereas combination therapies showed more promising results (-13.5 mm Hg for SBP and –3.4 mm Hg for DBP). More recently, Linden and Chambers (1999) conducted a meta-analysis comparing 90 randomized controlled studies on stress-reduction in the treatment of HTN with 30 pharmacological and 47 behavioral interventions. Similar to previous reviews, results showed only small or no effects on BP reductions from the single-component stress-reducing therapies while the multi-component stress management interventions reduced BP to a greater degree and over a longer period of time (-9.7/-7.2 mm Hg). Individualized cognitive stress management therapy showed the largest BP reductions, with BP reductions on average of 15.2/9.2 mm Hg.

In summary, many early studies that investigated the effect of biofeedback, relaxation techniques and/or cognitive behavioral therapy in the treatment of HTN suffered from serious methodological limitations such as small sizes, unsatisfactory controls, or unstable baseline BP values. Randomized controlled studies using single component interventions such as relaxation and biofeedback generally have shown little to no effect on BP reduction. Given the inconsistency of the findings to date, stress management therapy cannot be recommended routinely for patients with HTN. There is some evidence that individualized multi-component cognitive behavioral stress therapy can have a significant BP lowering effect among hypertensive patients, and perhaps that patients with high stress levels or who demonstrate elevated BPs in response to stress may benefit from stress management and relaxation therapies. Thus, in certain patient groups, such approaches might be a valuable complementary method of lowering BP, improving quality of life, and reducing cardiovascular risk. In addition, even if stress reducing techniques have not proven to have direct BP lowering effects, stress management may still prove to be a useful method in multi-component behavioral interventions by improving quality of life and increasing compliance to lifestyle modification and medical therapy.

Adherence to Lifestyle Behavior Changes

Despite the documented benefits of both pharmacological and lifestyle interventions, noncompliance with treatment recommendations is a significant problem in the management of HTN. Up to 50% of patients who are prescribed anti-hypertensive medications discontinue taking these medications within one year (Jones, Gorkin, Lian, Staffa, & Fletcher, 1995). Patients also have difficulty initiating regular exercise programs and modifying their dietary habits. Although many of the studies reviewed above report good compliance with treatment protocols, adherence typically declines over time, and long-term maintenance of lifestyle behavioral change remains a significant challenge.

Efforts to improve adherence to diet and exercise programs have been guided by a number of psychological theories of behavior change. The health belief model (Rosenstock, 1974) suggests that the adoption of new health-related behaviors is determined by an individual's beliefs about his or her health and about the behavior being considered. These beliefs include perceptions of susceptibility to an illness, severity of the illness, benefits of the behavior, and barriers to performing the behavior. Social cognitive theory (Bandura, 1986) proposes that behavior change can be predicted from two types of expectancies: *outcome expectancy* represents an individual's belief about the degree to which a given behavior will lead to a desired outcome, while *self-efficacy* represents the belief in one's ability to perform the behavior. Self-efficacy is proposed to be a stronger predictor of behavior change, and is determined by mastery experiences, modeling, social persuasion, and somatic and emotional states. The Theory of Planned Behavior (Azjen, 1991) suggests that the primary predictor of behavior change is an individual's intention to perform a given behavior. Intention is influenced by attitudes toward the behavior, perceived social norms, and perceived behavioral control.

The Transtheoretical Model (Prochaska & DiClemente, 1983) is a stage-based theory of behavior change that classifies an individual's motivation or readiness for behavior change based on current behavior and intentions for future behavior. The five stages of change are: precontemplation (not considering behavioral change), contemplation (considering behavior change but no action taken), preparation (making small or intermittent behavioral changes), action (engaging in behavioral change for less than six months), and maintenance (engaging in the behavior for six months or longer). Individuals may move back and forth among these stages, and progression is influenced by self-efficacy for behavior change, perceived benefits and costs of behavior change (decisional balance), and use of cognitive and behavioral strategies affecting readiness to change (processes of change).

Many of the psychological constructs proposed in these theories have received empirical support as predictors of dietary and exercise behaviors. For example, exercise self-efficacy was associated with adherence to both home-based and supervised exercise programs in a study of healthy, sedentary adults (Oman & King, 1998). Perceived barriers predicted adherence to dietary fiber goals in a six-month diet and exercise program for healthy men with IHD risk factors (Naslund,

Fredrikson, Hellenuis, & de Faire, 1996). Behavioral intentions significantly predicted adherence to prescribed exercise among patients in a phase II cardiac rehabilitation program (Blanchard et al., 2003).

Other predictors of adherence include mood, social support, environmental factors, and intervention characteristics. Depressive symptoms have been associated with poor adherence to a low-salt diet among hypertensive African American men (Kim, Han, Hill, Rose, & Roary, 2003) as well as lower exercise session attendance and less improvement in VO_{2max} among patients participating in a cardiac rehabilitation program (Glazer, Emery, Frid, & Banyasz, 2002). Spousal support has been shown to predict greater adherence to a low-fat diet among men with hypercholesterolemia (Bovbjerg et al., 1995), and instrumental support predicted the number of weeks exercised among women who had previously completed a cardiac rehabilitation program (Moore, Dolansky, Ruland, Pashkow, & Blackburn, 2003).

Enviromental factors that may affect dietary adherence include social situations, eating out, and diet difficulty (Jeffery, French, & Schmid, 1990), while factors such as availability of home exercise equipment, actual and perceived access to exercise facilities, and satisfaction with facilities have been shown to affect exercise adherence (Trost, Owen, Bauman, Sallis, & Brown, 2002). Examples of intervention characteristics that appear to enhance diet and exercise adherence include provision of prepared meals versus self-selected meals (Metz et al., 1997), and exercise prescriptions of moderate rather than vigorous intensity (Perri et al., 2002). With regard to the maintenance of any type of behavior change, the strongest and most consistent predictor of long-term adherence is initial adherence.

Meta-analyses of diet and exercise interventions have found that these programs can effectively promote behavior change (Brunner et al., 1997; Dishman & Buckworth, 1996). Specific strategies that have been shown to increase adherence to exercise, dietary changes, and pharmacotherapy have been summarized in several reviews (Brownell & Cohen, 1995; Burke, Dunbar-Jacob, & Hill, 1997; Dunbar-Jacob & Schlenk, 2001) and include behavioral contracting, behavioral skills training, self-monitoring, social support, self-efficacy enhancement, positive reinforcement, stimulus control, contingency contracting, telephone/mail contact, cognitive aids (e.g., reminders), and persuasive communication.

Diet and exercise interventions guided by social cognitive theory or the transtheoretical model appear to be particularly effective in promoting adherence. For example, an intervention designed to enhance exercise self-efficacy in a sample of sedentary adults resulted in increased frequency, duration, and distance walked over five months compared with a control group (McCauley, Courneya, Rudolph, & Lox, 1994). Patients receiving tailored educational information based on their stage of change significantly reduced dietary fat intake compared with the controls (no information), whereas patients receiving non-tailored information were not significantly different from controls (Campbell et al., 1994). Exercise consultation matched to patients' stage of change also increased physical activity during a phase

IV cardiac rehabilitation program compared with standard exercise information (Hughes et al., 2002).

The techniques used in behavior change interventions vary widely across studies, making it difficult to determine the relative efficacy of individual components. Multicomponent programs incorporating both education and behavioral strategies are generally recommended in order to promote the adoption of new health behaviors. In addition, individualized interventions appear to be more effective in enhancing adherence to diet and exercise than generic interventions (Bock, Marcus, Pinto, & Forsyth, 2001; Dalgard, Thuroe, Haastrup, Haghfelt, & Stender, 2001). Relapse prevention, which involves helping patients to identify high-risk situations, develop solutions, and manage lapses, is important to include in order to maximize long-term maintenance of behavior change.

Future Research Directions

Although there have been numerous studies that documented a relationship between lifestyle factors and elevated BP, there have been few randomized controlled trials of lifestyle modification in individuals with HTN. Additionally, inattentiveness to key methodological details has impeded progress in this area. Rigorous randomized controlled designs including careful medical screening, precise documentation of hypertensive status, reproducible interventions, and adequately powered samples are imperative. Consideration of individual differences should also be included, as there appears to be considerable variability in response to treatment. That is, the most important lifestyle behavior to modify may be different for different patient populations, and thus identifying the treatment that will be most effective for each patient is an important area for future research. In addition, consideration of mechanisms by which lifestyle modifications may reduce BP should be considered. Finally, it is important that the impact of the interventions on appropriate endpoints be carefully evaluated. HTN may represent a marker for underlying cardiovascular pathophysiology, and thus reliance solely on BP as an endpoint may provide only limited clinical value. Figure 6 suggests that inclusion of relevant intermediate structural and pathophysiologic endpoints may serve as useful targets for intervention studies because of their prognostic value and potential for change with therapy. Ultimately, development, implementation, and evaluation of lifestyle modification strategies is critically important for the treatment and prevention of HTN and its complications.

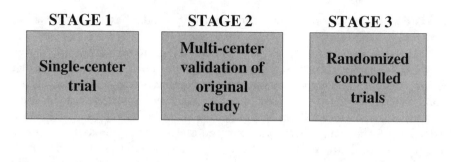

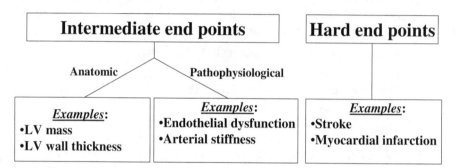

Figure 6. Research strategy for developing lifestyle interventions for treating HTN. Stage 1 consists of a single center evaluation of a specific behavioral intervention on BP and relevant intermediate endpoints. If successful, this intervention would be repeated at multiple centers, to assess the reproducibility of findings (Stage 2). In both stages, intermediate endpoints, such as changes in arterial stiffness or left ventricular mass would be used to minimize necessary sample size and follow-up time. If reproducible results are obtained during stage 2, a multi-center interventional trial would be performed in stage 3, during which subjects would be observed for the occurrence of hard clinical events such as MI and death. Adapted from Rozanski, Blumenthal et al. Journal of the American College of Cardiology (2005), 45, 637-651. Reprinted with permission.

References

Agras, W. S., & Jacob, R. G. (1979). Hypertension. In O. F. Pomerleau & J. P. Brady (Eds.), *Behavioral medicine theory and practice* (pp. 205-232). Baltimore, MD: Williams & Wilkins.

Aguilera, M. T., de la Sierra, A., Coca, A., Estruch, R., Fernandez-Sola, J., & Urbano-Marquez, A. (1999). Effect of alcohol abstinence on blood pressure: Assessment by 24-hour ambulatory blood pressure monitoring. *Hypertension, 33,* 653-657.

Alderman, M. H., Madhavan, S., Cohen, H., Sealey, J. E., & Laragh, J. H. (1995). Low urinary sodium is associated with greater risk of myocardial infarction among treated hypertensive men. *Hypertension, 25,* 1144-1152.

Allender, P. S., Cutler, J. A., Follmann, D., Cappuccio, F. P., Pryer, J., & Elliott, P. (1996). Dietary calcium and blood pressure: A meta-analysis of randomized clinical trials. *Archives of Internal Medicine, 124,* 825-831.

American College of Sports Medicine. (1994). Position stand. Physical activity, physical fitness, and hypertension. *Medicine & Science in Sports and Exercise, 25,* i-x.

Appel, L. J., Moore, T. J., Obarzanek, E., Vollmer, W. M., Svetkey, L. P., Sacks, F. M., et al. (1997). A clinical trial of the effects of dietary patterns on blood pressure. *New England Journal of Medicine, 336,* 1117-1124.

Arroll, B., & Beaglehole, R. (1992). Does physical activity lower blood pressure: A critical review of the clinical trials. *Journal of Clinical Epidemiology, 45,* 439-447.

Avenell, A., Broom, J., Brown, T. J., Poobalan, A., Aucott, L., Stearns, S. C., et al. (2004). Systematic review of the long-term effects and economic consequences of treatments for obesity and implications for health improvement. *Health Technology Assessment, 8,* 21.

Azjen, I. (1991). The theory of planned behavior. *Organizational Behavior and Human Decision Processes, 50,* 179-211.

Bandura, A. (1986). *Social foundations of thought and action: A social cognitive theory.* Englewood Cliffs, NJ: Prentice Hall.

Batey, D. M., Kaufmann, P. G., Raczynski, J. M., Hollis, J. F., Murphy, J. K., Rosner, B., et al. (2000). Stress management intervention for primary prevention of hypertension: Detailed results from phase I of Trials of Hypertension Prevention (TOHP-I). *Annals of Epidemiology, 10,* 45-58.

Beilin, L. J., Puddey, I. B., & Burke, V. (1996). Alcohol and hypertension—kill or cure? *Journal of Human Hypertension, 10 (Suppl 2),* S1-S5.

Berlowitz, D. R., Ash, A. S., Hickey, E. C., Friedman, R. H., Glickman, M., Kader, B., et al. (1998). Inadequate management of blood pressure in a hypertensive population. *New England Journal of Medicine, 339,* 1957-63.

Blair, S. N., Goodyear, N. N., Gibbons, L. W., & Cooper, K. W. (1984). Physical fitness and incidence of hypertension in healthy normotensive men and women. *Journal of the American Medical Association, 252,* 487-490.

Blair, S. N., & Holder., S. (2002). Exercise in the management of obesity. In C. G. Fairburn & K. D. Brownell (Eds.), *Eating disorders and obesity: A comprehensive handbook* (2nd ed., pp. 43-49). New York: Guilford.

Blanchard, C. M., Courneya, K. S., Rodgers, W. M., Fraser, S. N., Murray, T. C., Daub, B., et al. (2003). Is the theory of planned behavior a useful framework for understanding exercise adherence during phase II cardiac rehabilitation? *Journal of Cardiopulmonary Rehabilitation, 23,* 29-39.

Blanchard, E. B., Eisele, G., Vollmer, A., Payne, A., Gordon, M., Cornish, P., & Gilmore, L. (1996). Controlled evaluation of thermal biofeedback in treatment of elevated blood pressure in unmedicated mild hypertension. *Biofeedback & Self Regulation, 21,* 167-90.

Blumenthal, J. A., Sherwood, A., Gullette, E. C. D., Babyak, M., Waugh, R., Georgiades, A., et al. (2000). Exercise and weight loss reduce blood pressure in men and women with mild hypertension: Effects on cardiovascular, metabolic, and hemodynamic functioning. *Archives of Internal Medicine, 160,* 1947-1958.

Blumenthal, J. A., Sherwood, A., Gullette, E. C. D., Georgiades, A., & Tweedy, D. (2002). Biobehavioral approaches to the treatment of essential hypertension. *Journal of Consulting and Clinical Psychology, 70,* 569-89.

Bock, B. C., Marcus, B. H., Pinto, B. M., & Forsyth, L. H. (2001). Maintenance of physical activity following an individualized motivationally tailored intervention. *Annals of Behavioral Medicine, 23,* 79-87.

Bouchard, C., Bray, G. A., & Hubbard, V.S. (1990). Basic and clinical aspects of regional fat distribution. *American Journal of Clinical Nutrition, 52,* 946-950.

Bovbjerg, V. E., McCann, B. S., Brief, D. J., Follette, W. C., Retzlaff, B. M., Dowdy, A. A., Walden, C. E., & Knopp, R. H. (1995). Spouse support and long-term adherence to lipid-lowering diets. *American Journal of Epidemiology, 141,* 451-460.

Breckenridge, A. (1991). Angiotensin converting enzyme inhibitors and quality of life. *American Journal of Hypertension, 4,* 79S-82S.

Brownell, K. D. (2004). *The LEARN program for weight management* (10th ed). USA: American Health Publishing Co.

Brownell, K. D., & Cohen, L. R. (1995). Adherence to dietary regimens 2: components of effective interventions. *Behavioral Medicine, 20,* 155-164.

Brunner, E., White, I., Thorogood, M., Bristow, M., Curle, D., & Marmot, M. (1997). Can dietary interventions change diet and cardiovascular risk factors? A meta-analysis of randomized controlled trials. *American Journal of Public Health, 87,* 1415-1422.

Burke, L. E., Dunbar-Jacob, J. M., & Hill, M. N. (1997). Compliance with cardiovascular disease prevention strategies: A review of the research. *Annals of Behavioral Medicine, 19,* 239-263.

Burt, V. L., Cutler, J. A., Higgins, M., Horan, M. J., Labarthe, D., Whelton, P., et al. (1995). Trends in the prevalence, awareness, treatment, and control of hypertension in the adult US population. Data from the health examination surveys, 1960 to 1991. *Hypertension, 26,* 60-69. [erratum appears in *Hypertension, 27,* 1192].

Campbell, M. K., DeVellis, B. M., Strecher, V. J., Ammerman, A. S., DeVellis, R. F., & Sandler, R. S. (1994). Improving dietary behavior: The effectiveness of tailored messages in primary care settings. *American Journal of Public Health, 84,* 783-787.

Cappuccio, F. P., Elliott, P., Allender, P. S., Pryer, J., Follman, D. A., & Cutler, J. A. (1995). Epidemiologic association between dietary calcium intake and blood pressure: A meta-analysis of published data. *American Journal of Epidemiology, 142,* 935-945.

Casale, P. N., Devereux, R. B., Milner, M., Zullo, G., Harshfield, G. A., Pickering, T. G., & Laragh, J. H. (1986). Value of echocardiographic measurement of left ventricular mass in predicting cardiovascular morbid events in hypertensive men. *Annals of Internal Medicine, 105,* 173-178.

Collins, R., Peto, R., MacMahon, S., Hebert, P., Fiebach, N., Eberlein, K., et al. (1990). Blood pressure, stroke and coronary heart disease. Part 2, short-term reductions in blood pressure: Overview of randomised drug trials in their epidemiological context. *Lancet, 335,* 827-838.

Conlin, P. R., Chow, D., Miller, E. R., Svetkey, L. P., Lin, P. H., Harsha, D. W., et al. (2000). The effect of dietary patterns on blood pressure control in hypertensive patients: Results from the Dietary Approaches to Stop Hypertension (DASH) Trial. *American Journal of Hypertension, 13,* 949-55.

Cooper, Z., Fairburn, C. G., & Hawker, D. M. (2003). *Cognitive-behavioral treatment of obesity: A clinician's guide.* New York: Guildford Press.

Craighead, L. W., & Blum, M. D. (1989). Supervised exercise in behavioral treatment for moderate obesity. *Behavior Therapy, 20,* 49-59.

Cutler, J. A., Follmann, D., & Allender, P. S. (1997). Randomized trials of sodium reduction: An overview. *American Journal of Clinical Nutrition, 65 (2 Suppl.),* 643S-651S.

Dalgard, C., Thuroe, A., Haastrup, B., Haghfelt, T., & Stender, S. (2001). Saturated fat intake is reduced in patients with ischemic heart disease 1 year after comprehensive counseling but not after brief counseling. *Journal of the American Dietetic Association, 101,* 1420-1424.

Dengel, D. R., Galecki, A. T., Hagberg, J. M., & Pratley, R. E. (1998). The independent and combined effects of weight loss and aerobic exercise on blood pressure and oral glucose tolerance in older men. *American Journal of Hypertension, 11,* 1405-1412.

Dishman, R. K., & Buckworth, J. (1996). Increasing physical activity: a quantitative synthesis. *Medicine & Science in Sports & Exercise, 28,* 706-719.

Dunbar-Jacob, J., & Schlenk, E. (2001). Patient adherence to treatment regimen. In A. Baum, T. A. Revenson, & J. E. Singer (Eds.), *Handbook of health psychology* (pp. 571-580). Mahwah, NJ: Lawrence Erlbaum Associates.

Dyckner, T., & Wester, P. O. (1983). Effect of magnesium on blood pressure. *British Medical Journal (Clinical Research Ed)., 286,* 1847-1849.

Egan, B. M., Weder, A. B., Petrin, J., & Hoffman, R. G. (1991). Neurohumoral and metabolic effects of short-term dietary NaCl restriction in men: Relationship to salt-sensitivity status. *American Journal of Hypertension, 4,* 416-421.

Eisenberg, D. M., Delbanco, T. L., Berkey, C. S., Kaptchuk, T. J., Kupelnick, B., Kuhl, J., et al. (1993). Cognitive behavioral techniques for hypertension: Are they effective? *Annals of Internal Medicine, 118,* 964-972.

Flegal, K. M., Carroll, M. D., Ogden, C. L., & Johnson, C. L. (2002). Prevalence and trends in obesity among US adults, 1999-2000. *Journal of the American Medical Association, 288,* 1723-1727.

Glazer, K. M., Emery, C. F., Frid, D. J., & Banyasz, R. E. (2002). Psychological predictors of adherence and outcomes among patients in cardiac rehabilitation. *Journal of Cardiopulmonary Rehabilitation, 22,* 40-46.

Gordon, T., & Doyle, J. T. (1986). Alcohol consumption and its relationship to smoking, weight, blood pressure, and blood lipids: The Albany Study. *Archives of Internal Medicine, 146,* 262-265.

Gordon, T., & Kannel, W. B. (1983). Drinking and its relation to smoking, BP, blood lipids and uric acid. *Archives of Internal Medicine, 143,* 1366-1374.

Gordon, N. F., Scott, C. B., & Levine, B. D. (1997). Comparison of single versus multiple lifestyle interventions: Are the antihypertensive effects of exercise training and diet-induced weight loss additive? *American Journal of Cardiology, 79,* 763-767.

Graudal, N. A., Galloe, A. M., & Garred, P. (1998). Effects of sodium restriction on blood pressure, renin, aldosterone, catecholamines, cholesterols, and triglyceride: A meta-analysis. *Journal of the American Medical Association, 279,* 1383-1391.

Grimm, R. H., Flack, J. M., Grandits, G. A., Elmer, P. J., Neaton, J. D., & Cutler, J. A. (1996). Long-term effects on plasma lipids of diet and drugs to treat hypertension. *Journal of the American Medical Association, 275,* 1549-1556.

Hagan, R. D., Upton, S. J., Wong, L., & Whittam, J. (1986). The effects of aerobic conditioning and/or caloric restriction in overweight men and women. *Medicine and Science in Sports and Exercise, 18,* 87-94.

Halbert, J. A., Silagy, C. A., Finucane, P., Withers, R. T., Hamdorf, P. A., & Andrews, G. R. (1997). The effectiveness of exercise training in lowering blood pressure: A meta-analysis of randomized controlled trials of 4 weeks or longer. *Journal of Human Hypertension, 11,* 641-649.

Hall, W. D., Ferrario, C. M., Moore, M. A., Hall, J. E., Flack, J. M., & Cooper, W. (1997). Hypertension-related morbidity and mortality in the southeastern United States. *American Journal of the Medical Sciences, 313,* 195-209.

He, J., & Whelton, P. K. (1997). Role of sodium reduction in the treatment and prevention of hypertension. *Current Opinion in Cardiology, 12,* 202-207.

Henderson, R. J., Hart, M. G., Lal, S. K. L., & Hunyour, S. N. (1998). The effect of home training with direct blood pressure biofeedback of hypertensives: A placebo-controlled study. *Journal of Hypertension, 16,* 771-778.

Hughes, A. R., Gillies, F., Kirk, A. F., Mutrie, N., Hillis, W. S., & MacIntyre, P. D. (2002). Exercise consultation improves short-term adherence to exercise during phase IV cardiac rehabilitation: A randomized controlled trial. *Journal of Cardiopulmonary Rehabilitation, 22,* 421-425.

Hunyor, S. P., Henderson, R. J., Lal, S. K. L., Carter, N. L., Kobler, H., Jones, M., et al. (1997). Placebo-controlled biofeedback blood pressure effect in hypertensive humans. *Hypertension, 29,* 1225-1231.

Israili, Z. H., & Hall, W. D. (1992). Cough and angioneurotic edema associated with angiotensin-converting enzyme inhibitor therapy: A review of the literature and pathophysiology. *Annals of Internal Medicine, 117,* 234-42.

Jacob, R. G., Chesney, M. A., Williams, D. M., Ding, Y., & Shapiro, A. P. (1991). Relaxation therapy for hypertension: Design effects and treatment effects. *Annals of Behavioral Medicine, 13*, 5-17.

Jeffery, R. W. (1991). Weight management and hypertension. *Annals of Behavioral Medicine, 13*, 18-22.

Jeffery, R. J., French, S. A., & Schmid, T. L. (1990). Attributions for dietary failures: Problems reported by participants in the hypertension prevention trial. *Health Psychology, 9*, 315-329.

Joint National Committee on Prevention, Detection, Evaluation, and Treatment of High Blood Pressure. (2003). The seventh report of the Joint National Committee on Prevention, Detection, Evaluation, and Treatment of High Blood Pressure (JNC VII). *Journal of the American Medical Association, 289*, 2560-2572.

Joint National Committee on Detection, Evaluation, and Treatment of High Blood Pressure. (1997). The sixth report of the Joint National Committee on Detection, Evaluation, and Treatment of High Blood Pressure (JNC VI). *Archives of Internal Medicine, 157*, 2413-2445.

Jones, J. K., Gorkin, L., Lian, J. F., Staffa, J. A., & Fletcher, A. P. (1995). Discontinuation of and changes in treatment after start of new courses of antihypertensive drugs: A study of a United Kingdom population. *British Medical Journal, 311*, 293-295.

Kaufman, P. G., Jacob, R. G., Ewart, C. K., Chesney, M. A. Muenz, L.R., Doub, N., et al. (1988). Hypertension intervention pooling project. *Health Psychology, 7 (Suppl.)*, 209-224.

Kawano, Y., Matsuoka, H., Takishita, S., & Omae, T. (1998). Effects of magnesium supplementation in hypertensive patients: Assessment by office, home, and ambulatory blood pressures. *Hypertension, 32*, 260-265.

Keil, U., Liese, A., Filipiak, B., Swales, J. D., & Grobbee, D. E. (1998). Alcohol, blood pressure and hypertension. *Novartis Foundation Symposium, 216*, 125-144.

Kelley, G. A. (1999). Aerobic exercise and resting blood pressure among women: A meta-analysis. *Preventive Medicine, 28*, 264-275.

Kelley, G., & McClellan, P. (1994). Antihypertensive effects of aerobic exercise: A brief meta-analytic review of randomized controlled trials. *American Journal of Hypertension, 7*, 115-119.

Kim, M. T., Han, H-R, Hill, M. N., Rose, L., & Roary, M. (2003). Depression, substance use, adherence behaviors, and blood pressure in urban hypertensive black men. *Annals of Behavioral Medicine, 26*, 24-31.

Kochanek, K.D., Smith, B. L., & Anderson, R. N. (2001). Deaths: Preliminary data for 1999. *National Vital Statistics Report, 49*, 1-48.

Kromhout, D., Bosschieter, E. B., & Coulander, C. L. (1985). Potassium, calcium, alcohol intake and blood pressure: The Zutphen study. *American Journal of Clinical Nutrition, 41*, 1299-1304.

Lee, I-M., Hsieh, S., & Paffenbarger, R.S. (1995). Exercise intensity and longevity in men. The Harvard Alumni Health Study. *Journal of the American Medical Association, 273,* 1179-1184.

Levy, D., Garrison, R. J., Savage, D. D., Kannel, W. B., & Castelli, W. P. (1990). Prognostic implications of echocardiographically determined left ventricular mass in the Framingham Heart Study. *New England Journal of Medicine, 322,* 561-1566.

Linden, W., & Chambers, L. (1994). Clinical effectiveness of non-drug treatment for hypertension: A meta-analysis. *Annals of Behavioral Medicine, 16,* 35-45.

Lithell, H., Pollare, T., & Vessby, B. (1992). Metabolic effects of pindolol and propranolol in a double-blind cross-over study in hypertensive patients. *Blood Pressure, 1,* 92-101.

MacMahon, S., Cutter, J., Brittain, E., & Higgins, M. (1987). Obesity and hypertension: Epidemiological and clinical issues. *European Heart Journal, 8(Suppl. B),* 57-70.

MacMahon, S., Peto, R., Cutler, J., Collins, R., Sorlie, P., Neaton, J., et al. (1990). Blood pressure, stroke, and coronary heart disease. Part 1, prolonged differences in blood pressure: Prospective observational studies corrected for the regression dilution bias. *Lancet, 335,* 765-74.

McCauley, E., Courneya, K. S., Rudolph, D. L., & Lox, C. L. (1994). Enhancing exercise adherence in middle-aged males and females. *Preventive Medicine, 23,* 498-506.

Metz, J. A., Kris-Etherton, P. M., Morris, C. D., Mustad, V. A., Stern, J. S., Oparil, S., et al. (1997). Dietary compliance and cardiovascular risk reduction with a prepared meal plan compared with a self-selected diet. *American Journal of Clinical Nutrition, 66,* 373-385.

Midgley, J. P., Matthew, A. G., Greenwood, C. M., & Logan, A. G. (1996). Effect of reduced dietary sodium on blood pressure: A meta-analysis of randomized controlled trials. *Journal of the American Medical Association, 275,* 1590-1597.

Miller, E. R., Erlinger, T. P., Young, D. R., Jehn, M., Charleston, J., Rhodes, D., et al. (2002). Results of the Diet, Exercise, and Weight Loss Intervention Trial (DEW-IT). *Hypertension, 40,* 612-618.

Moore, S. M., Dolansky, M. A., Ruland, C. M., Pashkow, F. J., & Blackburn, G. G. (2003). Predictors of women's exercise maintenance after cardiac rehabilitation. *Journal of Cardiopulmonary Rehabilitation, 23,* 40-49.

Motoyama, T., Sano, H., & Fukuzaki, H. (1989). Oral magnesium supplementation in patients with essential hypertension. *Hypertension, 13,* 227-232.

Mulrow, C. D., Chiquette, E., Angel, L., Cornell, J., Summerbell, C., Anagnostelis, B., et al. (2002). Dieting to reduce body weight for controlling hypertension in adults. *The Cochrane Library, Cochrane Hypertension Group, Cochrane Database of Systematic Reviews, Issue 4,* Art. No.: CD000484. DOI: 10.1002/14651858.CD000484.

Naslund, G. K., Fredrickson, M., Hellenius, M. L., & de Faire, U. (1996). Determinants of compliance in men enrolled in a diet and exercise intervention trial: A randomized, controlled study. *Patient Education and Counseling, 29,* 247-256.

Neter, J. E., Stam, B. E., Kok, F. J., Grobbee, D. E., & Geleijnse, J. M. (2003). Influence of weight reduction on blood pressure: A meta-analysis of randomized controlled trials. *Hypertension, 42,* 878-884.

Oman, R. F., & King, A. C. (1998). Predicting the adoption and maintenance of exercise participation using self-efficacy and previous exercise participation rates. *American Journal of Health Promotion, 12,* 154-161.

Paffenbarger, R. S., Thorne, M. C., & Wing, A. L. (1968). Chronic disease in former college students. VIII. Characteristics in youth predisposing to hypertension in later years. *American Journal of Epidemiology, 88,* 25-32.

Paffenbarger, R. S., Wing, A. L., Hyde, R. T., & Jung, D. L. (1983). Physical activity and incidence of hypertension in college alumni. *American Journal of Epidemiology, 117,* 245-257.

Pahor, M., Guralnik, J. M., Furberg, C. D., Carbonin, P., & Havlik, R. (1996). Risk of gastrointestinal hemorrhage with calcium channel antagonists in hypertensive persons over 67 years old. *Lancet, 347,* 1061-1065.

Patel, C. (1991). *The complete guide to stress management.* New York: Plenum Press.

Patel, C., & North, W. R. S. (1975). Randomized controlled trial of yoga and biofeedback in management of hypertension. *The Lancet, 2,* 93.

Pérez-Stable, E. J., Coats, T. J., Baron, R. B., Biró, B. S., Hauck, W. W., McHenry, K. S., et al. (1995). Comparison of a lifestyle modification program with propranololuse in the management of diastolic hypertension. *Journal of General Internal Medicine, 10,* 419-428.

Perri, M. G., Anton, S. D., Durning, P. E., Ketterson, T. U., Sydeman, S. J., Berlant, N. E., et al. (2002). Adherence to exercise prescriptions: Effects of prescribing moderate versus higher levels of intensity and frequency. *Health Psychology, 21,* 452-458.

Pollare, T., Lithell, H., & Berne, C. (1989). A comparison of the effects of hydrochlorothiazide and captopril on glucose and lipid metabolism in patients with hypertension. *New England Journal of Medicine, 321,* 868-73.

Pratley, R. E., Hagberg, J. M., Dengel, D. R., Rogus, E. M., Muller, D. C., & Goldberg, A. P. (2000). Aerobic exercise training-induced reductions in abdominal fat and glucose-stimulated insulin responses in middle-age and older men. *Journal of the American Geriatric Society, 48,* 1055-61.

PREMIER Collaborative Research Group. (2003). Effects of comprehensive lifestyle modification on blood pressure control: Main results of the PREMIER clinical trial. *Journal of the American Medical Association, 289,* 2083-2093.

Prochaska, J. O., & DiClemente, C. C. (1983). Stages and processes of self-change of smoking: Toward an integrative model of change. *Journal of Consulting and Clinical Psychology, 51,* 390-395.

Rozanski, A., Blumenthal, J. A., Davidson, K. W., Saab, P. G., & Kubzansky, L. (2005). The epidemiology, pathophysiology, and management of psychosocial risk factors in cardiac practice. *The Journal of the American College of Cardiology, 45,* 637-651.

Rosenstock, I. M. (1974). Historical origins of the health belief model. *Health Education Monographs, 2,* 328-335.

Sacks, F. M., Svetkey, L. P., Vollmer, W. M., Appel, L. J., Bray, G. A., Harsha, D., et al. (2001). A clinical trial of the effects on blood pressure of reduced dietary sodium and the DASH dietary pattern. *New England Journal of Medicine, 344,* 3-10.

Saunders, J. B., Beevers, D. G., & Paton, A. (1981). Alcohol-induced hypertension. *Lancet, 2,* 653-656.

Shapiro, D., Tursky, B., Gershon, E., & Stern, M. (1969). Effects of feedback and reinforcement on the control of human systolic blood pressure. *Science, 163,* 388.

Siegel, W. C., & Blumenthal, J. A. (1991). The role of exercise in the prevention and treatment of hypertension. *Annals of Behavioral Medicine, 13,* 23-30.

Smutok, M. A., Reece, C., Kokkinos, P. F., Farmer, C., Dawson, P., Shulman, R., et al. (1993). Aerobic versus strength training for risk factor intervention in middle-aged men at high risk for coronary heart disease. *Metabolism, 42,* 177-84.

Staessen, J., Bulpitt, C. J., Fagard, R., Lijnen, P., & Amery, A. (1989). The influence of menopause on blood pressure. *Journal of Human Hypertension, 3,* 427-33.

Staessen, J., Fagard, R., & Amery, A. (1988). The relationship between body weight and blood pressure. *Journal of Human Hypertension, 2,* 207-217.

Suissa, S., Bourgault, C., Barkun, A., Sheehy, O., & Ernst, P. (1998). Antihypertensive drugs and the risk of gastrointestinal bleeding. *American Journal of Medicine, 105,* 230-235.

Svetkey, L. P., Simons-Morton, D., Vollmer, W. M., Appel, L. J., Conlin, P. R., Ryan, D. H., et al. (1999). Effects of dietary patterns on blood pressure: Subgroup analysis of the Dietary Approaches to Stop Hypertension (DASH) randomized clinical trial. *Archives of Internal Medicine, 159,* 285-93.

Systolic Hypertension in the Elderly Program Cooperative Research Group. (1991). Prevention of stroke by anti-hypertensive drug treatment in older persons with isolated systolic hypertension. *Journal of the American Medical Association, 265,* 3255-3264.

Tipton, C. M. (1991). Exercise training and hypertension: An update. In J. O. Holloszy (Ed.), *Exercise and Sport Sciences Reviews,* (pp. 447-505). Baltimore: Williams & Wilkins.

Trost, S. G., Owen, N., Bauman, A. E., Sallis, J. F., & Brown, W. (2002). Correlates of adults' participation in physical activity: Review and update. *Medicine & Science in Sports & Exercise, 34,* 1996-2001.

Wadden, T. A., Foster, G. D., & Brownell, K. D. (2002). Obesity: Responding to the global epidemic. *Journal of Consulting and Clinical Psychology, 70,* 510-525.

Wallace, M. B., Mills, B. D., & Browning, C. L. (1997). Effects of cross-training on markers of insulin resistance/hyperinsulinemia. *Medicine and Science in Sports and Exercise, 29,* 1170-1175.

Weingerger, M. H. (1985). Antihypertensive therapy and lipids: Evidence, mechanisms, and implications. *Archives of Internal Medicine, 145,* 1102-1119.

Whelton, P. K., Appel, L. J., Espeland, M. A., Applegate, W. B., Ettinger, W. H., Kostis, J. B., et al. (1998). Sodium reduction and weight loss in the treatment of hypertension in older persons: A randomized controlled trial of nonpharmacologic interventions in the elderly (TONE). *Journal of the American Medical Association, 279,* 839-846.

Whelton, S. P., Chin, A., Xin, X., & He, J. (2002). Effect of aerobic exercise on blood pressure: A meta-analysis of randomized controlled trials. *Annals of Internal Medicine, 136,* 493-503.

Whelton, P. K., He, J., Cutler, J. A., Brancati, F. L., Appel, L. J., Follmann, D., et al. (1997). Effects of oral potassium on blood pressure: Meta-analysis of randomized controlled clinical trials. *Journal of the American Medical Association, 277,* 1624-1632.

Widman, L., Wester, P. O., Stegmayr, B. K., & Wirell, M. (1993). The dose-dependent reduction in blood pressure through administration of magnesium. A double blind placebo controlled cross-over study. *American Journal of Hypertension, 6,* 41-45.

Wilfley, D. E., & Brownell, K. D. (1994). Physical activity and diet in weight loss. In R. K. Dishman (Ed.), *Advances in exercise adherence* (pp. 361-393). Champaign, IL: Human Kinetics Press.

Wilmore, J. H. (1983). Body composition in sport and exercise: Directions for future research. *Medicine and Science in Sports and Exercise, 15,* 21-31.

Windhauser, M., Karanja, N., McCullough, M., Lin, P. H., Swain, J., Hoben, K., et al. (1999). Dietary adherence in the DASH multi-center controlled feeding trial. *Journal of the American Dietetic Association, 99,* S76-83.

Wing, R. R., & Klem, M. (2002). Characteristics of successful weight maintainers. In C. G. Fairburn & K. D. Brownell (Eds.), *Eating disorders and obesity: A comprehensive handbook* (2nd ed., pp. 588-592). New York: Guilford.

Yamamoto, M. E., Applegate. W, B., Klag, M. J., Borhani, N. O., Cohen, J. D., Kirchner, K. A., et al. (1995). Lack of blood pressure effect with calcium and magnesium supplementation in adults with high-normal blood pressure. Results from Phase I of the Trials of Hypertension Prevention (TOHP). Trials of Hypertension Prevention (TOHP) Collaborative Research Group. *Annals of Epidemiology, 5,* 96-107.

Author's Note

Correspondence: James A. Blumenthal, Department of Psychiatry and Behavioral Sciences, Box 3119, Duke University Medical Center, Durham, NC 27710; tel: (919) 684-3828; fax: (919) 684-8629; email: Blume003@mc.duke.edu

Chapter 6

Psychosocial and Behavioral Issues in the Management of Diabetes in Children and Adolescents

Alan M. Delamater
University of Miami School of Medicine

The chapter summarizes key findings from the literature addressing psychosocial and behavioral issues in children with type 1 diabetes mellitus. The review considers specific issues such as sociodemographic factors, family functioning, psychosocial adjustment and psychiatric disorders, stress and coping, neurocognitive functioning, quality of life, and psychosocial and behavioral interventions. Implications for clinical practice will also be discussed. In addition, the chapter also considers the emerging public health problem of type 2 diabetes in children, including a review of factors affecting obesity in children, a major risk factor for type 2 diabetes, as well as interventions that address obesity in children.

Type 1 Diabetes Mellitus

A substantial literature exists on psychosocial and behavioral factors related to diabetes management in children and adolescents (Delamater et al., 2001; Johnson, 1995). Although much of this research has focused on the relationship of behavioral and psychosocial factors to diabetes-related outcomes such as regimen adherence and metabolic control, some studies have specifically focused on the impact of diabetes on psychosocial functioning. This section will highlight some of the most important findings in this area, including the role of demographic factors.

Sociodemographic Factors

Research has shown that regimen adherence declines over time, and is especially poor among many adolescents (Jacobson et al., 1990; Johnson et al., 1992). Studies also indicate that metabolic control tends to be worse in children from single-parent families, demonstrated in studies both in the United States (e.g., Overstreet et al., 1995; Thompson et al., 2001), and Sweden (e.g., Forsander et al., 2000). Ethnicity has also been examined in relation to regimen adherence and metabolic control. Studies consistently have shown that African American youths exhibit poorer metabolic control than Caucasian youths (Auslander et al., 1997; Delamater et al., 1991; Delamater et al., 1999). These findings may be explained in part by the greater prevalence of single parent families and lower adherence to diet and glucose testing among African Amercians (Auslander et al., 1997).

Family Functioning

Studies have shown that families of youths in poor metabolic control have more conflict and financial problems, and less cohesion and stability than those of youths in good metabolic control (Anderson et al., 1981; Hanson, Henggeler, & Burghen, 1987). Good metabolic control has been associated with better family communication and conflict resolution skills (Wysocki, 1993), agreement about family responsibilities and appropriate involvement of parents in diabetes management tasks (Anderson et al., 1990; Anderson et al., 1997) and more structured and controlling family environments (Weist et al., 1993). Significant family dysfunction for the majority of families has been observed in clinical studies of adolescents selected for chronically poor metabolic control (Orr et al., 1983; White et al., 1984).

Family relationships are also associated with regimen adherence. Adherence has been related with both general and regimen-specific family support (Schafer et al., 1983; La Greca et al., 1995) as well as communication skills (Bobrow et al., 1985) and conflict (Miller-Johnson et al., 1994). In a study of parenting styles in relation to regimen adherence of young children with diabetes, parental warmth was predictive of better adherence (Davis et al., 2001). While youths receive instrumental support from their families, they also receive considerable emotional support from their friends (La Greca et al., 1995).

Studies indicate that many mothers are at risk for psychological adjustment problems after their children are diagnosed with type 1 diabetes, with clinically significant depression noted in approximately one-third of mothers. However, most of these adjustment problems are resolved within the first year after the child's diagnosis (Kovacs et al., 1985). Few studies have addressed the role of fathers in diabetes management. In a recent study by Landolt et al. (2002), 24% of mothers and 22% of fathers met diagnostic criteria for post-traumatic stress disorder six weeks after their child had been diagnosed. Other recent studies indicate that fathers typically are not really involved in diabetes management tasks (Seiffge-Krenke, 2002), and suggest that psychological maladjustment of fathers predicts poor glycemic control in children five years after diagnosis (Forsander et al., 1998).

Psychological Adjustment

Adjustment after Diagnosis. The diagnosis of type 1 diabetes is a considerable stressor for children and their families. Several longitudinal studies have addressed this issue. Kovacs and colleagues (1985) found 36% of newly diagnosed children had diagnosable psychiatric disorders soon after diabetes onset, most commonly being adjustment disorders with depression and anxiety. However, most children's adjustment problems had resolved within the first year after diagnosis. Jacobson and colleagues (1986) also investigated the psychosocial outcomes of children with newly diagnosed diabetes. Five months after diagnosis there were no differences between diabetic children and a medical control group on a variety of behavioral and psychological measures, with the exception of decreased school-related competence in children with diabetes. Grey and colleagues (1995) observed that mild adjustment problems had dissipated by the end of the first year after diagnosis, but some problems reappeared by the end of the second year. Studies suggest that while the majority of children's adjustment problems appear to resolve within the first year, children who do not may be at risk for poor adaptation to diabetes, including regimen adherence problems, poor metabolic control, and continued psychosocial difficulties (Grey et al., 1995; Jacobson et al., 1994; Kovacs et al., 1995).

Long-term Adjustment. Earlier studies comparing children with diabetes to other groups generally did not reveal significant differences in psychological adjustment (Johnson, 1995), although one report found boys with later onset of diabetes to have more behavioral problems (Rovet, Ehrlich, & Hoppe, 1987). More recent findings, however, suggest that children with diabetes, like children with other chronic diseases, may be at increased risk for psychological problems (Lavigne & Faier-Routman, 1992). For example, Blanz, Rensch-Riemann, Fritz-Sigmund, and Schmidt (1993) found that one-third of their sample of 93 diabetic adolescents had psychiatric disorders (mostly internalizing symptoms), compared with 10% of the subjects in a control group. Kovacs and colleagues (1997), in a ten-year follow-up study of newly diagnosed youth, found that nearly half of the study sample had a psychiatric diagnosis, the most frequent being major depression, conduct disorder, and generalized anxiety disorder. In another 10-year follow-up study of newly-diagnosed children and adolescents, Jacobson and colleagues (1997) found that as young adults, patients reported lower self-esteem relative to control participants. Wysocki, Hough, Ward, & Green (1992) found that poorer adjustment to diabetes during adolescence may persist into early adulthood. In a more recent longitudinal study of 76 adolescents, Bryden et al. (2001) reported that patients with behavioral problems during their teen years had significantly poorer glycemic control as young adults.

Psychological factors have been associated with glycemic control within samples of children with diabetes. In an early study of this type, Anderson et al. (1981) found increased anxiety and lower self-concept in youths with poor glycemic control. La Greca et al. (1995) observed that girls were more likely than boys to be depressed, and that depression was associated with poorer glycemic control.

Eating Disorders. There is evidence that diabetic youths, especially girls, are at increased risk for eating disorders, and that eating disorders are associated with poor glycemic control (Rodin & Daneman, 1992). Both eating disorders and sub-clinically disordered eating attitudes and behaviors (e.g., severe dietary indiscretion and repeated insulin omissions) have been noted in adolescent girls with diabetes, and have been associated with worse glycemic control (Daneman et al., 1998; Jones et al., 2000; Neumark-Sztainer et al., 2002). It is estimated that at least 10% of adolescent girls with type 1 diabetes may meet diagnostic criteria for an eating disorder, a rate twice as common as in girls without diabetes (Jones et al., 2000). Without intervention, disordered eating and insulin manipulation may worsen over time and increase the risk of serious health complications (Rydall et al., 1997). Results from recent studies indicate that disordered eating in girls with diabetes is associated with problems in the mother-daughter relationship (Maharag et al., 2001;

Mahoney et al., 2001) and less perceived control (Schwartz et al., 2002). Although not all studies have found increased rates of eating disorders in samples of adolescents with diabetes, glycemic control has been observed to worsen with increasing numbers of symptoms of eating disorder (Bryden et al., 1999; Meltzer et al., 2001).

Stress and Coping

Studies indicate that children with high life stress tend to have worse glycemic control (Hanson, Henggeler, & Burghen, 1987; Hanson & Pichert, 1986; Kager & Holden, 1992). Research examining attributional and coping styles has revealed that youths in poor metabolic control are more likely to use the learned helplessness style (Kuttner, Delamater, & Santiago, 1990) and engage in avoidance and wishful thinking in response to stress (Delamater et al., 1987), while youths in good glycemic control have high levels of self-efficacy (Grossman, Brink, & Hauser, 1987). Maladaptive coping has also been related with poor regimen adherence (Hanson et al., 1989).

Studies of the health belief model in adolescents have shown that specific health beliefs related to the serious of diabetes, personal vulnerability to complications, costs of regimen adherence, and beliefs in the efficacy of treatment, have been associated with both regimen adherence and glycemic control (Bond, Aiken, & Somerville, 1992; Brownlee-Duffeck et al., 1987; Palardy et al., 1998). Skinner and Hampson (2001) showed that personal models of diabetes, i.e., specific illness beliefs, were associated with psychological adjustment and regimen adherence. These investigators found that greater impact of diabetes was related to increased anxiety, while beliefs about the effectiveness of treatment predicted better dietary self care. In a study of adolescents and young adults, Skinner et al. (2002) found that personal model beliefs about diabetes mediated the relationship between personality variables (emotional stability and conscientiousness) and self care behaviors. Health belief research has also been conducted with younger children with diabetes. In a study by Charron-Prochownick et al. (1993), youngsters' beliefs regarding barriers and self efficacy were related with adherence, and beliefs regarding severity of diabetes were related to glycemic control.

Neurocognitive Functioning

Neurocognitive functioning in children with diabetes has been examined in a number of studies. Findings indicate that children with early onset of diabetes and a history of hypoglycemic episodes have significantly poorer cognitive performance, particularly for visual-spatial functioning (Rovet et al., 1988; Ryan et al., 1985). Other studies suggest that children who develop diabetes early in life are at increased risk for later neurocognitive deficits, both verbal and visual-spatial (Holmes & Richman, 1985; Ryan et al., 1984). Ryan, Longstreet, & Morrow (1985) found that children with diabetes missed twice as much school as their non-diabetic peers, and lower reading achievement was associated with more school absences. Research also indicates that diabetic youths are more likely to have learning problems, with such problems more likely among boys than girls: in one study, 40% of boys and 16% of girls had learning problems (Holmes et al., 1992). Rovet and Alvarez (1997) reported lower verbal intelligence and poorer attentional functioning in diabetic children and adolescents, which was associated with a history of hypoglycemic seizures.

In a neuropsychological study of newly diagnosed children, Kovacs, Goldston, and Iyengar (1992) found that verbal intelligence and school grades were average shortly after diagnosis, but decreased significantly over time. Memory dysfunction in part predicted the decline in verbal skill (Kovacs et al., 1994). In another prospective study of newly-diagnosed children, mild neuropsychological deficits were observed two years after diagnosis, with reduced speed of information processing and decrements in conceptual reasoning and acquisition of new knowledge (Northam et al., 1998). Predictors of these changes in neurocognitive function included early onset of diabetes (prior to age four years) which was related to poorer visuospatial functioning, and both recurrent severe hypoglycemia and hyperglycemia, which was related to decreased memory and learning capacity (Northam et al., 1999). These same investigators evaluated neuropsychological functioning six years after diagnosis and found that children with diabetes performed more poorly on measures of intelligence, attention, processing speed, and long-term memory than control children. Children with early diabetes onset (before age four years) showed weaknesses in attention, processing speed, and executive functioning, while those with recurrent severe hypoglycemia had lower intellectual abilities (Northam et al., 2001).

Quality of Life

Management of type 1 diabetes imposes considerable challenges and demands that may potentially interfere with children's ability to negotiate important developmental tasks and achieve good psychosocial adjustment. This is especially the case in the post-DCCT era when the expectation is to initiate intensive insulin regimens in order to achieve and maintain optimal levels of glycemic control in order to reduce the risk of later health complications (DCCT Research Group, 1994). Despite improvements in diabetes care, it is clear that many youth with type 1 diabetes continue to be at risk for short-term adverse events, including severe hypoglycemia and emergency room visits (Levine et al., 2001).

Diabetes-related quality of life (DQOL) refers to those aspects of child and adolescent functioning that are directly affected by diabetes and its treatment. This construct includes disease state and physical symptoms, functional status, psychological functioning, social functioning, as well as academic functioning (Spieth & Harris, 1996).

Ingersoll and Marrero (1991) reported the first study on DQOL in youths. These investigators modified the QOL measure used in the DCCT so that it would be better suited for use by youths. The scale measures diabetes impact, worries, and satisfaction. Demographic and clinical correlates of DQOL were evaluated in 74 children and adolescents from culturally and socially diverse backgrounds. Girls reported more disease worries than boys. Age was not related with DQOL, but shorter diabetes duration was associated with greater disease impact. None of the DQOL scales was related with glycemic control.

Several studies examined DQOL using the measure developed by Ingersoll and Marrero (1991). For example, Grey and colleagues (1998) examined the personal and family correlates of DQOL in 52 adolescents, primarily a Caucasian sample from middle to upper socioeconomic status. Youths who reported greater disease impact and less satisfaction felt that diabetes was more upsetting and diabetes management was more difficult. Those who reported more disease-related worries felt that diabetes was more upsetting and diabetes management more difficult. Greater disease-related worries was associated with lower levels of self-efficacy, higher levels of depression, and less family support. Multiple regression analyses revealed that DQOL was bested predicted by depression, and to a lesser extent, difficulty coping with diabetes. Glycemic control was not associated with any aspect of DQOL.

Guttmann-Bauman, Flaherty, Sturgger, and McEvoy (1998) evaluated the relationship between metabolic control and DQOL in a sample of 69 youths. Minority youth (Hispanic and African American) comprised one-third of the study sample, but the socioeconomic status (SES) of the sample was not reported. Metabolic control was assessed both by glycohemoglobin and by the frequency of acute events such as diabetes-related emergency room visits or hospital admissions. Significant correlations were obtained between DQOL and glycohemoglobin, as well as between DQOL and acute events, such that youths who reported better DQOL had better glycemic control and fewer acute events. Analyses of the three DQOL scales revealed significant associations of glycohemoglobin with satisfaction and disease impact, but not with worries; acute events were significantly related to impact and worries.

Because minority youths are at increased risk for metabolic control problems (Auslander et al., 1997; Delamater et al., 1991; Delamater et al., 1999), it is important to focus on their DQOL. Delamater and colleagues (1998) studied DQOL in a culturally diverse (Caucasian, African American, and Hispanic) sample of 96 youths comprising the full range of socioeconomic status (SES). The results revealed significantly lower DQOL (i.e., greater impact and worries) in youths from single parent families and those with lower SES status. African American youths reported more disease worries than did Caucasian youths, but when SES was controlled for, this effect was attenuated. A number of psychosocial factors were significantly related with lower DQOL, including maladaptive coping, increased diabetes-related stress, more behavior problems, and greater levels of non-supportive family behavior. Multivariate analyses identified SES and diabetes-related stress to be the best predictors of DQOL impact and worry scores. However, age, gender, diabetes duration, and glycohemoglobin were unrelated with DQOL.

Hoey and colleagues from the Hvidore Study Group on Childhood Diabetes (2001), studied over 2000 adolescents using the DQOL measure modified by Ingersoll and Marrero (1991), and found that better glycemic control (measured by glycosylated hemoglobin A1c) was associated with lower impact, fewer worries, and greater satisfaction. In addition, girls reported more worries and less satisfaction than boys, and patients from ethnic minority groups had more impact and worries.

More recent studies have utilized both a generic QOL measure and a diabetes-specific module. Varni et al. (2003) developed such a measure (the PedsQL) and found it to be reliable for use in studies of diabetic youths. Laffel and colleagues (2003), using the PedsQL, found that diabetic youths reported a similar quality of life as youth without diabetes. In addition, they found that greater diabetes-specific family conflict was associated with less favorable DQOL.

Psychosocial and Behavioral Interventions

A number of controlled studies have examined the efficacy of various psychosocial and behavioral interventions for children and adolescents with type 1 diabetes. Review of these studies indicates that the effects of these interventions are positive, although generally modest in effect size (Delamater et al., 2001; Hampson et al., 2000). Most of these interventions have included the family as an integral part of treatment. It is important to include the family in diabetes management interventions, as studies have shown that when parents allow older children and adolescents to have self-care autonomy without sufficient cognitive and social maturity, youths are more likely to have problems with diabetes management (Ingersoll et al., 1986; Wysocki et al., 1996).

The results of controlled intervention studies indicate that family-based behavioral intervention techniques such as goal-setting, self-monitoring, positive reinforcement, behavioral contracts, supportive parental communications, and appropriately shared responsibility for diabetes management have improved regimen adherence and glycemic control (Anderson et al., 1999; Satin et al., 1989). In addition, such interventions can improve the parent-adolescent relationship (Anderson et al., 1999; Delamater et al., 1991; Wysocki et al., 1999, 2000). Wysocki and colleagues (2001) showed that improvements in parent-teen relationships were maintained for one year, and that the family intervention had positive, delayed effects on regimen adherence. Laffel and colleagues (2003) demonstrated that a family-focused teamwork intervention increased family involvement without impacting family conflict or youth quality of life, and helped prevent worsening of glycemic control. Psycho-educational interventions with children and their families that promote problem-solving skills and increase parental support early in the disease course have been shown to improve long-term glycemic control of children (Delamater et al., 1990). In a randomized trial, youth who received psycho-educational interventions delivered by a case manager at regular outpatient visits were shown to increase visit frequency, and have reduced acute adverse outcomes such as hypoglycemia and emergency department visits (Svoren et al., 2003).

The efficacy of group interventions for diabetic youth has also been studied. Research findings have shown that peer group support and problem-solving have improved short-term glycemic control (Anderson et al., 1989; Kaplan et al., 1985). Grey and colleagues (Boland et al., 1999; Grey et al., 1998) evaluated the effect of group coping skills training, and found that it improved glycemic control and quality of life for adolescents involved in intensive insulin regimens, effects which were maintained after the intervention was completed (Grey et al., 2000). In a peer group intervention study targeting problem-solving, Cook et al. (2002) found that problem-solving and glucose monitoring increased, while glycemic control improved for treated youths. Studies have also shown that stress management and coping skills training delivered in small groups of youths has reduced diabetes-related stress (Boardway et al., 1993; Hains et al., 2000) and improved social interaction (Mendez & Belendez, 1997).

A recent study by Greco et al. (2001) examined the effects of an intervention involving diabetic youths and their best friends who did not have diabetes. The intervention, focused on increasing diabetes knowledge, problem solving, and self-management, was delivered in small groups of patients and their friends in four weekly sessions. The findings showed increased knowledge and peer support for diabetes management, although measures of glycemic control were not reported. While this study is limited by the lack of a control group and the small sample size, it is noteworthy for the innovative approach.

Another innovative intervention approach was reported by Couper and colleagues (1999). In this randomized study, adolescents in poor glycemic control received either usual care or usual care plus a home based intervention targeting knowledge and goal-setting, consisting of six monthly sessions with telephone contact between home sessions. Results showed gains in knowledge and improved glycemic control after six months, although these gains were not maintained over the following year. Other innovative intervention studies have shown the potential benefits of computer-assisted approaches (Marrero et al., 1989; Horan et al., 1990), telecommunication technology (Marrero et al., 1995), and telephone-delivered support (Howells et al., 2002) to improve diabetes management.

Although recent research has not addressed the role of physical activity in diabetes management, studies reported during the 1980's demonstrated that increasing the physical activity of diabetic children and adolescents through structured exercise programs (conducted three times per week) improved glycemic control (Campaigne et al., 1984; Stratton et al., 1987). However, less frequent exercise (once per week) did not achieve improved glycemic control (Huttunen et al., 1989).

Clinical Implications

Psychological and family factors are essential to consider for optimal diabetes management for children and adolescents. Besides the attainment and maintenance of good metabolic control, the goals of diabetes management are to ensure that youth develop optimally in all areas of their life: psychologically, socially, academically, and physically. Therefore, clinicians should routinely assess youths' developmental progress in these areas, as well as disease-related skills, regimen adherence, and metabolic control. It is very important to maintain consistent contact with families, as studies have shown children who have infrequent and irregular visits with the health care team are more likely to have significant problems with metabolic control (Jacobson et al., 1997; Kaufman et al., 1999). Efforts to intensify regimens with insulin pumps, multiple daily injections, and more frequent glucose monitoring are very important, but many youths and their families may be unable to commit to and succeed with this type of regimen. Tercyak and colleagues (1998) reported that only 57% of adolescents agreed to participate in a trial of intensive therapy, with the major reasons for refusal being not wanting to have more frequent clinic visits, injections, and glucose monitoring. A recent study suggests that regimen intensification should not be limited to youth with high self-care competence, as those with low self-care competence may derive the most benefit in terms of glycemic control (Wysocki, et al., 2003).

Given that research findings indicate that quality of life is associated with depression and stress related to diabetes management, interventions to reduce depression and stress through improvement in coping abilities are indicated. As discussed previously, empirical support for such clinical approaches has been demonstrated (e.g., Boardway et al., 1993; Grey et al., 1998, 2000; Mendez & Belendez, 1997). Research has shown that youths who do not manage diabetes well are more likely to have psychological problems, eating disorders, family conflict, and less than optimal parental involvement and support for diabetes tasks. Therefore, interventions must also consider these psychosocial issues.

As they become older, many children are given self-care autonomy without sufficient cognitive and emotional maturity. Interventions to appropriately involve parents are essential, as research has shown that 25% of youths admitted to missing insulin injections, 29% fabricated blood glucose test results, and 81% ate inappropriately (Weissberg-Benchell et al., 1995). Parental involvement in children's diabetes care should be evaluated routinely, and interventions delivered to promote teamwork so that good control of diabetes can be achieved. There is empirical support for these approaches. Controlled studies have shown that interventions to improve parent-adolescent teamwork in diabetes management resulted in less conflict (Anderson et al., 1999), and family-based behavioral intervention utilizing communication skills, goal-setting with behavioral contracts, and problem-solving strategies resulted in improvements in adherence and parent-teen relationships (Delamater et al., 1991; Wysocki et al., 2001). Interventions to improve these kinds of psychosocial factors are also likely to improve the quality of life of children and adolescents with diabetes.

Summary

Research findings indicate youths with type 1 diabetes are at risk for adjustment problems during the initial period of adaptation after diagnosis. To the degree that there are such problems, the risks for continued adjustment difficulties may be increased. Diabetic youths, especially girls, appear to have a greater incidence of depression and eating disorders, and when present, these conditions are associated with poor glycemic control. Poor metabolic control has been associated with a number of psychosocial problems including anxiety, depression, poor self-esteem, high levels of stress, and maladaptive coping styles. Studies of neuropsychological functioning and school performance indicate that diabetic youths are also at risk for learning problems, especially with early diabetes onset, history of significant hypoglycemia, and chronic poor metabolic control. All of these factors are important components of quality of life and indicate the challenges that diabetic youths face in coping with diabetes management in the context of normal developmental tasks. Research findings indicate that quality of life is lower among youths from single-parent families, ethnic minority and lower SES groups, as well as girls, youths with shorter disease duration, and in those with diabetes-related family conflict. Less favorable quality of life also appears to be related with youths' perceptions that diabetes is upsetting, difficult to manage, and stressful, and is related to higher levels of self-reported depression. There is some evidence that better quality of life is associated with good glycemic control, but the relationship between glycemic control and quality of life appears modest.

The research literature has demonstrated that family factors are integral to the management of diabetes in children. A number of cross-sectional and prospective studies have shown that high levels of family cohesion, agreement about diabetes management responsibilities, and supportive behaviors are associated with better regimen adherence and glycemic control, while conflict, diffusion of responsibilities and regimen-related conflict have been associated with worse regimen adherence and glycemic control. In addition, studies have shown socio-demographic factors such as single-parenthood, lower SES, and ethnic minority status are related to greater risk for poor control of diabetes. Controlled intervention research has shown that family-based interventions utilizing positive reinforcement and behavioral contracts, communication skills training, negotiation of diabetes management goals, and problem-solving skills training, have led not only to improved regimen behaviors and glycemic control, but also to improved family relationships.

Type 2 Diabetes and Obesity

Epidemiologic Aspects and Clinical Features

Recent studies have shown a high incidence of type 2 diabetes in children, particularly among Native American Indian, Hispanic, African American, as well as Caucasian children (Fagot-Campagna et al., 2000; Rosenbloom et al., 1999). Pinhas-Hamiel et al. (1996) reported a 10-fold increase in the number of children diagnosed with type 2 diabetes at the diabetes clinic of a large urban hospital in Cincinnati during the years 1990-1994. Prior to 1990 these rates had been very low and stable. In this report as well as one from Arkansas (Scott et al., 1997), African-Americans accounted for almost 75% of youth presenting with type 2 diabetes. During the period 1990-1994, type 2 diabetes was diagnosed among 45% of the Mexican American youth presenting with newly diagnosed diabetes at a pediatric diabetes clinic in Ventura California (Neufeld et al., 1998). Many Mexican American children show risk factors for type 2 diabetes at young ages (Trevino et al., 1999).

These reports suggest that the appearance of type 2 diabetes in youth has recently begun to increase dramatically, and that it is children from minority ethnic groups that are particularly affected (Bloomgarden, 2004). It is also clear from these reports that obesity and a positive family history of type 2 diabetes, as well as markers of insulin resistance, are nearly always present in children and adolescents with type 2 diabetes (American Diabetes Association, 2000). In almost all cases of newly-diagnosed type 2 diabetes in youth, there is a family history of type 2 diabetes (Dabelea et al., 1999), so it is reasonable to view family history as a risk factor for insulin resistance. The mean age at diagnosis for new cases of type 2 diabetes is 13 years (Rosenbloom et al., 1999).

Obesity and Metabolic Risk

Obesity is considered to be of great importance to the development of type 2 diabetes. The increased risk of diabetes as weight increases has been shown in prospective studies in several adult studies (e.g., Knowler et al., 1981; Vanhala et al., 1999). From a metabolic standpoint, obesity is believed to increase the risk of type 2 diabetes in adults, particularly when it is centrally distributed, by increasing tissue resistance to insulin action (Reaven, 1988).

Studies indicate that the prevalence of overweight and obesity in children is very high (about 25-30%), and the incidence is increasing (Gortmaker et al., 1987; Hedley et al., 2004; Troiano & Flegal, 1998). Obesity in childhood is also associated with a high risk of continued obesity into adolescence and adulthood (Charney et al., 1976; Mossberg, 1989; Stark, 1981; Whitaker et al., 1997; Zack et al., 1979). In addition, obesity rates are higher in minority African-American and Hispanic children (Berenson et al., 1989; Kumianyika & Helitzer, 1985) and also increasing in incidence (Malina, 1993). Studies indicate African-American children have more obesity than whites, which track well into later adolescence (Berenson et al., 1989). Similarly, Hispanic children (Bradfield & Staeling,, 1984) and adolescents (Kumianyika & Helitzer, 1985) have shown greater prevalence of obesity than non-Hispanic whites, and their incidence is also increasing (Malina, 1993).

Studies of insulin action in obese children have revealed impaired insulin-stimulated glucose uptake in both pre-adolescent and adolescent subjects, as occurs in adults (Caprio & Tamborlane, 1999; Gower et al., 1999). However, unlike in most adult studies, obesity-related insulin resistance was not associated with visceral fat accumulation in pre-pubertal children (Gower et al., 1999). One study showed that obese children had fasting hyperinsulinemia and a 40% decrease in insulin stimulated glucose disposal compared with non-obese children; furthermore, visceral fat was inversely correlated with insulin sensitivity (Caprio & Tamborlane, 1999). Recent studies show reduced insulin sensitivity associated with obesity in African American (Klein et al., 2004; Young-Hyman et al., 2001) and Hispanic children (Cruz et al., 2004; Delamater et al., 2001; Goran et al., 2004). In another study, 25% of obese children and 21% of obese adolescents had impaired glucose tolerance (Sinha et al., 2002). In a community study of Native American Indians in Canada, very high rates of obesity were observed, and were associated with increased risk of having either IGT or type 2 diabetes (Young et al., 2000). Significant numbers of obese children have been demonstrated to have several risk factors for the metabolic syndrome (Cruz et al., 2004; Csabi et al., 2000; Weiss et al., 2004).

Public Health Significance

This new epidemic of diabetes among young people is of great public health significance. Diabetes is the leading cause of end-stage renal disease, visual loss and non-traumatic lower extremity amputation, and is a major risk factor for atherosclerotic vascular disease among adults (Harris, 1998). Although the long-term consequences of type 2 diabetes are unknown in children, it is expected that they will be susceptible to all of these complications, and based on adult studies, individuals from ethnic minority groups are likely to suffer greater morbidity and mortality (e.g., Cowie et al., 1989; Dorman & LaPorte, 1985; Haffner et al., 1988, 1989; Rosenman, 1985).

Determinants of Pediatric Obesity

Studies of the determinants of obesity in children have shown there is a relationship between child and parental obesity, which can be explained by genetic (Stunkard, 1986; Stunkard & Sorensen, 1986) and environmental/behavioral factors (Epstein et al., 1980; Epstein et al., 1987). Specific behavioral factors related to obesity involve consumption of high fat diets (Gortmaker et al., 1990) and physical inactivity (Berkowitz et al., 1985;). Excessive TV viewing has also been related to obesity (Dietz & Gortmaker, 1985; Kimm et al., 1996), presumably through its influence on diet and physical activity (Taras et al., 1989); there is also data suggesting the association of obesity and TV viewing may be related to a lowering of metabolic rate (Klesges et al., 1993). Epidemiologic studies have also shown that low levels of physical activity are associated with glucose intolerance and type 2 diabetes (Dowse et al., 1991; King et al., 1984). Familial aggregation of eating habits (Patterson et al., 1988) and physical activity (Sallis et al., 1988) have been observed in both Mexican-American and non-Hispanic families. Additionally, studies have shown Mexican-American youths engage in less physical activity and spend more time with adults (McKenzie et al., 1992), and spend less time outdoors and receive fewer parental prompts to be active (Sallis et al., 1993).

Interventions for High-Risk Children

Based on the above considerations it is becoming clear that obese children with a positive family history for type 2 diabetes represent a sub-group with an increased risk for the later development of type 2 diabetes. This risk is further compounded among minority youth who comprise an enlarging portion of the youth in this country. The advent of an increasingly frequent presentation among children and adolescents of a disease that appears to have similar characteristics to what has been observed in adults, adds a sense of urgency for the need to develop intervention programs targeted to those risk factors that are modifiable.

Which children should be targeted for prevention of type 2 diabetes? What type of intervention should be provided to children considered at high risk for developing type 2 diabetes? And when should intervention be given? When blood glucose levels are still normal or at the point when children have impaired glucose tolerance or impaired fasting glucose? As recommended by the American Diabetes Association (2000), early life-style interventions may have long-term health benefits. At present, data on the prevalence of impaired glucose tolerance is limited in pediatric populations (Fagot-Campagna et al., 2000), although recent findings indicate that up to 25% of obese children may have IGT (Sinha et al., 2002). Finding children who meet criteria for IGT would require a massive screening effort, and would likely result in very few students at any particular school. Furthermore it is likely that the phase of IGT as a precursor to conversion to diabetes may not last as long in children as it does in adults, where it constitutes the core element in screening strategies to identify subjects entered into prevention programs (The Diabetes Prevention Program Research Group, 2002). On the other hand, intervening with a high-risk group of children—those who are obese and who have a family history of type 2 diabetes—has the advantage of larger numbers of children who can be identified and receive intervention at an earlier age. Given that the mean age of onset is about 13 years of age (Rosenbloom et al., 1999), one reasonable strategy to prevent type 2 diabetes would be to intervene with high-risk pre-pubertal children.

According to the Consensus Statement of the American Diabetes Association (2000), "Lifestyle interventions focusing on weight management and increasing physical activity should be promoted in all children at high risk for the development of type 2 diabetes" (p. 388). While pharmacologic interventions are currently being used to prevent type 2 diabetes in adults with IGT, there is at present no evidence base for the use of drugs to prevent type 2 diabetes in children, especially those without IGT. As noted by the ADA Consensus Statement (2000), "Until the results of current trials with oral hypoglycemic agents in children are available, intervention using glucose-lowering drugs for prevention of diabetes in children is not recommended" (p.388). Furthermore, the ADA (2000) states that drug therapy to reduce weight is not recommended in children until more data concerning their safety and efficacy is available.

The results of the Diabetes Prevention Program Research Group (2002) recently demonstrated that a lifestyle intervention resulting in increased physical activity and at least a 7% reduction in weight decreased the risk of developing type 2 diabetes by 58%. A reasonable approach to prevent type 2 diabetes in children would be to focus on pre-pubertal children who are obese and who have a family history of type 2 diabetes, providing lifestyle interventions designed to promote habits of healthful eating and physical activity, in order to reduce weight and improve their metabolic risk profile.

Because both behavioral and physiological risk factors aggregate in families, the family unit should be targeted in health promotion intervention programs for children (Sallis & Nader, 1988). Studies of behavioral weight-reduction programs for children have shown that family involvement is a crucial component (Brownell et al., 1983; Epstein et al., 1987, 1990, 1998; Golan et al., 1998, 1999; Jelalian & Mehlenbeck, 2003; Jelalian & Saelens, 1999; Israel et al., 1994). Furthermore, when parents are involved in weight loss efforts along with their child, better results are obtained for children (Epstein et al., 1990). Exercise is also a critical component of weight loss programs, but in terms of physical activity, lifestyle change appears to be superior to programmed structured exercise for maintenance of weight loss in children (Epstein et al., 1982; Epstein & Goldfield, 1999), with better and sustained weight loss when individuals engage in habitual low intensity physical activity such as walking more (Kriska et al., 1986). Both proper dietary intake and physical activity are necessary for weight loss, but the key to these behavioral changes in children is involving the parent in their own as well as their child's weight loss, by behavioral methods including modeling, self-monitoring, appropriate goal-setting, and reinforcement.

School-based Health Promotion

School-based programs without direct parental involvement have been evaluated, but have not demonstrated significant long-term effects (Botvin et al., 1979; Brownell & Kaye, 1982; Parcel et al., 1987; Perry et al., 1990; Simons-Morton et al., 1991; Walter et al., 1989). A number of studies have examined the effects of broad-based school health education interventions targeting a variety of cardiovascular risk behaviors; the weakest effects of these school-based interventions have been on obesity (Resnicow & Robinson, 1997). However, the school site, because of it's accessibility to the community, may be an optimal place for delivery of family-based weight control programs (Healthy People 2000, 1991; Story, 1999; Williams, 1984). Family-based approaches at the school site hold particular promise for interventions with lower-income children, whose families may otherwise not have access to a health care team. It has already been demonstrated to be feasible and effective in a family-based cardiovascular risk reduction education program for Mexican-American youths (Nader et al., 1992). However, even when weight control programs are available at neighborhood sites such as the school, there may still be some barriers for many families that may limit their ability to participate or complete such programs. Interventions delivered at the homes of families may offer some advantages.

Home-based Interventions

There is an emerging literature documenting the effectiveness of health promotion interventions delivered at homes of pediatric patients with a variety of conditions (Aronen & Kurkela, 1996; Ciliska et al., 1996; Cooper et al., 1996; Margolis et al., 1996; Olds et al. 1997). Studies have not yet addressed the feasibility and efficacy of pediatric weight control programs delivered in the homes of minority families with obese children, but studies have utilized home-based interventions to modify dietary intake of children (e.g., Perry et al., 1988; Shannon et al., 1994; Vandongen et al., 1995). However, in the CATCH study (Luepker et al., 1996), home interventions provided only modest benefits in dietary knowledge over the school-based program, suggesting that family-based programs may need to be more involved than they were in that trial. A more intensive approach was used in the

Dietary Intervention Study for Children (DISC; Obarzanek et al., 1995). The DISC targeted reduction in dietary fat to reduce LDL-cholesterol in 8-10 year-old children with elevated LDL-cholesterol. Results of the DISC showed significant reductions dietary fat and LDL-cholesterol for children in the intervention group over three years (Obarzanek et al., 2001).

Cultural Issues

What strategies should be used to control weight in ethnically diverse children? It seems reasonable to apply an empirically validated behavioral weight loss program (Epstein et al., 1990, 1994) in working with obese, culturally diverse youths. However, the implementation must take into account culturally unique factors that characterize minority families (Hansen, Pepitone, & Greene, 2000; Sue & Sue, 1990). Studies have shown that cultural barriers of Hispanics to effective diabetes management include specific beliefs about causation and prevention, reliance on family influence, inadequate comprehension of the disease, less healthy behaviors with regard to diet and physical activity, and difficulties with the English language (Ernst & Harland, 1991; Tamez & Vicalis, 1989; Urdaneta & Krehbiel, 1989). In light of such cultural differences, interventions with Hispanic families to reduce obesity in children must be culturally sensitive in order to be clinically effective. The same is true for working with African American families, who may have different perceptions about obesity and health risks than white families (Young-Hyman et al., 2000). Therefore, although the specific goals or targets of behavior change will be the same as previously validated programs in working with obese Hispanic and African American children, the strategies employed to engage families in behavior change may need to be modified accordingly.

There are several examples from the literature of weight control programs for minority youth. For example, research with African American girls has shown the importance of working with the mother-child dyad to achieve changes in diet and physical activity (Stolley & Fitzgibbon, 1997). Studies of African American adolescent girls demonstrated the importance of mother participation (Wadden et al., 1990) and experiential physical activity and dietary activities during group sessions (Resnicow et al., 2000). Obesity prevention studies with African American and Hispanic children are ongoing and highlight the need to engage parents in promoting healthful dietary and physical activity habits (Fitzgibbon et al., 2002; Stolley et al., 2003). Reviews of programs for minorities indicate that few controlled, long-term studies are available, that barriers to change must be recognized, and that the cultural context and social networks play a prominent role in relation to dietary and physical activity habits (Foreyt, 2002; Kumanyika, 2002).

Summary

Type 2 diabetes is a significant health problem, especially among Hispanic and African American individuals, and is likely due, in part, to their greater rates of obesity, as well as genetic predisposition. Even in children, available evidence indicates obesity carries some metabolic risk factors for type 2 diabetes, including elevated insulin and abnormal glucose tolerance, particularly in those with a family history of type 2 diabetes. There is evidence for both genetic and environmental or behavioral factors in the development of obesity and type 2 diabetes. Given the fact that obese children and adolescents generally become obese adults, prevention of type 2 diabetes should intervene with obesity in childhood, focusing on those with family history of type 2 diabetes. In these high-risk children, behavioral interventions to improve dietary and physical activity habits should not only reduce body mass index, but also improve their metabolic risk profile, thereby reducing their risk for later development of type 2 diabetes. Of course, it is essential for public health approaches to be delivered to the entire pediatric population in order to prevent obesity by promoting healthy dietary behaviors, increased physical activity, and reduction of body mass index.

General Conclusions

A substantial amount of behavioral science research has demonstrated that psychosocial factors play an integral role in the management of type 1 diabetes in children and adolescents. Diabetic youth appear to be at increased risk for psychosocial difficulties, and when present, such difficulties are likely to be associated with problems with diabetes management. Family factors have consistently been related to regimen adherence and glycemic control, with the best outcomes attained for children with families that communicate well, provide support, and are appropriately involved in diabetes care. Research has demonstrated the efficacy of a number of psychosocial therapies that have been shown to improve regimen adherence and glycemic control, as well as psychosocial functioning and quality of life. More research is needed to develop psychosocial intervention programs for specific patient populations, and to demonstrate the cost-effectiveness of these approaches.

Type 2 diabetes has emerged as a significant health problem in the pediatric population, especially among Hispanic and African American youth. This is likely due, in part, to their greater rates of obesity, as well as genetic predisposition. Even in children, available evidence indicates obesity carries some metabolic risk factors for type 2 diabetes, including elevated insulin and abnormal glucose tolerance, particularly in those with a family history of type 2 diabetes. There is evidence for genetic and environmental or behavioral factors in the development of obesity and type 2 diabetes. Given the fact that obese children and adolescents generally become obese adults, prevention of type 2 diabetes should intervene with obesity in childhood, focusing on those with a family history of type 2 diabetes.

References

American Diabetes Association (2000). Type 2 diabetes in children and adolescents. *Diabetes Care, 23*(3), 381-389.

Anderson, B. J., Auslander, W. F., Jung, K. C., Miller, J. P., & Santiago, J. V. (1990). Assessing family sharing of diabetes responsibility. *Journal of Pediatric Psychology, 15,* 477-492.

Anderson, B. J., Brackett, J., Ho, J., & Laffel, L. (1999). An office-based intervention to maintain parent-adolescent teamwork in diabetes management: Impact on parent involvement, family conflict, and subsequent glycemic control. *Diabetes Care, 22,* 713-721.

Anderson, B. J., Ho, J., Brackett, J., Finkelstein, D., & Laffel, L. (1997). Parental involvement in diabetes management tasks: Relationships to blood glucose monitoring adherence and metabolic control in young adolescents with insulin-dependent diabetes mellitus. *Journal of Pediatrics, 130,* 257-265.

Anderson, B. J., Miller, J. P., Auslander, W. F., & Santiago, J. V. (1981). Family characteristics of diabetic adolescents: Relationship to metabolic control. *Diabetes Care, 4,* 586-594.

Anderson, B. J., Wolf, R. M., Burkhart, M. T., Cornell, R. G., & Bacon, G. E. (1989). Effects of peer-group intervention on metabolic control of adolescents with IDDM: Randomized outpatient study. *Diabetes Care, 12,* 179-183.

Aronen, E. T., & Kurkela, S. A. (1996). Long term effects of an early home-based intervention. *Journal of the American Academy of Child & Adolescent Psychiatry, 35,* 1665-1672.

Auslander, W. F., Thompson, S., Dreitzer, D., White, N. H., & Santiago, J. V. (1997). Disparity in glycemic control and adherence between African-American and Caucasian youths with diabetes: Family and community contexts. *Diabetes Care, 20,* 1569-1575.

Berenson, G. S., Srinivasan, S. R., Hunter, S. M., Nicklas, T. A., Freedman, D. S., Shear, C. L., et al. (1989). Risk factors in early life as predictors of adult heart disease: The Bogalusa Heart Study. *American Journal of Medical Science, 298,* 141-151.

Berkowitz, R. I., Agras, J. A., Korner, A. F., Kraemer, H. C., & Zeanah, C. H. (1985). Physical activity and adiposity: a longitudinal study from birth to childhood. *Journal of Pediatrics, 106,* 734-738.

Blanz, B., Rensch-Riemann, B., Fritz-Sigmund, D., & Schmidt, M. (1993). IDDM is a risk factor for adolescent psychiatric disorders. *Diabetes Care, 16,* 1579-1587.

Bloomgarden, Z. (2004). Type 2 diabetes in the young: The evolving epidemic. *Diabetes Care, 27,* 998-1010.

Boardway, R. H., Delamater, A. M., Tomakowsky, J., & Gutai, J. P. (1993). Stress management training for adolescents with diabetes. *Journal of Pediatric Psychology, 18,* 29-45.

Bobrow, E. S., AvRuskin, T. W., & Siller, J. (1985). Mother-daughter interaction and adherence to diabetes regimens. *Diabetes Care, 8,* 146-151.

Boland, E. A., Grey, M., Oesterle, A. L., Fredrickson, L., & Tamborlane, W. V. (1999). Continuous subcutaneous insulin infusion: A new way to lower risk of severe hypoglycemia, improve metabolic control, and enhance coping in adolescents with type 1 diabetes, *Diabetes Care, 22,* 1779-1784.

Bond, G. G., Aiken, L. S., & Somerville, S. C. (1992). The health belief model and adolescents with insulin-dependent diabetes mellitus. *Health Psychology, 11,* 190-198.

Botvin, G. J., Cantlon, A., Carter, B. J., & Williams, C. L. (1979). Reducing adolescent obesity through a school health program. *Journal of Pediatrics, 95,* 1060-1062.

Bradfield, R. B., & Staehling, N. (1984). The size of California nonmigrant Mexican-American children. *American Journal of Clinical Nutrition, 38,* 873-874.

Brownell, K. D., & Kaye, F. S. (1982). A school-based behavior modification, nutrition education and physical activity program for obese children. *American Journal of Clinical Nutrution, 35,* 277-283.

Brownell, K. D., Kelman, J. H., & Stunkard, A. J. (1983). Child and parent weight loss in family-based behavior modification programs. *Pediatrics, 71,* 515-523.

Brownell, K. D., Kelman, J. H., & Stunkard, A. J. (1983). Treatment of obese children with and without their mothers: Changes in weight and blood pressure. *Pediatrics, 71,* 515-523.

Brownlee-Duffeck, M., Peterson, L., Simonds, J. F., Goldstein, D., Kilo, C. & Hoette, S. (1987). The role of health beliefs in the regimen adherence and metabolic control of adolescents and adults with diabetes mellitus. *Journal of Consulting and Clinical Psychology, 55,* 139-144.

Bryden, K. S., Neil, A., Mayou, R. A., Peveler, R. C., Fairburn, C. G., & Dunger, D. B. (1999). Eating habits, body weight, and insulin misuse: A longitudinal study of teenagers and young adults with type 1 diabetes. *Diabetes Care, 22,* 1956-1960.

Bryden, K. S., Peveler, R. C., Stein, A., Neil, A., Mayou, R. A., & Dunger, D. B. (2001). Clinical and psychological course of diabetes from adolescence to young adulthood: A longitudinal cohort study. *Diabetes Care, 24,* 1536-1540.

Campaigne, B. N., Gilliam, T. B., Spencer, M. L., Lampman, R. M., & Schork, M. A. (1984). Effects of a physical activity program on metabolic control and cardiovascular fitness in children with IDDM. *Diabetes Care, 7,* 57-62.

Caprio, S., & Tamborlane, W. V. (1999). Metabolic impact of obesity in childhood. Pediatric Endocrinology, *28*(4), 731-747.

Charney, E., Goodman, H. C., & McBride, M. (1976). Childhood obesity antecedents of adult obesity. *New England Journal of Medicine, 295*(6), pp. 6-9.

Charron-Prochownik, D., Becker, M. H., Brown, M. B., Liang, W., & Bennett, S. (1993). Understanding young children's health beliefs and diabetes regimen adherence. *The Diabetes Educator, 19,* 409-418.

Ciliska, D., Hayward, S., Thomas, H., Mitchel, A., Dobbins, M., Underwood, J., et al. (1996). A systematic overview of the effectiveness of home visiting as a delivery strategy for public health nursing interventions. *Canadian Journal of Public Health, 87,* 193-198.

Cook, S., Herold, K., Edidin, D. V., & Briars, R. (2002). Increasing problem solving in adolescents with type 1 diabetes: The Choices Diabetes Program. *The Diabetes Educator, 28,* 115-124.

Cooper, W. O., Kotagal, U. R., Atherton, H. D., Lippert, C. A., Bragg, E., Donovan, E. F., et al. (1996). Use of health care services by inner-city infants in an early discharge program. *Pediatrics, 98,* 686-691.

Couper, J. J., Taylor, J., Fotheringham, M. J., & Sawyer, M. (1999). Failure to maintain the benefits of home-based intervention in adolescents with poorly controlled type 1 diabetes. *Diabetes Care, 22,* 1933-1937.

Cowie, C. C., Port F. K., Wolfe, R. A., Savage, P. J., Moll, P. P., & Hawthorne, V. M. (1989). Disparities in incidence of diabetic end-stage renal disease according to race and type of diabetes. *New England Journal of Medicine, 321,* 1074-1079.

Cruz, M., Weigensberg, M., Huang, T., Ball, G., Shaibi, G., & Goran, M. (2004). The metabolic syndrome in overweight Hispanic youth and the role of insulin sensitivity. *Journal of Clinical Endocrinology and Metabolism, 89,* 108-113.

Csabi, G., Torok, K., Jeges, S., & Monar, D. (2000). Presence of metabolic cardiovascular syndrome in obese children. *European Journal of Pediatrics, 159,* 91-94.

Dabalea, D., Pettitt, D. J., Jones, K., & Arslanian, S. A. (1999). Type 2 diabetes mellitus in minority children and adolescents: An emerging problem. *Endocrinol Metab Clin North Am, 28,* 709-729.

Daneman, D., Olmsted, M., Rydall, A., Maharaj, S., & Rodin, G. (1998). Eating disorders in young women with type 1 diabetes: Prevalence, problems and prevention. *Hormone Research, 50* (Suppl 1), 79-86.

Davis, C. L., Delamater, A. M., Shaw, K. H., La Greca, A. M., Eidson, M. S., Pewrez-Rodriguez, J. E., et al. (2001). Parenting styles, regimen adherence, and glycemic control in 4- to 10-year-old children with diabetes. *Journal of Pediatric Psychology, 26,* 123-129.

Delamater, A. M., Albrecht, D. R., Postellon, D. C., & Gutai, J. P. (1991). Racial differences in metabolic control of children and adolescents with Type I diabetes mellitus. *Diabetes Care, 14,* 20-25.

Delamater, A., Brito, A., Applegate, B., Casteleiro, V., Patino, A., Sabogal, C., et al. (1989). Obesity and family history increase metabolic risk in Hispanic children. *Annals of Behavioral Medicine, 23*(Supplement), S130.

Delamater, A. M., Bubb, J., Davis, S., Smith, J., Schmidt, L., White, N., et al. (1990). Randomized, prospective study of self-management training with newly diagnosed diabetic children. *Diabetes Care, 13,* 492-498.

Delamater, A. M., Jacobson, A. M., Anderson, B., Cox, D., Fisher, L., Lustman, P., et al. (2001). Psychosocial therapies in diabetes: Report of the Psychosocial Therapies Working Group. *Diabetes Care, 24,* 1286-1292.

Delamater, A. M., Kurtz, S. M., Bubb, J., White, N. H., & Santiago, J. V. (1987). Stress and coping in relation to metabolic control of adolescents with type I diabetes. *Journal of Developmental and Behavioral Pediatrics, 8,* 136-140.

Delamater, A. M., Shaw, K., Applegate, B., Pratt, I., Eidson, M., Lancelotta, G., et al. (1999). Risk for metabolic control problems in minority youth with diabetes. *Diabetes Care, 22,* 700-705.

Delamater, A. M., Smith, J., Bubb, J., Davis, S., Gamble, T., White, N., et al. (1991). Family-based behavior therapy for diabetic adolescents. In J. Johnson & S. B. Johnson (Eds.), *Advances in child health psychology: Proceedings of the Florida Conference* (pp. 363-391). Gainesville, FL: University of Florida Press.

Delamater, A. M., Tercyak, K., Applegate, B., Eidson, M., & Nemery, R. (1998). Quality of life in minority youths with diabetes. *Psychosomatic Medicine, 60,* 131.

Diabetes Control and Complications Trial Research Group. (1994). Effect of intensive diabetes treatment on the development and progression of long-term complications in adolescents with insulin-dependent diabetes mellitus, Diabetes Control and Complications Trial. *Journal of Pediatrics, 125,* 177-188.

Diabetes Prevention Program Research Group. (2002). Reduction in the incidence of type 2 diabetes with lifestyle intervention or Metformin. *New England Journal of Medicine, 346,* 393-403.

Dietz, W. H., & Gortmaker, S. L. (1985). Do we fatten our children at the television set?: Obesity and television viewing in children and adolescents. *Pediatrics, 75*(5), 807-812.

Dorman, J. S., & LaPorte, R. E. (1985). Mortality in insulin-dependent diabetes. In Diabetes in America. Washington, D.C.: US Government Printing Office (NIH publ. no. 85-1468).

Dowse, G. K., Zimmet, P. Z., Gareeboo, H., Alberti, K. G., Tuomilehto, J., Finch, C. F., et al. (1991). Abdominal obesity and physical inactivity are risk factors for NIDDM and impaired glucose tolerance in Indian, Creole, and Chinese Mauritians. *Diabetes Care, 14,* 271-282.

Epstein, L., & Goldfield, G. (1999). Physical activity in the treatment of childhood overweight and obesity: Current evidence and research issues. *Medicine & Science in Sports & Exercise,31,* S553-S559.

Epstein, L. H., Myers, M., Raynor H., & Saelens, B. (1998). Treatment of pediatric obesity. *Pediatrics, 101,* 554-570.

Epstein, L. H., Valoski, A., Wing, R., & McCurley, J. (1990). Ten-year follow-up of behavioral family based treatment for obese children. *Journal of American Medicine, 264,* 2519-2523.

Epstein, L. H., Valoski, A., Wing, R. R., & McCurley, J. (1994). Ten-year outcomes of behavioral family-based treatment for childhood obesity. *Health Psychology, 13,* 373-383.

Epstein, L. H., Wing, R. R., Koeske, R., & Valoski, A. (1987). Long-term effects of family-based treatment of childhood obesity. *Journal of Clinical and Consulting Psychology, 55,* 91-95.

Epstein, L. H., Wing, R. R., Koeske, R., Osssip, D. J., & Beck, S. (1982). A comparison of lifestyle change and programmed aerobic exercise on weight and fitness changes in obese children. *Behavior Therapy, 13,* 651-665.

Epstein, L. H., Wing, R. R., Steranchak, L., Dickson, B., & Michelson, J. (1980). Comparison of family-based behavior modification and nutrition education for childhood obesity. *Journal of Pediatric Psychology, 5,* 25-36, 1980.

Ernst, N., & Harland, W. R. (1991). Obesity and cardiovascular disease in minority populations. *American Journal of Clinical Nutrition, 53,* 1507S-1511S.

Fagot-Campagna, A., Pettitt, D., Engelgan, M. M., Burrows, N. R., Geiss, L. S., Valdez, R., et al. (2000). Type 2 diabetes among North American children and adolescents: An epidemiologic review and a public health perspective. *Journal of Pediatrics*, *136*, 664-672.

Fitzgibbon, M., Stolley, M., Dyer, A., VanHorn, L., & KauferChristoffel, K. (2002). A community-based obesity prevention program for minority children: Rationale and study design for Hip-Hop to Health Jr. *Preventive Medicine, 24*, 289-297.

Foreyt, J. P. (2002). Weight loss programs for minority populations. In C. G. Fairburn & K. D. Brownell (Eds.), *Eating Disorders and Obesity: A Comprehensive Handbook* (2nd edition) (pp. 583-587). New York: Guilford Press.

Forsander, G.A., Persson, B., Sundelin, J., Berglund, E., Snellman, K., & Hellstrom, R. (1998). Metabolic control in children with insulin-dependent diabetes mellitus 5 y after diagnosis: Early detection of patients at risk for poor metabolic control. *Acta Paediatr, 87*, 857-864.

Forsander, G. A., Sundelin, J., & Persson, B. (2000). Influence of the initial management regimen and family social situation on glycemic control and medical care in children with type 1 diabetes mellitus. *Acta Paediatr, 89*, 1462-1468.

Golan, M., Weizman, A., Apter, A., & Fainaru, M. (1998). Parents as the exclusive agents of change in the treatment of childhood obesity. *American Society for Clinical Nutrition, 67*, 1130-1135.

Golan, M., Weizman, A., & Fainaru, M. (1999). Impact of treatment for childhood obesity on parental risk factors for cardiovascular disease. *Preventive Medicine, 29*, 519-526.

Goran, M. I., Bergman, R. N., Avila, Q., Watkins, M., Ball, G. D. C., Shaibi, Q., et al. (2004). Impaired glucose tolerance and reduced beta-cell function in overweight Latino children with a positive family history for type 2 diabetes. *The Journal of Clinical Endocrinology & Metabolism, 89*, 207-212.

Gortmaker, S. L., Dietz, W. H., & Cheung, L. W. (1990). Inactivity, Diet, and the Fattening of America. *Journal of the American Dietetic Association, 90*, 1247-1255.

Gortmaker, S. L., Dietz, W. H., Sobol, A. M., & Wehler, C. A. (1987). Increasing pediatric obesity in the United States. *American Journal of Diseases of children, 141*, 535-540.

Gower, B. A., Nagy, T. R., & Goran, M. I. (1999). Visceral fat, insulin sensitivity, and lipids in prepubertal children. *Diabetes, 48*, 1515-1521.

Greco, P., Shroff Pendley, J., McDonell, K., & Reeves, G. (2001) A peer group intervention for adolescents with type 1 diabetes and their best friends. *Journal of Pediatric Psychology, 26*, 485-490.

Grey, M., Boland, E. A., Davidson, M., Yu, C., Sullivan-Bolyai, S., & Tamborlane, W. V. (1998). Short-term effects of coping skills training as adjunct to intensive therapy in adolescents. *Diabetes Care, 21*, 902-908.

Grey, M., Boland, E., Davidson, M., Yu, C., & Tamborlance, W. (2000). Coping skills training for youth on intensive therapy has long-lasting effects on metabolic control and quality of life. *Journal of Pediatrics, 137*, 107-113.

Grey, M., Boland, E. A., Yu, C., Sullivan-Bolyai, S., & Tamborlane, W.V. (1998). Personal and family factors associated with quality of life in adolescents with diabetes. *Diabetes Care, 21,* 909-914.

Grey, M., Cameron, M., Lipman, T., & Thurber, F. (1995). Psychosocial status of children with diabetes in the first 2 years after diagnosis. *Diabetes Care, 18,* 1330-1336.

Grossman, H. Y., Brink, S., & Hauser, S. T. (1987). Self-efficacy in adolescent girls and boys with insulin-dependent diabetes mellitus. *Diabetes Care, 10,* 324-329.

Guttmann-Bauman, I., Flaherty, B. P., Strugger, M., & McEvoy, R. C. (1998). Metabolic control and quality-of-life self-assessment in adolescents with IDDM. *Diabetes Care, 21,* 915-918.

Haffner, S. M., Fong, D., Stern, M. P., Pugh, H. P., Hazuda, J. K., Patterson, J. K., et al. (1988). Diabetic retinopothy in Mexican Americans and Non-Hispanic Whites. *Diabetes, 37,* 878-884.

Haffner, S. M., Mitchell, B. D., Pubh, G. A., Stern, M. P., Kozlowski, M. K., Hazuda, H. P., et al. (1989). Proteinuria in Mexican Americans and Non-Hispanic Whites with NIDDM. *Diabetes Care, 12,* 530-536.

Hains, A. A., Davies, W. H., Parton, E., Totka, J., & Amoroso-Camarata, J. (2000). A stress management intervention for adolescents with type 1 diabetes. *The Diabetes Educator, 26,* 417-424.

Hampson, S. E., Skinner, R. C., Hart, J., Storey L., Gage, H., Foxcroft, D., et al. (2000). Behavioral interventions for adolescents with type 1 diabetes: How effective are they? *Diabetes Care, 23,* 1416-1422.

Hanson, C. L., Cigrant, J. A., Harris, M, Carle, D. L., Relyea, G., & Burghen, G. A. (1989). Coping styles in youths with insulin-dependent diabetes mellitus. *Journal of Consulting and Clinical Psychology, 57,* 644-651.

Hanson, C. L., Henggeler, S. W., & Burghen, G. A. (1987). Model of associations between psychosocial variables and health-outcome measures of adolescents with IDDM. *Diabetes Care, 10,* 752-758.

Hanson, N. D., Pepitone, F., & Greene, A. (2000). Multicultural competence: Criteria and case examples. *Professional Psychology, 31,* 652-660.

Hanson, S. L., & Pichert, J. W. (1986). Perceived stress and diabetes control in adolescents. *Health Psychology, 5,* 439-452.

U.S. Department of Health and Human Services. (2000). *Healthy People 2000: National health promotion and disease prevention objectives.* (PHS, DHHS Publication No. 91-50212). Washington D.C.: U.S. Government Printing Office.

Hedley, A. A., Ogden, C. L., Johnson, C. L., Carroll, M. D., Curtin, L. R., & Flegal, K. M. (2004). Prevalence of overweight and obesity among US children, adolescents, and adults, 1999-2002. *The Journal of the American Medical Association, 291,* 2847-2850.

Hoey, H., Aanstoot, H., Chiarelli, F., Daneman, D., Danne, T., Dorchy, H., et al. (2001). Hvidore Study Group on Childhood Diabetes. Good metabolic control is associated with better quality of life in 2,101 adolescents with type 1 diabetes. *Diabetes Care, 24,* 1923-1928.

Holmes, C., Dunlap, W., Chen, R., & Cornwell, J. (1992). Gender differences in the learning status of diabetic children. *Journal of Consulting and Clinical Psychology, 60,* 698-704.

Holmes, C., & Richman, L. (1995). Cognitive profiles of children with insulin-dependent diabetes. *Developmental and Behavioral Pediatrics, 6,* 323-326.

Horan, P., Yarborough, M., Besigel, G., & Carlson, D. (1990). Computer-assisted self-control of diabetes by adolescents. *The Diabetes Educator, 16,* 205-211.

Howells, L., Wilson, A., Skinner, T., Newton R., Morris, A., & Grene, S. (2002). A randomized control trial of the effect of negotiated telephone support on glycaemic control in young people with type 1 diabetes. *Diabetic Medicine, 19,* 643-648.

Huttunen, N. P., Lankelaa, S. L., Knip, M., Lautala, P., Kaar, M. L., Laasonen, K., et al. (1989). Effect of once-a-week training program on physical fitness and metabolic control in children with IDDM. *Diabetes Care, 12,* 737-739.

Ingersoll, G. M., & Marrero, D. G. (1991). A modified quality-of-life measure for youths: Psychometric properties. *The Diabetes Educator, 17,* 114-120.

Ingersoll, G. M., Orr, D., Herrold, A., & Golden, M. (1986). Cognitive maturity and self-management among adolescents with insulin-dependent diabetes mellitus. *Journal of Pediatrics, 108,* 620-623.

Israel, A. C., Guile, C. A., Baker, J. E., & Silverman, W. K. (1994). An evaluation of enhanced self-regulation training in the treatment of childhood obesity. *Journal of Pediatric Psychology, 19,* 737-749.

Jacobson, A. M., Hauser, S. T., Lavori, P., et al. (1994). Family environment and glycemic control: a four-year prospective study of children and adolescents with insulin-dependent diabetes mellitus. *Psychosomatic Medicine, 56,* 401-409.

Jacobson, A. M., Hauser, S. T., Lavori, P., Wolfsdorf, J., Herskowitz, R., Milley, J., et al. (1990). Adherence among children and adolescents with insulin-dependent diabetes mellitus over a four-year longitudinal follow-up: I. The influence of patient coping and adjustment. *Journal of Pediatric Psychology, 15,* 511-526.

Jacobson, A. M., Hauser, S. T., Wertlieb, D., Woldsdorf, J., Orleans, J. & Viegra, M. (1986). Psychological adjustment of children with recently diagnosed diabetes mellitus. *Diabetes Care, 9,* 323-329.

Jacobson, A. M., Hauser, S. T., Willett, J., Wolfsdor, J., & Herman, L. (1997). Consequences of irregular versus continuous medical follow-up in children and adolescents with insulin-dependent diabetes mellitus. *Journal of Pediatrics, 131,* 727-733.

Jacobson, A. M., Hauser, S. T., Willett, J., Wolfsdorf, J. I., Herman, L., & de Groot, M. (1997). Psychological adjustment to IDDM: 10-year follow-up of an onset cohort of child and adolescent patients. *Diabetes Care, 20,* 811-818.

Jelalian, E., & Mehlenbeck, R. (2003). Pediatric obesity. In M. C. Roberts (Ed.), *Handbook of Pediatric Psychology* (3rd edition) (pp. 529-543). New York: Guilford.

Jelalian, E., & Saelens, B. (1999). Empirically supported treatments in pediatric psychology: pediatric obesity. *Journal of Pediatric Psychology, 24,* 223-248.

Johnson, S. B. (1995). Insulin-dependent diabetes mellitus in childhood. In M. C. Roberts (Ed.), *Handbook of Pediatric Psychology* (pp. 263-285). New York: Guilford.

Johnson S. B., Kelly, M., Henretta J. C., Cunningham W. R., Tomer A., & Silverstein, J. H. (1992). A longitudinal analysis of adherence and health status in childhood diabetes. *Journal of Pediatric Psychology, 17*, 537-553.

Jones, J. M., Lawson, M. L., Daneman, D., Olmsted, M. P., & Rodin, G. (2000). Eating disorders in adolescent females with and without type 1 diabetes: Cross sectional study. *British Medical Journal, 320*, 1563-1566.

Kager, V., & Holden, W. (1992). Preliminary investigation of the direct and moderating effects of family and individual variables on the adjustment of children and adolescents with diabetes. *Journal of Pediatric Psychology, 17*, 491-502.

Kaplan, R. M., Chadwick, M. W., & Schimmel, L. E. (1985). Social learning intervention to promote metabolic control in Type I diabetes mellitus: Pilot experimental results. *Diabetes Care, 8*, 152-155.

Kaufman, F. R., Halvorson, M., & Carpenter, S. (1999). Association between diabetes control and visits to a multidisciplinary pediatric diabetes clinic. *Pediatrics, 103*, 948-951.

Kimm, S. Y., Obarzanek, E., Barton, B. A., Aston, C. E, Similo, S. L., Morrison, J. A., et al. (1996). Race, socioeconomic status, and obesity in 9- to 10-year-old girls: The NHLBI Growth and Health Study. Annals of Epidemiology, 6, 266-275.

King, H., Taylor, R., Zimmet, P., Raper, L., & Balkau, B. (1984). Risk Factors for Diabetes in Three Pacific Populations. *American Journal of Epidemiology, 119*, 396-409.

Klein, D., Friedman, L., Harlan, W., Barton, B., Schreiber, G., Cohen, R., et al. (2004). Obesity and the development of insulin resistance and impaired fasting glucose in black and white adolescent girls. *Diabetes Care, 27*, 378-383.

Klesges, R. C., Eck, L. H., Hanson, C. L., Haddock, C. K., & Klesges, L. M. (1993). Effects of Obesity, Social Interactions, and Physical Environment on Physical Activity in Preschoolers. *Health Psychology, 9*, 435-449.

Knowler, W. C., Pettitt, D. J., Savage, P. J., & Bennet, P. H. (1981). Diabetes incidence in Pima Indians: contributions of obesity and parental diabetes. *American Journal of Epidemiology, 113*, 144-156.

Kovacs, M., Feinberg, T. L., Paulauskas, S., Finkelstein, R., Pollock, M. & Crouse-Novak, M. (1985). Initial coping responses and psychosocial characteristics of children with insulin-dependent diabetes mellitus. *Journal of Pediatrics, 106*, 827-834.

Kovacs, M., Finkelstein, R., Feinberg, T. L., Crouse-Novak, M., Paulauskas, S., & Pollock, M. (1985). Initial psychologic responses of parents to the diagnosis of insulin dependent diabetes mellitus in their children. *Diabetes Care, 8*, 568-575.

Kovacs, M., Goldston, D., & Iyengar, S. (1992). Intellectual development and academic performance of children with insulin-dependent diabetes mellitus: A longitudinal study. *Developmental Psychology, 28,* 676-684.

Kovacs, M., Goldston, D., Obrosky, D., & Bonar, L. (1997). Psychiatric disorders in youths with IDDM: Rates and risk factors. *Diabetes Care, 20,* 36-44.

Kovacs, M., Ho, V., & Pollock, M. H. (1995). Criterion and predictive validity of the diagnosis of adjustment disorder: a prospective study of youths with new-onset insulin-dependent diabetes mellitus. *American Journal of Psychiatry, 152,* 523-528.

Kovacs, M., Ryan, C., & Obrosky, D. S. (1994). Verbal intellectual and verbal memory performance of youths with childhood-onset insulin-dependent diabetes mellitus. *Journal of Pediatric Psychology, 19,* 475-483.

Kriska, A. M., Bayles, C., Cauley, J. A., LaPorte, R. E., Sandler, R. B., & Pambianco, G. A. (1986). Randomized exercise trial in older women: Increased activity over two years and the factors associated with compliance. *Medicine & Science in Sports & Exercise, 23,* 557-562.

Kumanyika, S. K. (2002). Obesity in minority populations. In C. G. Fairburn & K. D. Brownell (Eds.), *Eating Disorders and Obesity: A Comprehensive Handbook* (2nd edition) (pp. 583-587). New York: Guilford Press.

Kumanyika, S. K., & Helitzer, D. L. (1985). Nutrition Report of the Secretary's Task Force on Black and Minority Health - Volume II Cross Cutting Issues in Minority Health. Washington, D.C., U.S. Department of Health and Human Services.

Kuttner, M. J., Delamater, A. M., & Santiago, J. V. (1990). Learned helplessness in diabetic youths. *Journal of Pediatric Psychology, 15,* 581-594.

La Greca, A. M., Auslander, W. F., Greco, P., Spetter, D., Fisher, E. B., & Santiago, J. V. (1995). I get by with a little help from my family and friends: Adolescents' support for diabetes care. *Journal of Pediatric Psychology, 20,* 449-476.

La Greca, A. M., Swales, T., Klemp, S., Madigan, S., & Skyler, J. (1995). Adolescents with diabetes: Gender differences in psychosocial functioning and glycemic control. *Children's Health Care, 24,* 61-78.

Laffel, L., Connell, A., Vangsness, L., Goebel-Fabbri, A., Mansfield, A., & Anderson, B. J. (2003). General quality of life in youth with type 1 diabetes: Relationship to patient management and diabetes-specific family conflict. *Diabetes Care, 26,* 3067-3073.

Laffel, L., Vangsness, L., Connell, A., Goebel-Fabbri, A., Butler, D., & Anderson, B. J. (2003). Impact of ambulatory, family-focused teamwork intervention on glycemic control in youth with type 1 diabetes. *Journal of Pediatrics, 142,* 409-416.

Landolt, M. A., Ribi, K., Laimbacher, J., Vollrath, M., Gnehm, H. E., & Sennhauser, F. H. (2002). Posttraumatic stress disorder in parents of children with newly diagnosed type 1 diabetes. *Journal of Pediatric Psychology, 27,* 647-652.

Lavigne, J., & Faier-Routman, J. (1992). Psychological adjustment to pediatric physical disorders: A meta-analytic review. *Journal of Pediatric Psychology, 17*, 133-157.

Levine, B., Anderson, B. J., Butler, D., Antisdel, J., Brackett, J., & Laffel, L. (2001). Predictors of glycemic control and short-term adverse outcomes in youth with type 1 diabetes. *Journal of Pediatrics, 139*, 197-203.

Luepker, R. V., Perry, C. L., McKinlay, S. M., Nader, P. R., Parcel, G. S, Stone, E. J, et al. (1996). Outcomes of a field trial to improve children's dietary patterns and physical activity: The Child and Adolescent Trial for Cardiovascular Health (CATCH). *Journal of the American Medical Association, 275*, 768-776.

Maharag, S., Rodini, G., Olmsted, M., Connolly, J., & Daneman, D. (2001). Eating problems and the observed quality of mother-daughter interactions among girls with type 1 diabetes. *Journal of Consulting and Clinical Psychology, 69*, 950-958.

Malina, R. (1993). Ethnic variation in the prevalence of obesity in North American children and youth. *Critical Reviews in Food Science and Nutrition, 33*, 389-396.

Margolis, P. A., Lannon, C. M., Stevens, R., Harlan, C., Bordley, W. C., Carey, T., et al. (1996). Linking clinical and public health approaches to improve access to health care for socially disadvantaged mothers and children: A feasibility study. *Archives of Pediatrics & Adolescent Medicine, 150*, 815-821.

Marrero, D. G., Kronz, K. K., Golden, M. P., Wright, J. C., Orr, D. P., Fineberg, N. S., et al. (1989). Clinical evaluation of computer-assisted self-monitoring of blood glucose system. *Diabetes Care, 12*, 345-350.

Marrero, D. G., Vandagriff, J., Kronz, K., Fineberg, N., Golden, M., Bray, D., et al. (1995). Using telecommunication technology to manage children with diabetes: The computer-linked outpatient clinic (CLOC) Study. *The Diabetes Educator, 21*, 313-319.

McKenzie, T. L., Sallis, J. F., Nader, P. R., Broyles, S. L., & Nelson, J. A. (1992). Anglo- and Mexican-American preschoolers at home and at recess: Activity patterns and environmental influences. *Developmental and Behavioral Pediatrics, 13*, 173-180.

Meltzer, L. J., Johnson, S. B., Prine, J. M., Banks, R. A., Desrosiers, P. M., & Silverstein, J. H. (2001). Disordered eating, body mass, and glycemic control in adolescents with type 1 diabetes. *Diabetes Care, 24*, 678-682.

Mendez, F., & Belendez, M. (1997). Effects of a behavioral intervention on treatment adherence and stress management in adolescents with IDDM. *Diabetes Care, 20*, 1370-1375.

Miller-Johnson, S., Emery, R., Marvin, R., Clarke, W., Lovinger, R., & Martin, M. (1994). Parent-child relationships and the management of insulin-dependent diabetes mellitus. *Journal of Consulting and Clinical Psychology, 62*, 603-610.

Mossberg, H. O. (1989). Forty-year follow up of overweight children. *Lancet, 2*, 491-493.

Nader, P. R., Sallis, J. F., Abramson, I. S., Broyles, S. L., Patterson, T. L., Senn, K., et al. (1992). Family-based cardiovascular risk reduction education among Mexican- and Anglo-Americans. *Family Community Health, 15*, 57-74.

Neufeld, N., Raffel, L., Landon, C., Chen, Y., & Vadheim, C. (1998). Early presentation of type 2 diabetes in Mexican-American youth. *Diabetes Care, 21*, 80-86.

Neumark-Sztainer, D., Patterson, J., Mellin, A., Ackard, D., Utter, J., Story, M., et al. (2002). Weight control practices and disordered eating behaviors among adolescent females and males with type 1 diabetes: Associations with sociodemographics, weight concerns, familial factors, and metabolic outcomes. *Diabetes Care, 25*, 1289-1296.

Northam, E. A., Anderson, P. J., Jacobs, R., Hughes, M., Warne, G. L., & Werther, G. A. (2001). Neuropsychological profiles of children with type 1 diabetes 6 years after disease onset. *Diabetes Care, 24*, 1541-1546.

Northam, E., Anderson, P., Werther, G., Warne, G., Adler, R., & Andrewes, D. (1998). Neuropsychological complications of IDDM in children 2 years after disease onset. *Diabetes Care, 21*, 379-384.

Northam, E., Anderson, P., Werther, G., Warne, G., Adler, R., & Andrewes, D. (1999). Predictors of change in the neuropsychological profiles of children with type 1 diabetes 2 years after disease onset. *Diabetes Care, 22*, 1438-1444.

Obzarzanek, E., Hunsberger S., Van Horn, L., Hartmuller, V. V., Barton, B. A., Stevens, V. J., et al. (1997). Safety of a fat-reduced diet: The dietary intervention study in children. *Pediatrics, 100*, 51-59.

Obzarzanek, E., Kimm, S., Barton, B., Van Horn, L., Kwiterovich, P. O., Simons-Morton, D. G., et al. (2001). Long-term safety and efficacy of a cholesterol-lowering diet in children with elevated low-density lipoprotein cholesterol: Seven-year results of the Dietary Intervention Study in Children. *Pediatrics, 107*, 256-264.

Olds, D., Kitzman, H., Cole, R., Robinson, J., Sidora, K., Luckey, D. W., et al. (1997). Long-term effects of home visitation on maternal life course and child abuse and neglect: Fifteen-year follow-up of a randomized trial. *Journal of the American Medical Association, 278*, 637-643.

Orr, D., Golden, M. P., Myers, G., & Marrero, D. G. (1983). Characteristics of adolescents with poorly controlled diabetes referred to a tertiary care center. *Diabetes Care, 6*, 170175.

Overstreet, S., Goins, J., Chen, R. S., Holmes, C. S., Greer, T., Dunlap, W. P., et al. (1995). Family environment and the interrelation of family structure, child behavior, and metabolic control for children with diabetes. *Journal of Pediatric Psychology, 20*, 435-447.

Palardy, N., Greening, L., Ott, J., Holderby, A., & Atchison, J. (1998). Adolescents' health attitudes and adherence to treatment for insulin-dependent diabetes mellitus. *Developmental and Behavioral Pediatrics, 19*, 31-37.

Parcel, G. S., Simons-Morton, B. G., O'Hara, N. M., Baranowski, T., Kolbe, L. J., & Bee, D. E. (1987). School promotion of healthful diet and exercise behavior: an integration of organizational change and social learning theory interventions. *Journal of School Health, 57,* 150-156.

Patterson, T. L., Rupp, J. W., Sallis, J. F., Atkins, C. J., & Nader, P. R (1988). Aggregation of dietary calories, fats, and sodium in Mexican American and Anglo families. *American Journal of Preventive Medicine, 4,* 75-82.

Perry, C. L., Luepker, R. V, Murray, D. M., Kurth, C., Mullis, R., Crockett, S. et al. (1988). Parent involvement with children's health promotion: The Minnesota Home Team. *American Journal of Public Health, 78,* 1156-1160.

Perry, C. L., Stone, E. J., Parcel, G. S., Ellison, R. C., Nader, P. R., Webber, L. S., et al. (1990). School-based cardiovascular health promotion: The Child and Adolescent Trial for Cardiovascular Health (CATCH). *Journal of School Health, 60,* 406-413.

Pinhas-Hamiel, O., Dolan, L. M., Daniels, S. R., Standiford, D., Khoury, P. R., & Zeitler, P. (1996). Increased incidence of non-insulin-dependent diabetes mellitus among adolescents. *Journal of Pediatrics, 128,* 608-615.

Reaven, G. M. (1988). Role of insulin resistance in human disease. *Diabetes, 37,* 1595-1607.

Resnicow, K., & Robinson T. (1997). School-based cardiovascular disease prevention studies: Review and synthesis. *Annals of Epidemiology, 7,* S14-S31.

Resnicow, K., Yaroch, A. L., Davis, A., Wang, D. T., Carter, S., Slaughter, L., et al. (2000). GO GIRLS: Results from a nutrition and physical activity program for low-income, overweight African American adolescent females. *Health Education and Behavior, 27,* 616-631.

Rodin, F., & Daneman, D. (1992). Eating disorders and IDDM. *Diabetes Care, 15,* 1402-1412.

Rosenbloom, A., Joe, J., Young, R., & Winter, W. (1999). The emerging epidemic of type 2 diabetes mellitus in youth. *Diabetes Care, 22,* 345-354.

Rosenman, J. M. (1985). Diabetes in Black Americans. *Diabetes in America* (NIH Publication No. 85-1468). Washington, D.C.: U.S. Government Printing Office.

Rovet, J., & Alvarez, M. (1997). Attentional functioning in children and adolescents with IDDM. *Diabetes Care, 20,* 803-810.

Rovet, J., Ehrlich, R., & Hoppe, M. (1987). Behavior problems in children with diabetes as a function of sex and age of onset of disease. *Journal of Child Psychology and Psychiatry, 28,* 477-491.

Rovet, J., Ehrlich, R., & Hoppe, M. (1988). Specific intellectual deficits associated with the early onset of insulin-dependent diabetes mellitus in children. *Child Development, 59,* 226-234.

Ryan, C., Longstreet, C., & Morrow, L. (1985). The effects of diabetes mellitus on the school attendance and school achievement of adolescents. *Child Care, Health and Development, 11,* 229-240.

Ryan, C., Vega, A., & Drash, A. (1985). Cognitive deficits in adolescents who developed diabetes early in life. *Pediatrics, 75,* 921-927.

Ryan, C., Vega, A., Longstreet, C., & Drash, A. (1984). Neuropsychological changes in adolescents with insulin-dependent diabetes. *Journal of Consulting and Clinical Psychology, 52,* 335-342.

Rydall, A. C., Rodin, G. M., Olmsted, M. P., Devenyi, R. G., & Daneman, D. (1997). Disordered eating behavior and microvascular complications in young women with insulin-dependent diabetes mellitus. *New England Journal of Medicine, 336,* 1849-1854.

Sallis, J. F., & Nader, P. R. (1998). Family determinants of health behaviors. In D. S. Gochman (Ed.), *Health Behavior: Emerging Research Perspectives* (pp. 107-124). New York: Plenum.

Sallis, J. F., Nader, P. R., Broyles, S. L., Berry, C. C., Elder, J. P., McKenzie, T. L., et al. (1993). Correlates of Physical Activity at Home in Mexican-American and Anglo-American Preschool Children. *Health Psychology, 12,* 390-398.

Sallis, J. F., Patterson, T. L., Buono M. J., Atkins, C. J., & Nader, P. R. (1988). Aggregation of Physical Activity Habits in Mexican-American and Anglo Families. *Journal of Behavioral Medicine, 11,* 31-40.

Satin, W., La Greca, A., Zigo, M., & Skyler, J. (1989). Diabetes in adolescence. (1989). Effects of multifamily group intervention and parent simulation of diabetes. *Journal of Pediatric Psychology, 14,* 259-276.

Schafer, L. C., Glasgow, R. E., McCaul, K. D., & Dreher, M. (1983). Adherence to IDDM regimens: Relationship to psychosocial variables and metabolic control. *Diabetes Care, 6,* 493-498.

Schwartz, S. A., Weissberg-Benchell, J., & Perlmuter, L. C. (2001). Personal control and disordered eating in female adolescents with type 1 diabetes. *Diabetes Care, 25,* 1987-1991.

Scott, C. R., Smith, J. M., Cradock, M., & Pihoker, C. (1997). Characteristics of young-onset non-insulin-dependent diabetes mellitus and insulin-dependent diabetes mellitus at diagnosis. *Pediatrics, 100,* 84-91.

Seiffge-Krenke, I. (2002)."Come on, say something, Dad!": Communication and coping in fathers of diabeteic adolescents. *Journal of Pediatric Psychology, 27,* 439-450.

Shannon, B. M., Tershakovec, A. M., Martel, J. K., Achterberg, C. L., Cortner, J. A., Smiciklas-Wright, H. S., et al. (1994). Reduction of elevated LDL-cholesterol levels of 4- to 10-year-old children through home-based dietary education. *Pediatrics, 94,* 923-927.

Simons-Morton, B. G., Parcel, G. S., Baranowski, T., Forthofer, R., & O'Hara, N. M. (1991). Promoting physical activity and healthful diet among children: Results of a school based intervention study. *American Journal of Public Health, 81,* 986-991.

Sinha, R., Fisch, G., Teague, B., Tamborlane, W., Banyas, B., Allen, K., et al. (2002). Prevalence of impaired glucose tolerance among children and adolescents with marked obesity. *New England Journal of Medicine, 346,* 802-810.

Skinner, T. C., & Hampson, S. E. (2001). Personal models of diabetes in relation to self-care, well-being, and glycemic control: A prospective study in adolescence. *Diabetes Care, 24,* 828-833.

Skinner, T. C., Hampson, S. E., & Fife-Schaw, C. (2002). Personality, personal model beliefs, and self-care in adolescents and young adults with type 1 diabetes. *Health Psychology, 21,* 61-70.

Spieth, L. E., & Harris, C. V. (1996). Assessment of health-related quality of life in children and adolescents: An integrative review. *Journal of Pediatric Psychology, 21,* 175-193.

Stark, O., Atkins, E., & Wolff, O. H. (1981). Longitudinal study of obesity in the National Survey of Health and Development. *British Medical Journal, 283,* 13-17.

Stolley, M. R., & Fitzgibbon, M. L. (1997). Effects of an obesity prevention program on the eating behavior of African American mother and daughters. *Health Education Behavior, 24,* 152-164.

Stolley, M. R., Fitzgibbon, M. L., Dryer, A., Van Horn, L., KauferChristoffel, K., & Schiffer, L. (2003). Hip-hop to health jr., and obesity prevention program for minority preschool children baseline characteristics of participants. *Preventive Medicine. 36,* 320-329.

Story, M. (1999). School-based approaches for preventing and treating obesity. *International Journal of Obesity, 23*(2), S43-S51.

Stratton, R., Wilson, D. P., Endres, R. K., & Goldstein, D. E. (1987). Improved glycemic control after supervised 8 week exercise program in insulindependent diabetic adolescents. *Diabetes Care, 10,* 589-593.

Sue, D. W., & Sue, D. (1990). *Counseling the culturally different: Theory and practice* (2nd ed.). New York, NY: Wiley & Sons.

Svoren, B., Butler, D., Levine, B., Anderson, B. J., & Laffel, L. (2003). Reducing acute adverse outcomes in youths with type 1 diabetes: A randomized, controlled trial. *Pediatrics, 112,* 914-922.

Tamez, E. G., & Vacalis, T. D. (1989). Health beliefs, the significant other and compliance with therapeutic regimens among adult Mexican-American diabetics. *Health Education, 20,* 24-31.

Taras, H. L., Sallis, J. F., Patterson, T. L., Nader, P. R., & Nelson, J. A. (1989). Television's influence on children's diet and physical activity. *Developmental and Behavioral Pediatrics, 10,* 176-180.

Tercyak, K. P., Johnson, S. B., Kirkpatrick, K. A., & Silverstein, J. H. (1998). Offering a randomized trial of intensive therapy for IDDM to adolescents: Reasons for refusal, patient characteristics, and recruiter efforts. *Diabetes Care, 21,* 213-215.

Thompson, S. J., Auslander, W. F., & White, N. H. (2001). Comparison of single-mother and two-parent families on metabolic control of children with diabetes. *Diabetes Care, 24,* 234-238.

Trevino, R., Marshall, R., Hale, D., Rodriguez, R., Baker, G., & Gomez, J. (1999). Diabetes risk factors in low-income Mexican-American children. *Diabetes Care, 22,* 202-207.

Troiano, R., & Flegal, K. (1998). Overweight children and adolescents: Description, epidemiology, and demographics. *Pediatrics, 101*, 497-504.

Urdaneta, M. L., & Krehbiel, R. (1989). Cultural heterogeneity of Mexican-Americans and its implications for the treatment of diabetes mellitus type II. *Medical Anthropology, 11*, 269-282.

Vandongen, R., Jenner, D. A., Thompson, C., Taggart, A. C., Spickett, E. E, Burke, V., et al. (1995). A controlled evaluation of a fitness and nutrition intervention program on cardiovascular health in 10- to 12-year-old children. *Preventive Medicine, 24*, 9-22.

Vanhala, M. J, Vanhala, P. T., Keinanen-Kiukaanniemi, S. M., Kumpusalo, E. A., & Takala, J. K. (1999). Relative weight gain and obesity as a child predict metabolic syndrome as an adult. *International Journal of Obesity and Related Metabolic Disorders, 23*, 656-659.

Varni, J. W., Burwinkle, T., Jacobs, J., Gottschalk, M., Kaufman, R., & Jones, K. (2003). The PedsQL in type 1 and type 2 diabetes. *Diabetes Care, 26*, 631-637.

Wadden, T. A., Stunkard, A. J., Rich, L., Rubin, C. J., Sweidel, G., & McKinney, S. (1990). Obesity in black adolescent girls: A controlled clinical trial of treatment by diet, behavior modification, and parental support. *Pediatrics, 85*, 345-352.

Walter, H. J. (1989). Primary prevention of chronic disease among children: The School-Based Know Your Body Intervention Trials. *Health Education Quarterly, 16*, 201-214.

Weiss, R., Dziura, J., Burgert, T., Tamborlane, W., Taksali, S., Yeckel, C., et al. (2004). Obesity and metabolic syndrome in children and adolescents. *New England Journal of Medicine, 350*, 2362-2374.

Weissberg-Benchell, J., Glasgow, A. M., Tynan, W. D., Wirtz, P., Turek, J., & Ward, J. (1995). Adolescent management and mismanagement. *Diabetes Care, 18*, 77-82.

Weist, M., Finney, J., Barnard, M., Davis, C., & Ollendick, T. (1993). Empirical selection of psychosocial treatment targets for children and adolescents with diabetes. *Journal of Pediatric Psychology, 18*, 11-28.

Whitaker, R., Wright, J., Pepe, M., Seidel, K., & Dietz, W. (1997). Predicting obesity in young adulthood from childhood and parental obesity. *New England Journal of Medicine, 337*, 869-873.

White, K., Kolman, M., Wexler, P., Polin, G., & Winter, R. J. (1984). Unstable diabetes and unstable families: A psychosocial evaluation of diabetic children with recurrent ketoacidosis. *Pediatrics, 73*, 749-755.

Williams, C. L. (1984). Prevention and treatment of childhood obesity in a public school setting. (1984). *Pediatric Annals, 13*, 482-490.

Wysocki, T. (1993). Associations among teen-parent relationships, metabolic control, and adjustment to diabetes in adolescents. *Journal of Pediatric Psychology, 18*, 441-452.

Wysocki, T., Greco, P., Harris, M. A., Bubb, J., & White, N. H. (2001). Behavior therapy for families of adolescents with diabetes: Maintenance of treatment effects. *Diabetes Care, 24*, 441-446.

Wysocki, T., Harris, M. A., Greco, P., Bubb, J., Danda, C. E., Harvey, L. M., et al. (2000). Randomized, controlled trial of behavior therapy for families of adolescents with insulin-dependent diabetes mellitus. *Journal of Pediatric Psychology, 25*, 23-33.

Wysocki, T., Harris, M. A., Wilkinson, K., Sadler, M., Mauras, N., & White, N. (2003). Self-management competency as a predictor of outcomes of intensive therapy or usual care in youth with type 1 diabetes. *Diabetes Care, 26*, 2043-2047.

Wysocki, T., Hough, B. S., Ward, K. M., & Green, L. B. (1992). Diabetes mellitus in the transition to adulthood: Adjustment, self-care, and health status. *Journal of Developmental and Behavioral Pediatrics, 13*, 194-201.

Wysocki, T., Miller, K., Greco, P., Harris, M.A., Harvey, L., Taylor, A., et al. (1999). Behavior therapy for families of adolescents with diabetes: Effects on directly observed family interactions. *Behavior Therapy, 30*, 507-525.

Wysocki, T., Taylor, A., Hough, B., Linscheid, T., Yeates, K., & Naglieri, J. (1996). Deviation from developmentally appropriate self-care autonomy: Association with diabetes outcomes. *Diabetes Care, 19*, 119-125.

Young, T., Dean, H., Flett, B., & Wood-Steiman, P. (2000). Childhood obesity in a population at high risk for type 2 diabetes. *Journal of Pediatrics, 136*, 365-369.

Young-Hyman, D., Herman, L. J., Scott, D. L., & Schlundt, D. J. (2000). Care giver perception of children's obesity-related health risk: A study of African American families. *Obesity Research, 8*, 241-248.

Young-Hyman, D., Schlundt, D. G., Herman, L., De Luca, F., & Counts, D. (2001). Evaluation of the insulin resistance syndrome in 5- to 10-year old overweight/ obese African American children. *Diabetes Care, 24*, 1359-1364.

Zack, P. M., Harlan, W. R., Leaverton, P. E., & Cornoni-Huntley, J. (1979). A longitudinal study of body fatness in childhood and adolescence. *Journal of Pediatrics, 95*, 126-130.

Author Note

Correspondence to: Alan M. Delamater, Ph.D., Professor of Pediatrics, Department of Pediatrics (D-820), PO Box 016820, University of Miami School of Medicine, Miami, FL 33101, or via internet to adelamater@med.miami.edu.

Chapter 7

Self-Management of Chronic Illness & Disease Management

Thomas L. Creer

Professor Emeritus, Department of Psychology, Ohio University

The word "science" may elicit a number of attitudes ranging from what science can and cannot do to how it does what it does. Conflicting attitudes towards science emerge so that while we admire its theoretical achievements and the technological developments that improve our lives, we may be disappointed that desired discoveries are not readily forthcoming, dismayed when scientific discoveries threaten our beliefs about ourselves and our place in the universe, distrustful of what we perceive as scientist's elitism, or discouraged by the enormous costs of research (Haack, 2003). Our ambivalence may incline us to fail to recognize the uniquely human aspects of science and our own use of scientific methods. The reality of science led Haack (2003) to declare:

> "Science has managed to discover a great deal about the world and how it works, but it is a thoroughly human enterprise, messy, fallible, and fumbling; and rather than using a uniquely rational method unavailable to other inquirers, it is continuous with the most ordinary inquiry, 'nothing more than a refinement of our everyday thinking,' as Einstein once put it. There is no distinctive, timeless 'scientific method,' only the modes of inference and procedures common to all serious inquiry, and the multifarious 'helps' the sciences has gradually devised to refine our natural human cognitive capacities; to amplify the senses, stretch the imagination, extend reasoning power, and sustain respect for evidence" (pp. 9-10).

In support of her argument, Haack employs the metaphor of crossword puzzles. Crossword puzzles are rarely solved by acting on clues in numerical order with a pen, but by using a pencil and eraser so one can backtrack and work consequentially, with a willingness to return and make corrections. The best cognitive skill for doing science, therefore, is common sense; indeed, science is perceived as an extension of common sense. As a result of this position, science and scientists are, mostly, right. The metaphor of a crossword puzzle is applicable to many scientific activities, including the development and introduction of treatment guidelines for chronic diseases. Guidelines for the treatment of asthma, for example, categorize how attacks of different severity should be managed (National Asthma Education & Prevention Program, 1997; 2002), and indicate what medications, as well as the dose levels, should be taken by patients with differing severity of attacks. The guidelines provide a stepwise approach for the management of four levels of asthma: severe persistent, moderate persistent, mild persistent, and mild intermittent. The purpose of the stepwise approach is to provide assistance to health care personnel and patients in moving up or down treatment steps in order to match the severity of an attack.

Solomon (2004) conceded that the position taken by Haack (2003) was widely shared by many scientists, although those who have made major innovations in science may find it too conservative. These scientists may see common sense as "a flawed tool because it includes both the biases of everyday reasoning and the entrenched assumptions of a community" (Solomon, 2004, p. 44). Many scientific insights required the rejection of common sense, such as the results obtained by Amos Tversky and Daniel Kahneman on human reasoning and decision making (1974). Their research, familiar to many psychologists, repeatedly demonstrated that humans often reason with unseen and persistent biases. The writings of Longrino (2002) raised an important issue regarding the common sense view of science. She argued that the common sense value of simplicity in scientific reasoning often represents a preference for (or an inability to imagine) linear hierarchal theories over complex interactive theories. She suggested that instead of the traditional trio of values in science (that is, accepted theories, ontological simplicity, and hierarchal interaction), we also consider the use of an alternative set: novelty, ontological heterogeneity, and mutuality of interaction. Both sets of values, she contended, can deliver success; either alone is impoverished.

Complexity & Chaos

In the past few decades, the study of chaos and complexity has captured the imagination of scientists from a wide range of backgrounds, stretching from mathematics to economics and from biology to medicine (e.g., Gleick, 1987; Bar-Yam, 2000). Investigation of different sets of phenomena have been described in a large number of articles and books, most of which are beyond the pale of the ordinary reader and far beyond what might be considered as common sense. Explanations of breakthroughs are further hampered because of the language used to describe the two topics. Definitions of complexity, for example, are often too vague or too precise to be of value. To remedy this, Rolf Landauer (cited in Ball, 1999) cautioned: "A complex system is exactly that; there are many things going on simultaneously. If you search carefully, you can find your favorite toy; fractals, chaos, self-organized criticality, phase transition analogies, Lotka-Volterra predator-prey oscillations, etc., in some corner, in a relatively well-developed and isolated way. But do not expect any simple insight to explain it all" (p. 252). Waldrup (1992) suggested that the science of complexity is so new and wide ranging that nobody knows how to define it, or even where its boundaries lie. But then, he continued, that's the whole point.

"If a field seems poorly defined at the moment, it's because complexity research is trying to grapple with questions that defy all the conventional categories" (p. 9).

Definitions of chaos are equally ambiguous. Strevens (2003) provided what he referred to as the central insight of chaos theory:

"A system may behave in an extremely complicated manner, yet it may obey a simple deterministic dynamic law. Such a system has a hidden simplicity. The appeal of chaos theory is rooted in the hope of chaoticians that there is much hidden simplicity to be found, that is, that much complex behavior is generated by simple, and thus relatively ascertained, dynamic laws. If this is so, then it will have turned out that there is even more simple behavior, in my proprietary sense, than was previously supposed" (p. 6).

Strevens believes there is reason to think that all simple behavior is surprising, and in need of explanation, when it occurs in a simple system.

Most of the decisions we make in our daily life are unconscious choices based upon years of learning and performance. We do not make many complex decisions when, upon awakening in the morning, we take a shower, fix breakfast, or drive an automobile to work. These activities have been performed so much that they become almost automatic. We only realize the need to make choices when a sequence of behavior is disrupted or we have a number of choices to select from. The linearity of our decisions is effective in helping us grapple with our daily living. There are times, however, when linearity may be more a liability than an asset. Nowhere is this more notable than in patients and clinicians in their efforts to manage a chronic condition.

The present chapter reviews the scientific techniques that patients and health care providers bring to the management of a chronic condition, notably asthma. I describe the management of three topics–complexity, context, and uncertainty–by focusing on the strategies patients use, particularly in applying self-management skills to control their disorder. Their input suggests how they integrate the linear values of common sense with an alternative set of nonlinear elements found in complex adaptive theories.

Management of Complexity

Background

Definitions of complexity are pertinent to behavior; most are presented within the framework of a system. Bar-Yam (2000), for example, declared:

"To describe the behavior (actions) of a system acting in response to its environment, where the complexity of the environmental system are $C(e)$ and of the action is $C(a)$, we often try to describe the response function f, where $a = f(e)$. Unless simplifying assumptions are made, specifying the response to each environment requires an amount of information that grows exponentially with the complexity of the environment (a response must be specified for each possible environment). Specifically, C (f) = C (a) x 2^c (e). This is impossible for all but simple environments (e.g., less than a few tens of bits). This means that behaviorism in psychology, or strict phenomenology in any field, or testing the effects of multiple drugs, or testing computer chips with many input bits, is fundamentally impossible" (p. xxii).

This presents an impenetrable barrier in considering complexity and behavior; indeed, this may often be the case. However, Blumberg (1995) offered a different position in addressing the topic of complexity. He declared that models of complexity are important, "since very complex problems are being addressed: real problems, as they exist in the world, not constructions of experimentalists shorn of the richness of actual events" (p. x). These models harbor the promise that complex problems will be solvable, and the forms of synthesis of complexity will make an impact on patients and medical and behavioral scientists who must deal with "an embarrassing richness of variables." The definitions are widely desperate, but they serve as opposing poles as patients—a category that, from time to time, includes all of us—attempt to manage the massive array of variables involved with a chronic condition and its treatment. As we cannot possibly manage all variables—indeed, we don't know what all the variables are—we rely on simple rules and laws to help us navigate a path beginning with our limited knowledge through the frontier of complexity to the outer reaches of chaos.

Elements of Complexity

Although there is a debate over the definition of complexity, there is considerable agreement on elements involved in complexity. These properties are often described within a system as a group of related elements organized for a purpose. The purpose of a system in health care is to provide care, including that offered to patients with a chronic condition, in an effective and efficient manner. The system often recommended for use is a complex adaptive system (CAS). A complex adaptive system has been described as "a collection of individual agents that have the freedom to act in ways that are not always predictable and whose actions are interconnected such that one agent's actions changes the context for other agents" (Plsek, 2001, p. 313). Topics studied with CAS include immunology, insects, and economics; Plsek recommended that such a system be employed in changing the health care system of the United States. A number of systems can be developed here, but I focus on patients with chronic conditions and the clinicians who treat them. Key elements of CAS offer a way of thinking of complexity. As with other phenomena, the elements of complexity are relevant within the setting as patients attempt to manage their particular chronic disorder. Important elements include (e.g., Plsek, 2001):

Adaptable Elements

Systems are adaptive in that they do not passively respond to events the way a rock might, if dislodged, tumble down a mountain side (Waldrup, 1992). Systems actively try to turn whatever happens to their advantage. Elements of the system can, under the right conditions, change themselves through adaptation (Plsek, 2001). An example is anyone who learns. For example, patients, like effective clinicians, not only learn about their condition and treatment, but adapt the skills they have to control their disorder. They continue to accumulate a data base of knowledge and experience they can use to make decisions and improve their performance.

Simple Rules

Complex outcomes can emerge from a few simple rules (Plsek, 2001). Ball (1999) amplified the role of complexity and rules:

I wish to show in particular that pattern and organized complexity of form need not arise from something as complicated as life, but can be created by simple physical laws. This idea of complexity from simplicity has become almost a new scientific paradigm in recent years, and most probably a cliché too. Yet, I hope here to tie it down, to show that is not a recondite solution to all of life's mysteries, nor a result of a newly acquired facility for tricky computer-modeling, nor even a particularly new discovery—but a theme that has that has featured in scientific inquiry for centuries (p. 2).

Later, we will review how patients and physicians independently developed a set of simple rules for decision making that permitted them to manage asthma in a highly effective and efficient manner.

Nonlinearity

The property of complexity described the most is nonlinearity. Goerner (1995) elaborated three characteristics of nonlinearity:

(1) Despite its distressing name, nonlinearity is utterly simple. Technically, "a nonlinear system is any system in which input is not proportional to output, e.g., an increase in x does not mean a proportional increase or decrease in y"(p. 19). Goerner presented the treatment of headache as a nonlinear system. If you have a headache and take one aspirin, it will reduce your headache by a certain amount; if you take 2 aspirins, they will reduce it somewhat more, and 8 aspirins somewhat more. Sixty-four aspirins will not, however, reduce your headache 64 times as much as one tablet will. Treatment of a headache, therefore, is a nonlinear process.

(2) From a linear perspective, nonlinearity is a paradoxical beast. Our primary way of thinking is linear. If something works well, we do more of it; if it has a bad effect, less is better. This is a reasonable start, but the world is more complicated than this. The rise of nonlinear models offers a more subtle and, consequently, a more realistic version of the world.

(3) It is virtually impossible to pin down or link nonlinearity as a whole to any one type of effect. Nonlinearity can produce either positive or negative feedback. It can produce stability or instability. It may also produce coherence or divergence. The key to understanding nonlinearity is that, unlike linear systems, opposing systems can be build into a single system. This means a nonlinear world is extremely versatile. In general, nonlinear systems cannot be solved and cannot be added together (Gleick, 1987), but small changes can have large effects (Plsek, 2001). Nonlinearity can produce complex and frequently unexpected results (Coveney & Highfield, 1995), a point repeated throughout the chapter.

Emergent Behavior, Novelty

Continual creativity is a natural state of a complex adaptive system (Plsek, 2001). Casti (1997) added that emergent phenomena are the feature separating simple from complex systems. Coveney and Highfield (1995) offered a broader perspective on emergent behavior by suggesting that life itself is an emergent property that arises when physiochemical systems are organized and interact in certain ways. In this scheme, a human is viewed as an emergent property of huge numbers of cells. The study of complexity, through its emphasis on emergent properties, offers a way for patients to create or restore a balance between the psychological and physical sides of managing an illness and living a full life.

Not Predictable in Detail

As anyone knows who has been rained out at a picnic when the weatherman predicted clear and sunny skies, forecasting is inherently an inexact, yet bounded, art. Accurate long-range weather forecasting is fundamentally impossible. Every complex adaptive system is constantly making decisions based on its internal models of the world—its implicit or explicit assumptions about the way things are out there. The systems are far more than passive blueprints; they are active (Waldrop, 1992). This does not mean, as will be illustrated, that any decisions made by the system will produce totally accurate predictions.

Inherent Order

Systems can be orderly without central control (Plsek, 2001). Self-organization is an essential idea in complexity science. Systems undergo self-organization, often considered as spontaneous, in order to adapt to the world. From the perspective of chronic conditions, this means patients attempt to achieve and maintain an equilibrium in controlling their conditions vis-à-vis other demands in their lives.

How successful they are rests less on spontaneity than on their systematic ability to manage their disorder.

Complexity & Patients

Patients use elements of complexity to control a chronic disease. They use simple rules to manage and adapt to changing variables that may have an impact on their illness. In addition, they do not adhere to a strictly linear model in controlling their disorder, but often think in a nonlinear manner. The actions often result in emergent, creative outcomes, such as found in their attempts to predict exacerbations of a chronic illness. This will be illustrated with asthma.

Living with Asthma (Creer, Backiel, Leung, & Backial, 1985 a,b) was a self-management program developed and evaluated for pediatric asthma at the National Asthma Center in Denver. At intake, each child was taught self-monitoring skills: he or she was provided with a peak flow meter and asked to record in an asthma diary the highest of three values he or she blew in the morning and evening. The patients were then randomly assigned to a waiting or treatment group. Throughout the investigation, the children and their parents were monitored to insure that they faithfully wrote down their daily peak flow values.

Attempting to predict and control future attacks is always of paramount interest to patients. If you have asthma and can predict the likelihood of an attack, it permits you to plan your life in a more reliable manner. This was pointed out in the following example: in submitting peak flow data, a boy and his mother explained that they had learned to predict future attacks based on the peak flow data they gathered. They described how they had learned to compare a given flow value against peak flow rates they had obtained in the past to predict the likelihood of attacks occurring in the near future. The simple formula they used was formalized by Stirzaker (1999):

$$p\,(n) = \frac{r(n)}{n}$$

In treating their data, this meant that the patients performed the following:

$$p \text{ is approximately equal to } \frac{r(n)}{n} = \frac{\text{number of times a given peak flow value occurred 12 hours before an attack}}{\text{number of attacks that occurred in following 12 hour period}}$$

Using this approach, the boy and his mother were able to assign a probability as to whether or not an attack would occur within 12 hours.

Prompted by the observations of the child and his mother, Taplin and Creer (1979) analyzed morning and evening peak expiratory flow rates (PEFRs) obtained from the youngster and another child. After obtaining baseline data, conditional probabilities were calculated. These can be defined as the probability that event B (an asthma attack) will occur if you know that event A (a given peak flow value) has already occurred; it is called the conditional probability of B given A. The probability formula is (A)/PEFR $\leq$ B where A is the occurrence of asthma, and B is the critical PEFR value. The results determined that data gathered in the natural environment did increase the predictability of asthma episodes in an upcoming period of time, such as 12 hours.

The observation by the boy and his mother, as well as the subsequent study by Taplin and Creer, launched a series of studies on the analysis of risk factors in precipitating asthma attacks. These are described in Table 1.

Stimuli	Probability equation	Reference
PEFR	$P_t(A) = F(P_{t-k}, B_{t-k})$	Taplin & Creer (1979) Harm, Kotses, & Creer (1985) Kotses, Stout, Wigal, Carlson, Creer & Lewis (1991) Pinzone, Carlson, Kotses, & Creer (1991)
Medication compliance	$P_t(A) = F(B_{t-k})$	Creer (1979) Pinzone et al. (1991) Kotses, Winder, Stout, McConnaughy, & Creer (1996)
Environmental stimuli (Ragweed, Temperature change, Dust, Pollen, Humidity, Cigarette smoke, Heat, Odors, Wind, Animal dander, Air pollution, Mold)	$P_t(A) = F(E_{t-k})$	Stout, Kotses, Carlson, & Creer (1991) Kotses et al. (1996)
Emotional factors	$P_t(A) = F(Em_{t-k})$	Kotses et al. (1996)
Physiological (Exercise, Alcohol consumption, Fatigue)	$P_t(A) = F(P_{t-k}, B_{t-k})$	Kotses et al. (1991) Kotses et al. (1996) Pinzone et al. (1991)

Table 1. An analysis of risk factors for the precipitation of asthma. Note: PEFR=peak expiratory flow rate; $P_t(A)$=probability of asthma at a given time; F=function; P= physiological; B=behavior; E=environment; Em=emotion; $_{t-k}$=past history.

Harm, Kotses, & Creer (1985) analyzed peak flow data gathered by 25 children in the morning and evening. The procedure involved the calculation of conditional posterior probabilities, and the ratio of hits to misses in predicting the probability of asthma. The results showed that the average improvement in predictability from the prior probability to the highest posterior probability was 491 percent. However, the ratio of hits to misses and the number of episodes predicted decreased as the posterior probability increased. This suggested that the selection of the peak expiratory flow rate at lower posterior probabilities resulted in fewer prediction errors, and led to prediction of a higher number of episodes than selection of the PEFR at the highest posterior probabilities. Peak flow values also proved instrumental in tailoring asthma self-management programs for individual patients (Kotses, et al. 1991).

Our research in risk factor analysis was extended in two additional studies. Pinzone, Carlson, Kotses, and Creer (1991) analyzed medication compliance and exercise data to predict attacks in 10 children with asthma. The analysis featured individual logistic regression equations calculated for each child. The results indicated that peak flow rates predicted attacks in 9 of 10 patients. Exercise predicted attacks in 2 of the 5 children with exercise-induced asthma. No relationship was found between attacks and medication compliance (although Creer [1979] found that a missed medication dose predicted 100% of the attacks experienced by a child in an earlier analysis). Logistic regression equations were predictive of 1 of 10 attacks when a previous attack had occurred in the previous 12 hours. Whether an attack occurred in previous 12 hours was predictive of 1 of 10 attacks, but whether an attack occurred in previous 24 hours was predictive of 4 of 10 attacks experienced by the patients. Stout, Kotses, Carlson, and Creer (1991) determined the degree to which asthma episodes were associated with seven variables for 17 adults with asthma. Using stepwise regression procedures, cladosporium mold, ragweed pollen, and temperature change were found to be significant predictors of attacks. Stout and colleagues concluded that knowledge of the probability of the occurrence of known risk factors, unique to each person, predicted the likelihood they would experience asthma within a preset period of time. Such information would be invaluable in the control of asthma attacks by the patients.

Peak flow rates, medication compliance, environmental factors, and exercise have all been shown to be amenable to application of simple probability analysis in predicting the likelihood that an exacerbation would occur. Future research should not only focus on refining statistical analyses, but on determining the probabilities that patient responses, e.g., coughing, laughing, crying, and shouting, also precipitate an asthma attack.

Summary

Participants in Living with Asthma were taught to monitor and record peak flow readings as an outcome measure (Creer et al., 1988). This was anticipated to be a simple and linear process for subjects. However, patients looked at the data they were collecting in an unexpected and nonlinear manner: through a simple procedure, they were able to calculate the probabilities of future attacks. It was their way of perceiving the complexity of asthma. As a consequence of their action, my colleagues and I were able to conduct a series of studies on predicting factors that placed individual patients at risk for triggering their asthma. The studies not only increased our knowledge of asthma and its precipitants, but they would have value with other chronic conditions. However, it should be noted that studies on asthma were easy to conduct as there were observable data, peak flow readings, to use in calculating the probability of an attack. Measurable data using appropriate instruments can also be gathered with diabetes and hypertension. Such is not the case with many other chronic disorders, including pain or headache. Patients with these conditions must rely on matching internal changes they experience against an subjective standard to determine the likelihood of an exacerbation of their condition. Holroyd (2001) outlined approaches that can be taken to managing migraine headaches. Of importance here was the self-monitoring of accurate data on computer diaries supplied to patients. By carefully charting any headaches they experienced, patients were able to identify possible triggers or warning signs of headache. Reliable data on these topics permitted patients to take early action to prevent or abort an incipient migraine headache.

Context

Background

Black box theory relates input to output in a system by a formal description of the transformation rules that link the two, but without stating the nature of the process that embodies or gives realization to these rules (Bullock & Thombley, 1999). Black box theory is inherent to many disciplines, ranging from economics to biology and from philosophy to medicine. The theory has been widely accepted in psychology, particularly since the middle of the 20th century when there was a lively debate with respect to learning theory. A major point of contention centered on the role of intervening variables in learning and performance. The latter events were postulated as intraorganismic variables that occurred between the presentation of input (independent variables) and the subsequent output (dependent variables) which influenced the process (Tolman, 1959). For a period of time, intervening variables were utilized by a number of theorists to account for learning (Marx & Hillix, 1963). However, many intervening variables were hypothesized events that were difficult (if possible) to verify empirically, and thus were generally ignored from the 1960s onward.

Black box theory dominates medical and behavioral research, including investigations on the self-management of chronic conditions (Creer , Caplin & Holroyd,in press). The approach has applicability in analyzing studies according to the experimental design used across investigations (e.g., Gibson et al., 2003; Wolf, Guevara, Grum, Clark, & Cotes, 2003). However, the tradeoff in adopting this strategy has been the failure to examine behaviors that occur between input, teaching of self-management skills, and output, changes in medical or behavioral outcome measures. Consequently, a major determinant of behavior—the context within which often unknown behaviors occur—has been ignored.

Ironically, the significance of context is possibly the only issue where there is agreement across the spectrum of psychological thought ranging from the most cognitive to the most behavioral (Creer et al., in press). One end of the continuum is anchored by Engel (1999), a cognitive psychologist, who proclaimed that context is central to understanding any type of remembering. She pointed out that in conversations friends have about the past, "the interpersonal dynamic of the relationship, the situation in which you are talking, the topic that led you to reminisce, and your internal state at the moment of conversation taken together provide the context in which your memories find shape"(p. 124). At the other end of the continuum, Rachlin (2000), a behavioral psychologist, was equally adamant in declaring that "no particular act or pattern of acts can be judged by itself. An act or pattern of acts may be impulsive or self-controlled, depending on the behavioral context in which it is embedded. No single act or pattern or acts can be understood outside of its context"(p. 60). Rachlin argued that a behavior or act must be viewed within the broadest context, including the life span of an individual.

Previous attempts have been made to to examine behaviors and context in asthma self-management by examining the reports of asthma attacks (Creer, 1990; Creer et al., 1988; Burkhart & Ward, 2003). The studies provided useful insight into what patients do when they experience asthma exacerbations as they offer isolated snapshots of the patients' actions during specific episodes. Creer et al. (in press), however, examined the myriad of contextual events that occurred during asthma attacks in a large number of patients. Of particular interest was how embedded behaviors were within the contexts within which they occurred. In particular, the analysis permitted a determination of behavioral changes observed in intake/baseline and training/post-training contexts where individual patients performed self-management skills.

Context of Study

Kotses and colleagues (1995) described the development and implementation of an asthma self-management program for adults. Seventy-six subjects, whose asthma was medically controlled at the outset of intervention, were randomly assigned to either a treatment group or a waiting-list control group. Those in the treatment group were exposed to a 7-week program that incorporated proven features of effective training and establishment of behavioral control. Subsequently, subjects in the control group received the same treatment. Short-term evaluation of the intervention was made after the subjects in the experimental group were trained but before the control subjects were trained. Long-term evaluation was conducted after both groups of subjects were trained. In the short-term, results showed self-management training led to fewer asthma symptoms and physician visits, as well as to improvement in asthma management skills and cognitive abilities. In the long term, self-management training was related to lower asthma attack frequency, reduced medication use, improvement in cognitive measures, and increased use of self-management skills.

When subjects were enrolled in the study, they were given a peak flow meter and introduced to self-monitoring of their pulmonary functioning. The meter was demonstrated individually to each subject; patients, in turn, performed maneuvers until they displayed mastery of the technique of blowing flow values to the staff. Subjects were instructed how to interpret values obtained with the meters. They were also taught to compare peak flow scores to information contained on the asthma treatment plan they had developed with their health care provider. An asthma diary and report of attack of asthma were also introduced as components of self-monitoring. Subjects were taught how to observe and record information on themselves on both the diary and the report. Data were recorded daily by the patients in the diary; data on asthma attacks were gathered via reports completed following separate episodes. As self-monitoring is the core of self-management (Creer & Holroyd, 1997), staff members were certain that all subjects understood what was expected of them before leaving the intake interview. Periodic checks with patients throughout their participation showed that they continued to perform self-monitoring in a correct manner, thus ensuring the accuracy of the collected data.

The Report of Attack

A key measure used in the study was the Report of Asthma Attack. Patients were asked to complete the reports after each attack, and to provide data regarding 13 categories of information: (a) day and time of episode; (b) degree of severity of asthma (as operationally defined on the asthma diary); (c) use of the peak flow meter during the attack; (d) adherence to medication instructions; (e) where the attack occurred; (f) whether any early warning signs were observed; (g) factors that participant's thought precipitated a given attack; (h) the activity engaged in at the time of the attack; (i) whether the patient or others were upset over the episode; (j) a rank order listing of the steps a patient performed during an attack; and (k) medications taken to control an episode. The latter item was excluded from analysis in the current study as data on medications taken during attacks were statistically treated and reported by Kotses and colleagues (1995). Another category—other actions—was omitted from analysis as few patients provided such information.

Data Extraction

A total of 3,442 reports of attack were obtained from 90 subjects. These were submitted from the 76 patients described in the article by Kotses and colleagues, 9 who dropped out of the study, and 5 who served as pilot subjects. Not all subjects submitted attack reports throughout the study. Their response was likely due to the fact that some of the information was a duplication of data gathered on the asthma diary and was, therefore, considered redundant by some participants. The focus of the current analysis was, in particular, on the 63 subjects who submitted forms during two periods: intake/baseline and training/after training. This permitted a pre-post analysis of self-management behaviors performed to treat attacks over time. The number of reports completed by subjects ranged from 1 to 292; the average number of reports submitted by patients was 38. As information was obtained from both a diary and attack report, the data set was collected by comparing a participant's attack report information to relevant data reported on his or her weekly asthma diary. Only matched data from the two forms were included in the analysis. In addition, the investigators independently reviewed the resulting information and discarded any questionable entries.

Data Analysis

The average number of triggers patients perceived as correlated with their attacks, as well as the average number of steps they took to control the episodes before and during/after training, were presented. The remainder of the data were treated using the probability analysis according to the formula, described earlier, by Stirzaker (1999). In treating frequency data, it is advantageous to consider that the probability a response will occur ranges continuously between never occurs or always occurs ($0 \leqslant p \leqslant 1$). This means that A and B are independent if the occurrence of one does not imply anything about the chance of the other occurring. The approach also permits the analysis of the combined effect of more than one variable. Previous research on the probability of a relationship between specific stimuli or responses to asthma, described earlier, treated data by using sophisticated statistical procedures. These procedures are invaluable in determining the probability of frequency data, although the findings are rarely understood by those without a solid background in statistics. The assumption in the study was that the loss of statistical sophistication was offset by using a simple, but appropriate, method of considering probability as a relative frequency (Skinner, 1953).

Results

The Report of an Attack gathered information on 10 areas of responses. Highlights of the data include:

1. Time. The time of attack was essentially equal with the probability of an attack in the morning at $p = .52$ and the probability of an attack in the evening at $p = .48$. All patients experienced attacks in both the morning and evening although, as expected, some patients had more attacks in the morning than in the evening and vise versa.
2. Setting. The probability of attacks occurring at home was $p = .71$, followed by attacks occurring in other places at $p = .21$. The probability of attacks occurring at work was $p = .08$.
3. Activity. The probability of attacks occurring while patients were asleep was $p = .34$. This was followed, in descending order, by participation in a quiet activity ($p = .28$), other activities ($p = .20$), working ($p = .14$), and during or following exercise ($p = .04$).
4. Triggers. Patients were asked to note what factors they thought precipitated a given attack. The average number of triggers listed was 2.07 during

pretreatment and declined to 1.93 during treatment onward. The average number of triggers identified by individual patients per attack ranged from 0 to 4.81 triggers.

5. Adherence. A question asked of patients was if they had taken all prescribed medications as directed over the past 24 hours. The range of nonadherence was variable across subjects. Some patients reported they were nonadherent from 1 to 146 attacks, while other patients claimed they were always adherent. The probability that patients reported they had followed these medication instructions was $p = .78$ in the baseline phase, but rose to $p = .86$ during and after training.

6. Peak flow value. In the pretreatment period, the probability was $p = .62$ that the patients obtained a peak flow reading during an attack; from training onward, the probability increased to $p = .70$ that a peak flow value was obtained.

7. Early warning signs. The probability that early warning signs would be detected during baseline was $p = .37$ and $p = .51$ during and after training, respectively. Throughout the study, the number of attacks patients reported early warning signs ranged from never ($p = .00$) to always ($p = 1.00$). This finding could be anticipated, in part, because patients reported they never experienced early warning signs before being awakened by an asthma attack.

8. Upset. The probability of subjects reporting they were upset was $p = .20$ in both the baseline and during and after training. Although a decrease in being upset was reported by 62 percent of the subjects, 38 percent either showed no changes or an increase in being upset from baseline to training and beyond.

9. Severity of attack. In the baseline period, the severity of attacks reported as mild, moderate, or severe asthma showed a probability of $p = .34$, $p = .42$, and $p = .24$, respectively. The probabilities found in training and after were identical ($p = .34$ for mild, $p = .42$ for moderate, and $p = .24$ for severe asthma, respectively). Although a trend was found toward a decrease in reported attack severity over the baseline and during and after training in 86 percent of the subjects, the severity of attacks remained the same or slightly increased in the remaining 14 percent of the patients.

10. Action. A major component of the analysis was to determine the steps patients took to control their attacks. There were at least 13 steps patients could take; they were told to list, in rank order, the actions they took. Steps ranged from assessing peak flow values to using a quick relief drug to asking their health care provider for advice in treating an attack. The number of steps taken by subjects ranged from 1 to 9 during separate episodes. During the course of the study, the average number of steps taken by patients to control an episode was 3.36. The average number of actions reported by patients in the intake/baseline phase was 3.50; this decreased to 3.23 steps during and after training.

Of the actions that patients could take, three are possibly the most significant to the management of an episode: assessment of peak flow values, use of a quick relief inhaler, and watchful waiting. Overall, the probability that peak flow values would be obtained increased from p = .45 to p = .51, use of a quick relief inhaler increased from p = .83 to p = .84; and watchful waiting decreased from p = .48 to p = .45 in intake/baseline versus training/after training. The probability that patients would use one of the three steps in managing at least 85 percent of their attacks was p = .70 during baseline but rose to p = .87 during and following training. Data obtained from individual patients showed they took differing approaches to managing their attacks. Thirteen subjects did not perform any of the three steps during baseline, but did during and after training; one patient did the opposite in that the three steps were used during intake/baseline but not during or following training. Other variability among patients in attack management was reflected by the number and type of steps they performed: one end of the spectrum was anchored by a subject who treated 109 attacks by performing only one step, use of a quick relief inhaler, and another patient who treated 155 attacks with a combination of peak flow assessment and inhaler use. The other end of the spectrum was illustrated by a subject who used a combination of steps—breathing exercises, escaping the trigger of the attack, drinking warm liquids, resting, using a quick relief inhaler, and watchful waiting—to manage 64 episodes. Other prominent findings included:

(1) The time and place where an attack occurred prompted particular responses in many patients. For example, the probability that a quick relief inhaler would be the first or second step taken by subjects to treat an attack was p = .85 for nighttime asthma and p = .89 for work-time asthma over the course of the study. Longer sequences of actions were linked to patients being away from home without a quick relief inhaler or at home and having more time to treat an attack. When away from home, patients were apt to use a full arsenal of self-management skills including relaxation or drinking a cup of coffee, a xanthine compound in the same class as the asthma drug, theophylline. The patients' behavior suggested they reviewed the repertoire of responses they could make to the attack and systematically performed one step after another until an episode was aborted.

(2) Over time, it was found that thirteen percent of the subjects integrated peak flow readings into their determination of the severity of their episode. In the post-training stages, they were particularly adroit at analyzing data and making choices based upon the information. They likely referred to the asthma action or treatment plan they had developed with their health care provider to manage attacks; at other times, however, patients appeared to employ tactics in using the peak flow meter that were idiosyncratic to themselves and their experiences in classifying the severity of their episodes.

(3) Perhaps the most important finding was that there was a dichotomy across all subjects in the type of actions they performed to manage attacks before and during/after training. The patients' performance during intake/baseline was characterized by trial-and-error in their performance of management steps they had been

taught during intake. This began at intake when they were taught self-monitoring via peak flow meters, asthma diaries, and attack reports. Subjects employed different strategies to incorporate assessment of peak flow, correct use of a quick relief inhaler, and watchful waiting to abort or control asthma exacerbations. The results suggested that during this period, patients acquired self-management skills. During and after self-management training, however, the patients' management of individual attacks became more skilled and systematic. In short, they honed their performance of asthma self-management.

The purpose of the study by Creer et al. (in press) was to analyze the influence of context in determining how asthma patients managed their attacks. Two findings merit discussion. First, several processes comprise self-management, ranging from goal setting to appraisal of one's actions (Creer & Holroyd, 1997). Self-monitoring, the observation and recording of data on oneself, is the backbone of self-management. It merits the label. However, what emerged from both the current study and a previous investigation on self-management behaviors reported by individual patients (Creer, 1990) is the importance of two other processes—information collection and data processing, and decision making. When subjects were introduced to self-monitoring by use of peak flow meters, an asthma diary, and a report of an attack, they began using these tools, often in an experimental manner, to match the information they obtained to the actions they took. As a result, they acquired skills at self-monitoring prior to training. During and after training, however, patients demonstrated that they became highly skilled at processing and making decisions based on the data they collected. The information provided by patients in the current and past study (Creer, 1990) stresses the point that greater attention must be paid to information collection, data processing, and decision making in future self-management studies. Second, stimuli present during an attack evolved so as to evoke distinctive behavioral patterns whereby individual patients considered the reciprocal interaction of environmental, physiological, behavioral, and cognitive variables in order to prevent or control attacks. In this scenario, based on the work of Bandura (1986, 1997), a change in breathing might prompt use of a peak flow meter to determine if airway obstruction was occurring. Lower flow rates, in turn, could prompt the patient to consider the best action to take. He or she might decide to use a quick relief inhaler or the patient could take other actions such as to relax or just watch and wait. Hence, any action would be the result of careful data processing and evaluation, as well and systematic decision making, on the part of patients to select and perform those self-management skills expected to generate the best result for them.

Summary

The study by Creer et al. (in press) yielded unexpected findings not only with respect to the behavior of individual patients, but with regards to how behavior changed as a function of context. An analysis of context increases our knowledge of how to better design and implement self-management programs for patents with a chronic condition. These programs should enhance the effectiveness and efficiency with which patients use self-management skills. Enhanced knowledge of context will also improve our ability to control other behavioral reactions that occur across chronic illness with the exacerbation of a given condition. A common problem is increased anxiety, referred to as panic, that often accompanies such exacerbations. Creer (1979) chronicled attempts to operationally define panic that occurred concurrently with an asthma attack. Controlling the pattern was relevant as panic accompanying an asthma episode meant that patients would be unable to cooperate fully with treatment and exhaust themselves physically. Their breathing pattern when panicked also exacerbated ongoing attacks. The approach of including panic applying only to patients proved illusionary: the pattern was, in this case, in the eyes of the beholder. Two findings verify this comment:

First, the assumption was that panic referred to a well-defined behavioral pattern in that nurses and physicians independently identified children labeled as panickers when the youngsters experienced an asthma attack. A behavioral analysis shattered the assumption: some children, for example, were observed to be experiencing what was referred to as "fearful agitation" in that they found it difficult to remain in bed, were always pleading for higher doses of medications, and demanded more and more medical attention. As these responses were readily observable, it was thought that this was the pattern referred to as panic. However, a more detailed analysis of behaviors accompanying attacks revealed a pattern that was the antithesis of the above: these were children who exhibited what was referred to as a "frozen" pattern of panic. They were wide-eyed and immobile in their beds, stared at the ceiling, and did not signal for help although they required it. If not watched closely, they were apt to show symptoms of worsening asthma, a situation that frightened attending medical personnel as the children did not make their condition known on a busy pediatric ward.

Second, a more realistic approach to panic would have been to rely on physicians and nurses to identify the children who frightened them when the youngsters experienced asthma attacks. This is likely how they identified panic in the first place. This would have been the most efficient way of categorizing patients who panic during an exacerbation of a condition; in turn, it would permit behavioral scientists to readily remedy the problem through use of relaxation, systematic desensitization by reciprocal inhibition, or other behavioral techniques.

Uncertainty

A decision as to what action to take is subject to uncertainty if the probabilities of possible outcomes are unknown. With most choices in daily living, decision making presents no dilemma: if we decide to take cauliflower instead of broccoli when offered, there is little chance that we will question our choice. These choices do not require a great amount of conscious decision making and are almost automatic. The action we take reflects that most of our choices are based on our certainty concerning the likelihood that a particular outcome will occur, e.g., in the above case, cauliflower will taste better to us than broccoli. If it doesn't, we are not apt to be upset at the choice we made. Making decisions becomes a problem when there is a greater degree of uncertainty as to the outcome of our actions or we have too many choices from which to make a selection. This is a continuing issue to patients with a chronic illness in that they have to make many decisions, such as what medications to take in a given situation, whether to take more drugs, go to an ER, etc., in order to manage their condition. Excess choices, may lead patients to question their decisions before they make them, set up unrealistic expectations, and lead to their blaming themselves for any failures (Schwartz, 2004). The consequence of overload of choices is a dilemma: while enamored of freedom, personal determinism, variety of choice, and a reluctance to give up options, clinging to all available choices contributes to bad decisions, anxiety, dissatisfaction, and even depression.

Decisions are based on beliefs concerning the supposed likelihood of an event (Tversky & Kahneman, 1974). Humans have always sought certainty in predicting future events in their lives; as a result, belief systems evolved to help us make decisions. Many philosophical or religious systems thought to provide a degree of certainty with respect to life's adventures were grasped, often in a fanatical embrace, to combat the very notion of uncertainty. As a consequence, many of us spend our lives wrapped in a cocoon of beliefs and thoughts that we think will not only allow us to manage uncertainty in this life, but often throughout eternity. Scientists have not been immune from clinging to belief systems. The mission of modern scientists has been to break their subject matter down into the simplest elements that obey scientific rules, a process referred to as reductionism. In all science, a kind of Newtonian determinism was brought to bear to simplify the complex. However, as Gleick (1987) noted,

"There was always one small comprise, so small that working scientists usually forgot it was there, lurking in a corner of their philosophies like an unpaid bill. Measurements could never be perfect. Scientists marching under Newton's banner actually waved another flag that said something like this: Given an approximate knowledge of a system's initial conditions and an understanding of natural law, one can calculate the approximate behavior of the system. This assumption lay at the heart of science" (pp. 14-15).

Outside of death, everything is uncertain. No where this more evident than in considering how clinicians and patients deal with uncertainty on a daily basis.

Background

The importance of uncertainty in medical care was discussed by Gawande (2002). He warned that:

"The core predicament of medicine—the thing that makes being a patient so wrenching, being a doctor so difficult, and being a part of a society that pays the bills that run up so vexing—is uncertainty. With all that we know nowadays about people and diseases and how to diagnose and treat them, it can be hard to see this, hard to grasp how deeply uncertainty runs. As a doctor, you come to find, however, that the struggle in caring for people is more often with what you do not know than what you do. Medicine's ground state is uncertainty. And wisdom—for both patients and doctors— is defined by how one copes with it"(p. 229).

In recent years, a developing literature on medical decision making has emerged with books and a journal, *Medical Decision Making*, devoted to research on the topic. A major topic of research has centered on the identification of biases and errors in decision making, particularly among medical personnel (Arkes, 1981, 1991; Crosskerry, 2003; Dawson & Arkes, 1987). Dawson and Arkes (1987) pointed out that people generally use rules of thumb in situations where a judgment or prediction is necessary. The short cuts are called "heuristics." Heuristics are useful in that they save time and lessen the complex task of assessing probabilities in a simple judgment procedure. The disadvantage inherent in their use, continued Dawson and Arkes, is they can lead to systematic errors in judgment called cognitive biases. The use of heuristics and the tendency towards making biased assessments are not limited to the lay public as people with extensive research and statistical training are prone to the same biases when thinking intuitively (Tversky & Kahneman, 1974).

A number of errors and biases, described by Arkes (1981, 1991), Croskerry (2002; 2003), and Dawson and Arkes (1987), are enumerated in Table 2. The heuristics apply to both clinicians and patients. Readers will no doubt identify biases, or combinations of biases, that they or others have in making decisions in both their professional and personal life.

Context

Most studies on the self-management of chronic disorder have ignored decision making strategies taken by patients and clinicians in managing a particular condition. As the goal of self-management research has usually been on the impact that a given program has on outcomes of a disorder, the omission is understandable. However, the serendipitous collection of two sets of data—one from patients and the second from clinicians—demonstrates the significance of decision making in the overall management of a chronic condition, asthma. The two sets of data were obtained in the following manner:

Decision Making by Patients

An important measure in Living with Asthma (Creer et al., 1988) concerned how patients responded to attacks. The data was gathered via a standard Report of Attack described earlier. The questionnaire included information as to: (a) the stimuli thought to have triggered an attack; (b) where and when episodes occurred; and (c) the order of steps performed by a patient and his or her parents to abort an attack. A total of 84 families in the program completed Report of Attack forms; an average of 13.03 were submitted per family. Most children and their parents

Aggregate Bias

An aggregate bias occurs when clinicians believe that aggregate data, such as those used to develop clinical practice guidelines, do not apply to individual patients, particularly their own. As a consequence, both errors of commission, e.g., ordering tests when guidelines indicate none are required, or omission, e.g., ordering fewer tests to rule out equally possible diagnoses, may occur.

Anchoring Bias

This is the tendency to lock onto salient features in a patient's presentation too early in the diagnostic process, and then failing to adjust this initial impression in light of later information.

Ascertainment Bias

The bias that occurs when a clinician's thinking is shaped by prior expectations. Examples would include both stereotyping and gender bias. An ascertainment may occur when a clinician has limited experience with a particular condition and, therefore, does not have a useful base rate of experience.

Availability Bias

The availability heuristic is used when clinicians equate the ease of remembering specific instances with the probability that such instances will occur. Common events may be remembered more easily. Recent experience, for example, may inflate the likelihood of it being diagnosed. On the other hand, if a disease has not been seen for a long time, it may be underdiagnosed.

Base Rate Neglect

This is the tendency to ignore the true prevalence of a disease, either inflating or reducing its baserate, and distorting Bayesian reasoning. However, in some cases, a clinician may, consciously or otherwise, inflate the likelihood of a disease to avoid missing a rare but significant diagnosis.

Commission Bias

The heuristic results from an obligation towards beneficence, in that harm to the patient can only be prevented by active intervention. The tendency here is towards taking action instead of doing nothing or watchful waiting. Commission bias is more common than omission bias, and more often occurs in overconfident clinicians or patients.

Confirmation Bias

Clinicians and patients tend to seek only evidence that can be used to confirm a given diagnosis or event. They search for confirmatory evidence, including interpretation of information, rather than looking for disconfirmatory evidence to refute it, even though the latter may be more persuasive and definitive.

Diagnosis Momentum

Once diagnostic labels are introduced, they become stickier and more difficult to discard. What started out as a possible diagnosis gathers momentum among those making the decision, including patients, physicians, and other health care personnel, until it becomes definite and all other possibilities are excluded.

Ego Bias

Ego bias is the warping of probability estimates in a self-serving way. For example, clinicians may think that mortality rates for other patients may be higher than it is for their own patients (similar to what occurred in aggregate bias). Related to the influence of ego bias on estimating probabilities is its influence on the confidence with which diagnoses are made.

Framing Effect

How clinicians and patients perceive events may be strongly influenced by the way the problem is framed. What may seem to be inconsequential changes in the presentation of problems involving choices may cause major shifts in preferences. In making a diagnosis, for example, a clinician should be aware of how patients, nurses, and colleagues frame potential outcomes and contingencies of the clinical problem to them. In addition, how decisions are made by patients have been found to be influenced by how the choices are framed.

Fundamental Attribution Error

This is the tendency to be judgmental and blame patients for their illnesses (dispositional factors) rather than examining the circumstances (situational factors) that might be responsible. In particular, psychiatric patients, minorities, and other marginalized groups suffer from this bias. However, patients with a chronic condition such as migraine headache, chronic pain, and asthma are often blamed for causing their own illness. A problem observed across all chronic conditions, nonadherence to medication regimens, is inevitably blamed on the patient even when the clinician is at fault for not explaining when or how to take a particular drug.

Gambler's Fallacy

This is the bias that if a coin is tossed 10 times and is heads each time, the 11th toss has a greater chance of being tails even though the coin has no memory of past events. A clinician who sees a series of patients with chest pain at a hospital, for example, may diagnosis all of them with myocardial infarction and assume that the sequence will not continue. Or, on the other hand, if a certain number of cases of myocardial infarction occurs in a hospital in a period time, the clinician may believe they are overdue for such a case and anticipate that the next patient will present with symptoms of a myocardial infarction. In both cases, the pretest probability that a patient will have a particular diagnosis may be influenced by preceding, but independent, events.

Gender Bias

A gender bias is the tendency to believe that gender is a determining factor in the probability of a particular disease when no such pathological basis exists. The result is often an overdiagnosis of the favored gender and the underdiagnosis of the neglected gender. The diagnosis of breast cancer in women versus men would be an example.

Hindsight Bias

This bias occurs when knowing the outcome profoundly influences the perception of past events, and serves to avoid our making a realistic appraisal of what actually occurred. We are likely to say that we could have predicted the event beforehand as prediction is easier in hindsight than in foresight. With respect to diagnostic error, it may compromise learning through either an underestimation (illusion of failure) or overestimation (illusion of control) of our decision making abilities.

Ignoring Negative Evidence

Clinicians are often inept at using negative evidence or normal findings. For example, it seems easier to learn that the presence of moderate or severe acute cough increases the probability of pneumonia than to learn that the absence of rhinorrhea also increases the probability of pneumonia. In being short of breath following exercise, we may think we are only out of shape when, in reality, we are beginning to experience exercise-induced asthma. This tendency can be a barrier to clinicians and patients when coupled with the confirmatory bias.

Omission Bias

This is a tendency toward inaction; it is rooted in the principle of nonmalefience. In hindsight, for example, events that occurred through the natural progression of disease are more acceptable than those that may be attributed directly to the action of the clinician. While the bias may be associated with reinforcement associated with not doing anything, it may prove disastrous. Omission biases are thought to typically outnumber commission biases.

Order Effects

Order effects have long been recognized in psychology as a U-function: we tend to remember the beginning part (primacy effect) or the end (recency effect). In considering a diagnosis, clinicians should evaluate all information provided by patients, nurses, and others regardless of the order in which it was presented.

Overconfidence Bias

The bias is the universal tendency to believe we know more than we do. Our belief is often based on incomplete information, hunches, or intuition.

Posterior Probability Error

The bias occurs when a clinician's estimate of the likelihood of a conditions is unduly influenced by what has gone on before with a particular patient. If a patient presents to the clinician five times with a headache and it is correctly diagnosed each time as having a tension headache, there is the tendency to diagnose the sixth presentation as a tension headache; the diagnosis here is likely correct, but it could be incorrect. The problem occurs because the headaches were not considered as separate events.

Premature Closure

This is a powerful bias in that it accounts for a high proportion of missed diagnoses. The tendency is to close the decision making process and accepting a diagnosis before it has been fully verified. The consequence is that other potential diagnoses may be given sufficient consideration.

Representativeness Heuristic or Restraint

The representativeness heuristic is used to assess the likelihood that an object or person, A, belongs to a given class, B. The probability that A belongs to class B is directly related to the degree to which A resembles B. This bias prompts the clinician to look for a prototypical manifestation of a disease or, in the case of patients, the prototypical exacerbation of a condition.

Sunk Costs

The sunk cost heuristic is characterized by a willingness to continue spending after an investment of time, effort, or money have failed to prove the validity of a diagnosis. The more clinicians invest in a particular diagnosis, the less likely they may be to release it and consider alternatives even when they should. Confirmation bias may be a manifestation of an unwillingness to let go of a failing diagnosis.

Visceral Bias

The visceral bias is the influence of affective sources of error on decision making. A type of visceral or emotional bias are the outcome bias and regret error described earlier. Regret is a value-induced bias that may affect subjective estimates of probability. Clinicians or patients may distort probability estimates by combining two steps in the decision-making process, i.e., allowing the undesirability of a certain outcome or diagnosis to alter the estimate of its likelihood of occurrence. Emotional or visceral errors are greatly underestimated by clinicians.

Table 2. Errors and biases in medical decision making.

approached the treatment of attacks in a thoughtful and systematic manner. They reported they treated attacks in a sequential stepwise manner by selecting and applying what they thought was the most appropriate treatment, assessing the effect of their action, introducing a second step if needed, and so on; these instructions comply with treatment guidelines later issued for asthma. The families displayed not only adherence to medical instructions, but use of the common sense scientific method discussed at the outset. A subset of the families, referred to as Gold Standard patients, took the time to describe in detail how they made decisions in treating asthma. Data from the aggregate responses to the Report of Asthma Attacks were described by Creer and colleagues (1988). Specific comments offered by patients on strategies taken in decision making were reported in a subsequent publication (Creer, 1990).

Decision Making by Physicians

The second set of data came from an investigation conducted on decision making heuristics used by physicians and those learning to be physicians (Marion, 1983; Marion, Creer, Arkes, & Kotses, 1983). Three case scenarios regarding the treatment of asthma were composed by an allergist skilled in the treatment of the condition. The scenarios were presented to three groups of participants—30 second year medical students, 30 practicing allergists, and 8 allergists or pulmonary physicians labeled as the Gold Standard group. The eight physicians in the latter group were selected because: (a) they were both solid clinicians and investigators; (b) had published widely, including authorship of leading textbooks in the area; or (c) because of their election to the presidency of major professional organizations (most physicians in the Gold Standard group met all three criteria). After reading the scenarios, the Gold Standard group determined from a group of available asthma treatments the most beneficial treatments for each child. They then rank ordered the remaining alternatives according to the respective desirability of each alternative. A decision making matrix, constructed for each case history, utilized seven probabilities—peak flow rates, medication compliance, allergens, infections, behavior/emotions, physical exertion, and miscellaneous factors—as weights for each selection criteria and the available treatments as outcome alternatives. The 30 allergists and 30 medical students were randomly assigned to either a decision-aid condition or a no decision-aid condition. In the former conditions, participants were given the three case scenarios and supplied with a decision-making matrix to use with each case; in the latter condition, participants were given the same three scenarios, but not provided with the decision-making matrix. Subjects were instructed to use the matrix when determining the order of treatment importance for each patient.

Results showed that the decision-making matrix had little effect. It was also found that the medical students did not know how to treat asthma. Perhaps the topic had not yet been broached in their curriculum because, on average, their base of knowledge was likely below that of patients with asthma. The 30 allergists indicated they were highly skilled in the treatment of asthma; they indicated they would treat the attacks in an orderly, stepwise manner as later suggested by treatment guidelines for asthma (National Asthma Education & Prevention Program, 1997; 2002). The Gold Standard physicians were found to have a relatively low intercorrelation in making decisions; this lack of agreement was much stronger in this group than it was among the group of 30 allergists. Reasons suggested by the Gold Standard group as contributing to the lack of correlation included defects in the case scenarios, the context within which the fictional attacks occurred, and their attitudes towards participating in the study. Those physicians in the Gold Standard group differed from both medical students and the group of 30 allergists. They not only expressed their feelings about weaknesses in the study, but went to some length to describe the heuristics they used in treating asthma.

Discussion

In reviewing the comments on decision making made by the Gold Standard physicians, a deja vu occurred: there was remarkable overlap with the data collected from Gold Standard physicians with that gathered earlier from the Gold Standard patients. Both groups showed what Bandura (1987) referred to as advanced cognitive capabilities, coupled with remarkable flexibility and the ability to synthesize information to generate ideas, often original, to manage attacks. They not only treated attacks in a systematic and, overall, a linear stepwise manner, but they also were able to perceive events in a nonlinear manner when necessary.

The data gathered by Marion (1983) and Marion et al. (1983) were carefully reviewed and analyzed. The data were then compared to the information provided by the Gold Standard patients in the study by Creer et al. (1988). Emerging from the analysis were a set of common judgment heuristics used by both groups. Results of the analysis were reported by Creer (1990). Twelve judgment rules common to both Gold Standard patients and physicians were:

Considered each patient and/or asthma attack as a separate experiment. A common sense view of science was reflected in this heuristic. Gold Standard physicians recognized not only that patients differ from one another, but that the attacks they experience vary from episode to episode. Gold Standard patients also recognized that attacks fluctuate from episode to episode. If asthma is under medical control, attacks should be mild. Even if the asthma is basically controlled, however, there remains the potential for a severe episode to occur. Both Gold Standard groups recognized that individual attacks are like fingerprints in that they change from episode to episode; for this reason, they approach decision making and treatment action from an experimental perspective.

Showed greater awareness of attacks, treatments, and potential outcomes. Gold Standard physicians and patients were highly knowledgeable about asthma and its treatment. The Gold Standard physicians were not only skilled at treating asthma, but conducted research and wrote extensively on the topic. Gold Standard patients read everything they could find on childhood asthma. Today, these would be the patients knowledgeable about what information would be available via the internet and how to use it in planning treatment strategies with their child's clinician. In treating an attack, both groups of participants reported they took a stepwise approach in that they: (a) analyzed the attack and considered how it could be treated; (b) based decisions upon this analysis; (c) considered the best option for treating the episode; (d) selected and acted on the best option; and (e) evaluated the outcome of their action. Participants emphasized that they wanted to attain optimal control over an episode with a minimal amount of medication.

Avoided preconceived notions in the treatment of asthma and individual attacks. Both Gold Standard groups reported they avoided potential pitfalls created by such biases as availability errors or the confirmation heuristic. They used similar ploys in seeking more information, producing more treatment options, and in appraising the actions they took. While the actions they took were likely those they had taken during most previous episodes, they realized the potential for the occurrence of a more severe episode then normally experienced and were prepared to manage it.

Generated number of testable treatment alternatives. Gold Standard physicians requested more information than other physicians in the study reported by Marion et al. (1983). Based upon the additional data, they developed more treatment options. In doing so, they demonstrated the importance of two qualities of effective decision making (Arkes, 1981): First, they gave consideration to alternative strategies available for the treatment of a patient's asthma, including a given attack he or she experienced. Second, the physicians indicated that when able to do so, they made their final selection of the most appropriate treatment later in the course of attack. This extra time appeared to improve the accuracy of judgment and avoidance of bias. Gold Standard patients took a similar tactic: they often performed watchful waiting or relaxation exercises before using a quick-relief medication. However, they also realized that if immediately required, the administration of a quick-relief drug was the first step to take. They knew the available treatment alternatives they had at their disposal and took a systematic approach in their application.

Consistently referred to personal data base in making decisions. Past experience in treating asthma is invaluable in controlling future attacks. Gold Standard physicians and Gold Standard patients repeatedly emphasized the value of their past experiences in treating attacks. The combination of a data base of experience, coupled with their never ending quest for more and more knowledge of asthma, contributed to the status they attained in controlling the disorder.

Adjusted treatment to fit perceived severity of asthmatic episode. The 30 allergists studied by Marion et al. (1983) all reported they adjusted their treatment according to the severity of an attack. All essentially used a stepwise, sequential approach to treating attacks. This permitted them to make whatever changes, sometimes subtle, to establish control over an episode. A basic difference between the two physician groups were more requests for additional information and the generation of a wider range of treatment options by the Gold Standard physicians. Gold Standard patients were also sophisticated at matching the perceived severity of an episode to what would likely be the best treatment option to implement. Both groups of Gold Standard participants used dynamic rather than static decision-making strategies.

Kanfer and Busemeyer (1982) delineated these two approaches by noting that in a dynamic decision-making framework, a series of interdependent judgments is made so that the outcome of a decision, at one time or another, may influence the outcomes of later judgments. Dynamic decisions are reversible and rely on the continued monitoring of their action by physicians and patients.

Did not misperceive severity of asthma episode. Gold Standard physicians and patients indicated they did not misperceive or misjudge the severity of a given asthmatic exacerbation. They followed a stepwise approach to treatment, but were prepared to quickly make adjustments in order to control an attack that was increasing in severity. Gold Standard patients knew what skills they had in their treatment repertoire and were prepared, if necessary, to seek medical assistance.

Regarded events as correlated with, not causative of, asthma and asthmatic attacks. The exact cause of a given asthma attack is usually unknown. Although a patient may be exposed to a known precipitant of his or her asthmatic exacerbations, such as exposure to an allergen, the attack could have been triggered by another factor, such as exercise or an infection. Gold Standard physicians and patients were cognizant of the fact that a number of events may be correlated with the onset and course of an attack. By perceiving events as correlative rather than causative, both groups avoided particular decision making biases such as the availability heuristic, premature closure, and sunk costs.

Thought in terms of probabilities in making decisions and managing attacks. Gold Standard patients and physicians recognized that their actions had a probable, not certain, chance of success. Recognizing this factor permitted them to keep open the possibility that other treatment options might be required. Thinking in terms of probability also permitted patients to consider the risk of any treatment. Risk perception and the subsequent action of participants lead them to be prudent in making the best decision and, as a consequence, increased the likelihood that they would arrive at the safest solution to abort an asthmatic episode.

Did not rely on memory. A number of reviews have indicated that a reliance on memory can decrease judgmental accuracy (e.g., Arkes, 1981; Faust, 1986). For example, patients or physicians may remember what they perceived as past symptoms of an attack when, in actuality, the symptoms were not present. The process of filling in gaps in memory can lead to a misdiagnosis of the severity of an attack or to taking inappropriate action. Arkes (1981) warned that an excessive amount of reliance on memory may lead to poorer clinical judgment. He presented evidence that illusory correlations were often more pronounced when greater amounts of information were processed. The Gold Standard patients and physicians were cautious in not over relying on their memory to make decisions about the actions to take to control an asthmatic episode.

Were thoughtful and cautious. Gold Standard physicians and patients were thoughtful and cautious. They did not launch into automatically treating an attack without first considering whether their decisions and actions were the most appropriate for that given situation. They relied upon their past experiences, but not to the exclusion of new information that might bear on the management of an episode. They did not panic, but were able to include watchful waiting as a significant treatment strategy.

Were not overconfident. The Gold Standard participants were not overconfident about their ability to treat asthma. They all made concerted efforts to enhance their skills to control the condition. Overconfidence may result in many of the biases described in Table 2. This does not imply that either group lacked confidence in their ability to treat asthma; they were confident that they could. However, there clearly is a delicate line between confidence and overconfidence that was not breached by either Gold Standard physicians or patients.

Summary

The information supplied by the Gold Standard patients and physicians offer a empirical set of decision making tools that can be used to teach others about decision making. They should be incorporated into future self-management studies across all chronic conditions. Other ways to debase both physicians and patients were described by Arkes (1981; 1991), Croskerry (2003), Dawson and Arkes (1987), and Garb (1998). These sources are well worth reading for those concerned with both decision making and biases in such activity.

Discussion & Conclusions

Reality is a chaotic and complex beast. It is an entity that can never be fully understood or controlled. The chapter focused on how patients with asthma attempted to deal with three components of reality–complexity, context, and uncertainty. Patients with a chronic condition are likely more accepting of complexity with respect to their illness than others; they realize the infinite number of combinations and permutations of factors that can interact to influence their condition. They recognize that chaos can create an infinity of patterns over which they have no control. For these reason, they tend to generate solutions for controlling a chronic illness outside the context of a crossword puzzle because, after all, a crossword puzzle offers only a finite number of options. Because they realize there is a only probability of success in any action they take, patients are more apt to perceive their condition and its treatment more as a jigsaw puzzle that they know they can never totally put together (for that matter, neither medical nor behavioral scientists are apt to fully assemble the puzzle; we don't know what the pieces of the puzzle are any more than do patients). Patients just want to identify a few variables, such as the use of peak flow values they blow or the actions they find effective in managing an attack, to assist them that can help them control their condition within a given setting.

Patients have a far greater stake in management of a condition than do others: they not only live with the illness each day, but they provide almost all of the action needed to manage and control the condition. In learning and performing self-management skills, patients were very effective at managing their disorder. They not only used the linear, stepwise skills they could perform, but they used nonlinear and simple rules, within a probabilistic framework, to achieve their goal. By doing so, they not only brought a degree of order to controlling their asthma, but inspired my colleagues and I to conduct a number of studies on prediction of events related to asthma. Conducting a refined analysis of the context within which behaviors occurred showed that acquiring self-management skills was initiated by most patients when introduced to self-monitoring. They then used a trial-and-error approach to acquire and perform skills to match characteristics of their asthma. Finally, a number of children and their families became particularly skilled at managing unpredictability via the development and implementation of a series of effective decision making heuristics. That these rules were common with decision making strategies utilized by Gold Standard physicians, eminently knowledgeable and skilled at treating asthma, attests to the ability of the patients to use the scientific method to apply identical heuristics to control their asthma. The creation of procedures to manage complexity and uncertainty likely contributed to the solid findings in the study by Creer and colleagues (1988).

The program used in the adult version of Living with Asthma was described by Creer, Kotses, and Reynolds (1991). In developing the materials used in the program, attention was focused on the management of complexity and unpredictability based on the data on these topics discussed in the chapter. Was the program effective? As discussed, the findings described by Kotses and colleagues (1995) demonstrated we were decidedly effective in teaching patients to manage their asthma. In addition to the significance of these findings, however, Caplin and Creer (2001) conducted a long-term follow-up of the participants from the Kotses et al. (1995) study. We were able to contact 53 out of the 76 subjects from the study by 6 years after they had participated in the program or 7 years after training. The patients were interviewed using a 13-item questionnaire developed for the follow-up. Based on the data, subjects were divided into groups labeled as continuers or relapsers according to: (a) their estimates of time spent engaged in self-management behaviors; (b) a monitoring index based on performance of 5 monitoring behaviors; (c) ratings by participants of themselves as continuers or relapsers; and (d) behavior relapse. Using this criteria, 33 subjects were categorized as continuers and 20 subjects were classified as relapsers. A number of findings were common to both groups: (a) all participants remained motivated; (b) the degree of satisfaction was $p = .92$ and $p = .89$ for perceived self-efficacy for all participants; (c) all participants had controlled or could manage interfering factors; and (d) all subjects were flexible in managing their asthma. Differences occurred in that those categorized as continuers: (a) enumerated more reasons for using self-management skills; (b) continued to improve and refine self-management skills; (c) experienced fewer asthma symptoms; and (d) reported they received reinforcement in self-management ranging from avoidance of or escape from attacks to self-reinforcement. These reports were highly positive. However, half of the relapsers spontaneously commented that they no longer performed self-management on a regular basis because their asthma had gone into remission. The latter findings, also coupled with reports that they experienced fewer asthma symptoms by members of the continuer group, made us realize after the fact that we should have asked the question, "Has your asthma gone into remission for periods or totally remitted after you learned and began to perform self-management skills?" A conservative estimate is that the asthma of half of the participants in the study by Kotses and coworkers went into remission because of the patients' performance. Although it has long been thought that there is no cure for asthma, periods of remission of the condition, much as occurs with other chronic illnesses, does regularly occur. In the study by Caplin and Creer (2001), the findings indicate that optimal performance of self-management skills by patients, linked to sound medical care, leads to remission of asthma in many patients.

Disease management has been touted as the tool for managing health care in the future. Will it prove up to the challenge? If I were betting—certainly a well-practiced activity in Reno!– I'd bet heavily against disease management improving health care in the United States. The reason would not be because of the gravity of the problem, particularly of chronic illnesses. Chronic disease is the principal cause of disability; in addition, use of health services by patients with a chronic condition consumes 78% of health care expenditures in the U.S. (Holman, 2004). Thus, chronic disease is undoubtedly a heavy burden for all of us. My bet, therefore, would be based on the following factors:

First, Holman pointed out that "it is axiomatic that medical education should prepare students well for the clinical problems they will face in their future practice" (p. 1057). Medical education is currently oriented towards the treatment of acute conditions. These conditions are episodic and treated mainly by physicians. Chronic conditions, on the other hand, are continuous with, in many cases, occasional exacerbations of the illness. With chronic conditions, patients supply almost all of the the daily care of their condition, although they should do so in accordance with assistance from their physicians and other personnel. As Holman noted, "The patient usually lives indefinitely with the disease and its symptoms, with persistent treatment and with multiple consequences, including necessary behavioral changes to forestall worsening of the disease, social and economic dislocation, emotional turmoil, financial fear, lowered self-esteem, and depression. As a result, the patient becomes experienced, is often more knowledgeable than the physician about the effects of the disease and its treatment, and has an integral role in the treatment process" (p. 1057). Positive behavioral changes in patients with a chronic disease do not happen overnight; many patients need to overcome past conditioning where they were told by medical personnel and pharmaceutical companies not to take personal action without first consulting with a physician. This was epitomized by a manufacturer of a cough syrup who insisted that patients see their physician before purchasing one of several cough syrups the company had on the market. Unless medical education changes—there are no signs it will—the treatment of chronic conditions will remain the same as in the past.

Second, physicians are taught in medical school that they are the person in charge: everyone who assists them is referred to as "allied medical personnel." The approach is appropriate in treating acute disorders; physicians should be in control. However, the situation turns 180 degrees in treating a chronic asthma. Physicians can not retain, to use the words of Gawande (2002), a "tall in the saddle" approach to health care. They must recognize that a patient with a chronic illness must be treated via a team approach in which physicians are but members. Presently, most treatment teams comprised of members from different disciplines are described as multidisplinarian in nature. Members contribute to the team, headed by a physician, to develop and implement treatment plan for a given patient. The assumption is that the cooperative result will result in the best care, an outcome that may be achieved in some cases. It does not: better outcomes occur with an interdiscplinarian approach where each team member brings not only his or her knowledge to a team, but has a current and working knowledge about the condition and the skills of other team members (e.g., Creer, 1979). The team is truly collaborative with the membership serving collectively as the leader. The difference may seem insignificant, but interdisciplinarian teams permitted my colleagues and I to conduct the research in the 1960s and 1970s, which provided the basis for self-management programs for chronic illness (Creer & Christian, 1976; Creer, 1979), as well as our work in subsequent years to implement and test self-management in asthma patients (Creer et al.,1988; Kotses et al., 1995).

Third, a model that has been proposed for the management of chronic illness is collaborative management (e.g., Von Korff, Gruman, Schaefer, Curry, & Wagner, 1997). The model has considerable appeal; it could make a significance difference in the health care provided patients. However, at the same time, it could also create a layer of health care providers, with attendant bureaucracy, to further muddle what should be a partnership between patients and their physicians. This outcome would add further costs to what are finite resources for providing health care in the U.S.

In conclusion, health care personnel, a category that includes behavioral scientists, must share medical management responsibilities and decisions with patients. During visits, patients learn from each other, and physicians and behavioral scientists learn from the experiences of patients (Holman, 2004). It is an ideal situation when we and patients meet in groups, but this is not always feasible. The theme of the chapter has been that we can learn a lot from patients when they apply self-management skills to control chronic conditions. They often have a much more accurate perception of chaos, complexity, and unpredictability than medical and behavioral scientists. It constitutes the reality in which they live. If we continue to learn from patients, I'd hedge my bets regarding the viability of disease management as an approach to provide better health care at less cost. This will not happen, at least in our lifetime. The gridlock in Washington, created by health care interests, the pharmaceutical industry, and Congress, has been impervious to even hints of change. The ever increasing number of uninsured and partially insured in the United States has not budged the impasse. The only resolution to this impediment is if we, both as psychologists and as patients, learn to effectively manage our health, including taking a positive and strongly proactive approach with our care givers as did the patients I've described. A grassroots movement where we partner with our health care provider to care for our health, including any chronic condition we experience, offers us our only chance of attaining better health at a reduced cost. That is the reality, mainly illustrated by patients, in the chapter.

References

Arkes, H. R. (1981). Impediments to accurate clinical judgment and possible ways to minimize their impact. *Journal of Consulting and Clinical Psychology, 49*, 323-330.

Arkes, H. R. (1991). Costs and benefits of judgment errors: Implications for debiasing. *Psychological Bulletin, 110*, 486-498.

Ball, P. (1999). *The self-made tapestry. Pattern formation in nature.* Oxford: Oxford University Press.

Bandura, A. (1986). *Social foundations of thought and action: A social cognitive theory.* Englewood Cliffs, NJ: Prentice-Hall.

Bandura, A. (1997). *Self-efficacy. The exercise of control.* New York: W.H. Freeman & Company.

Bar-Yam, Y. (Ed.). (2000). *Unifying themes in complex systems. Proceedings of the international conference on complex systems.* Cambridge, MA: Perseus Books.

Bullock, A., & Thombley, S. (Eds.). (1999). *The Norton dictionary of modern thought.* New York: W.W. Norton.

Blumberg, B. (1995). Preface. In P. Covney, & P. Highfield (Eds.), *Frontiers of complexity: The search for order in a chaotic world* (pp. ix-xii). New York: Random House.

Burkhart, P. V., & Ward, M. J. (2003). Children's self-reports of characteristics of their asthma episodes. *Journal of Asthma, 40*, 909-916.

Caplin, D. L., & Creer, T. L. (2001). A self-management program for adult asthma. Part III. Maintenance and relapse of skills. *Journal of Asthma, 38*, 343-356.

Casti, J. L. (1997). *Would-be worlds: How simulation is changing the frontiers of science.* New York: John Wiley.

Coveney, P., & Highfield, R. (1995). *Frontiers of complexity. The search for order in a chaotic world.* New York: Random House.

Creer, T. L. (1979). *Asthma therapy: A behavioral health care system for respiratory disorders.* New York: Springer.

Creer, T. L. (1990). Strategies for judgment and decision-making in the management of childhood asthma. *Pediatric Asthma Allergy and Immunology, 4*, 253-264.

Creer, T. L., Backial, M., Burns, K., Leung, P., Marion, R., Miklich, D. R., et al. (1988). Living with Asthma. Genesis and development of a self-management program for childhood asthma. *Journal of Asthma, 25*, 335-362.

Creer, T. L., Backiel, M., Ullman, S., & Leung, P. (1985a). Living with asthma. Part I. In *Manual for teaching parents the self-management of asthma* (NIH Publication no. 86-2364). Washington, D.C.: U.S. Department of Health & Human Services.

Creer, T. L., Backiel, M., Ullman, S., & Leung, P. (1985b). Living with asthma. Part II. *Manual for teaching children the self-management of asthma.* (NIH Publication no. 86-2364). Washington, D.C.: U.S. Department of Health & Human Services.

Creer, T. L., Caplin, D. L., & Holroyd, K. A. (in press). A self-management program for adult asthma. Part IV. Analysis of context. *Journal of Asthma.*

Creer, T. L., & Christian, W. P. (1976). *Chronically-ill and handicapped children. Their management and rehabilitation.* Champaign, IL: Research Press.

Creer, T. L., & Holroyd, K. A. (1997). Self-management. In A. Baum, S. Newman, J. Weinman, R. West, & C. McManus (Eds.), *Cambridge handbook of psychology, health, and medicine* (pp. 255-258). Cambridge: Cambridge University Press.

Creer, T. L., Kotses, H., & Reynolds, R. V. C. (1991). *A handbook for asthma self-management: A patient's guide to living with asthma.* Athens, OH: Athens University Press.

Croskerry, P. (2002). Achieving quality in clinical decision making: Cognitive strategies and detection of bias. *Academy of Emergency Medicine, 9,* 1184-1204.

Croskerry, P. (2003). The importance of cognitive errors in diagnosis and strategies to minimize them. *Academic Medicine, 78,* 775-778.

Dawson, N. V., & Arkes, H. R. (1987). Systematic errors in medical decision making. Judgment limitations. *Journal of General Internal Medicine, 2,* 183-187.

Engel, S. (1999). *Context is everything: The nature of memory.* New York: W.H. Freeman.

Faust, D. (1986). Research on human judgment and its application to clinical practice. *Professional Psychology Research and Practice, 17,* 420-430.

Garb, H. N. (1998). *Studying the clinician. Judgment research and psychological assessment.* Washington, D.C.: American Psychological Press.

Gawande, A. (2002). *Complications: A surgeon's notes on an imperfect science.* New York: Metropolitan Books.

Gibson, P. G., Powell, H., Coughlan, J., Wilson, A.J., Abramson, M., Haywood, P., et al. (2003). Self-management education and regular practitioner review for adults with asthma. *Cochrane Library,* Issue 2. Oxford: Update Software.

Gleick, J. (1987). *Chaos. Making a new science.* New York: Penquin Books.

Goerner, S. (1995). Chaos, evolution, and deep ecology. In R. Robertson & A. Combs (Eds.), *Chaos theory in psychology and the life sciences* (pp. 17-38). Mahwah, NJ: Lawrence Erlbaum Associates.

Haack, S. (2003). *Defending science—within reason: Between scientism and cynicism.* Amhearst, NY: Promoetheus Books.

Harm, D. L., Kotses, H., & Creer, T. L. (1987). Improving the ability of peak expiratory flow rates to predict asthma. *Journal of Allergy and Clinical Immunology, 76,* 688-694.

Holman, H. (2004). Chronic disease—the need for a new clinical education. *Journal of the American Medical Association, 292,* 1057-1059.

Holroyd, K. A. (2001). *Behavioral management for migraine headaches.* Athens, OH: Ohio University & the National Institutes of Health.

Kanfer, F. H., & Busemeyer, J. R. (1982). The use of problem solving and decision making in behavior therapy. *Clinical Psychology Review, 1,* 239-266.

Kotses, H., Stout, C., Wigal, J. K., Carlson, B., Creer, T. L., & Lewis, P. (1991). Individualized asthma self-management: A beginning. *Journal of Asthma, 28,* 287-289.

Kotses, H., Bernstein, I. L., Bernstein, D.I., Reynolds, R.V., Korbee, L., Wigal, J., et al. (1995). A self-management program for adult asthma: Part I. Development and evaluation. *Journal of Allergy & Clinical Immunology, 95,* 529-540.

Kotses, H., Stout, C., McConnaughy, K., Winder, J. A., & Creer, T. L. (1996). Evaluation of individualized asthma self-management programs. *Journal of Asthma, 33,* 113-118.

Longrino, H. E. (2002). *The fate of knowledge.* Princeton, NJ: Princeton University Press.

Marion, R. J. (1983). *The treatment of asthma: A decision-making approach.* Unpublished Master's thesis, Ohio University, Athens, Ohio.

Marion, R. J., Creer, T. L., Arkes, H. R., & Kotses, H. (1983). *The treatment of asthma: A decision-making approach.* Paper presented at the World Congress on Behavior Therapy and the 17th Annual Convention, Association for the Advancement of Behavior Therapy, Washington, D.C.

Marx, M. H., & Hillix, W. A. (1963). *Systems and theories in psychology.* New York: McGraw-Hill.

National Asthma Education and Prevention Program (1997). *Expert Panel 2. Guidelines for the diagnosis and management of asthma.* (NIH Publication No. 97-4051). Washington, D.C: U.S. Department of Health and Human Services.

National Asthma Education & Prevention Program (2002). *Expert Panel Report: Guidelines for the diagnosis and management of asthma–Update on selected topics 2002.* (NIH Publication No. 02-5075). Washington, D.C.: U.S. Department of Health and Human Services.

Pinzone, H. A., Carlson, B. W., Kotses, H., & Creer, T. L. (1991). Prediction of asthma episodes in children using peak expiratory flow rates, medication compliance, and exercise data. *Annals of Allergy, 67,* 481-486.

Plsek, P. (2001). Appendix B. Redesigning health care with insights from the science of complex adaptive systems. In Institute of Medicine, *Crossing the quality chasm. A new health system for the 21st century* (pp. 309-322). Washington, D.C.: National Academy Press.

Rachlin, H. (2000). *The science of self-control.* Cambridge: Harvard University Press.

Schwartz, B. (2004). *The paradox of choice. Why more is less.* New York: HarperCollins.

Skinner, B. F. (1953). *Science and human behavior.* New York: Macmillan.

Solomon, M. (2004). Messing with common sense. *Science, 305,* 44-45.

Stirzaker, D. (1999). *Probability and random variables: A beginner's guide.* Cambridge: Cambridge University Press.

Stout, C., Kotses, H., Carlson, B. W., & Creer, T. L. (1991). Predicting asthma in individual patients. *Journal of Asthma, 28,* 41-47.

Strevens, M. (2003). *Bigger than chaos: Understanding complexity through probability.* Cambridge, MA: Harvard University Press.

Taplin, P. S., & Creer, T. L. (1979). A procedure for using peak expiratory flow rate data to increase the predictability of asthma episodes. *Journal of Asthma Research, 16,* 15-19.

Tolman, E. C. (1959). Principles of purposive behavior. In S. Koch (Ed.), *Psychology: A study of a science. Vol. 2. General systematic formulations, learning and special processes* (pp. 92-157). New York: McGraw-Hill.

Tversky, A., & Kahneman, D. (1974). Judgment under uncertainty: Heuristics and biases. *Science, 185,* 1124-1131.

Von Korff, M., Gruman, J., Schaefer, J., Curry, C. J., & Wagner, E. H. (1997). Collaborative management of chronic illness. *Annals of Internal Medicine, 127,* 1097-1102.

Waldrup, M. M. (1992). *Complexity. The emerging science at the edge of order and chaos.* New York: Touchstone.

Wolf, F. M., Guevara, J. P., Grum, C. H., Clark, N. M., & Cotes, C. J. (2003). Educational interventions for asthma in children. *Cochrane Library,* Issue 2. Oxford: Update Software.

Chapter 8

Psychopathology and Chronic Pain: Theoretical and Treatment Implications[1]

Robert J. Gatchel
Professor and Chair
Department of Psychology, College of Science
The University of Texas at Arlington

The comorbidity of psychopathology and chronic pain is well documented (e.g., Dersh, Polatin, & Gatchel, 2002; Gatchel & Epker, 1999). Kroenke and colleagues (1989, 1994) have also reported that patients with anxiety or depressive disorders have more physical symptoms such as pain, and that as the number of physical symptoms increases so does the likelihood of an anxiety or depressive disorder. This holds true for symptoms with and without a diagnosed etiology. For example, Katon, Sullivan and Walker (2001) evaluated medical symptoms without clearly identified pathology (such as irritable bowel syndrome, fibromyalgia, headache, etc.), and noted a close association with psychiatric disorders such as panic disorder, major depression and somatization disorder. In a larger scale study by the World Health Organization (WHO), Gureje, Simon and Von Korff (2001) assessed 5,438 patients from 15 primary care sites and 14 countries. Of the 22% of patients who reported persistent pain for more than 6 months, there was a 4-fold increase in associated anxiety or depressive disorders. These relationships were consistent across cultures. WHO also estimated that 450 million people worldwide have mental or psychosocial problems, most of which are not adequately diagnosed or properly treated (Goldberg, Privett, Ustun, Simon, & Linden, 1998).

In this country, pain is a pervasive medical problem: it accounts for more than 80% of all physician visits; it affects in excess of 50 million Americans; and it costs more than $70 billion annually in health care costs and lost productivity. Each year, an estimated 176,850 patients seek treatment in pain centers in the U.S. alone (Marketdata Enterprises, 1995). Also, the number of patient-visits to pain programs increased 26% in 2000, with new patients accounting for 16% of the total gain (Marketdata Enterprises, 2001). In addition to the pain and emotional suffering

[1] *The writing of this article was supported in part by Grants No. 5R01 MH046452, 1K05 MH71892-01 and 5R01 DE010713 (from the National Institutes of Health) and Grant No. DAMD17-03-1-0055 (from the Department of Defense).*

these patients experience, chronic pain presents enormous costs to society. Such costs include lost earnings, decreased productivity, and increased health care utilization expenses and disability benefits. One study calculated the annual cost of chronic low back pain to be between $20 billion and $60 billion, when measures such as lost productivity and social security disability insurance benefits were calculated along with treatment costs (Gatchel & Mayer, 2000). In another study by Frymoyer and Durett (1997), medical charges and hospitalization costs related to chronic pain were calculated to be in excess of $125 billion.

Thus, there is no doubt that the prevalence and cost of chronic pain is still a major health care problem in the U.S. Recently, several important organizations in the U.S. have developed new standards for the evaluation of pain. One such organization—the Joint Commission on Accreditation of Healthcare Organizations (2000)—now requires that physicians consider pain as the *"5th Vital Sign"* (added to the other vital signs of pulse, blood pressure, core temperature and respiration). As another example of this current interest in pain, Congress has designated 2001-2010 as the Decade of Pain Control and Research. In addition, for the first time ever, the National Institutes of Health convened a conference, attended by mental health and pain specialists, focused specifically on the problem of pain and its treatment (National Institute of Health Technology Assessment Panel, 1995).

Emergence of the Biopsychosocial Perspective

The most promising comorbid psychopathology and chronic pain research conducted to date has embraced a biopsychosocial perspective. The emergence of this biopsychosocial perspective of mental health and pain disorders has paralleled the evolution of scientific thought in medicine (Gatchel, 1999). During the Renaissance, increased scientific knowledge in the areas of anatomy, biology and physiology was accompanied by a *biomedical reductionism* or a "dualistic" viewpoint that mind and body function separately and independently. This perspective dominated medicine until quite recently, and affected our understanding of the relationships between mental health and pain. The *gate control theory of pain*, introduced by Melzack and Wall (1965), however, began to highlight the potentially significant role that psychosocial factors play in the perception of pain. As a result, pain is now viewed as a complex set of phenomena, rather than as a simple, specific or discrete entity. This view converged with a biopsychosocial approach to medicine that emerged during the 1970s and 1980s. In the past, organic pain was viewed as different from "psychogenic" pain. The term "psychogenic" suggested that the pain was due to psychological causes only, and that it was not "real" pain because no specific organic basis could be found. This perspective hindered the development of effective psychiatric and pain management strategies. Today, fortunately, the DSM-IV does not list "psychogenic pain" as a diagnostic entity. The assessment or diagnosis of organically caused pain does not rule out the important role that psychosocial factors can play for any particular patient. The general term "Pain Disorder" is used, with subtypes coded according to the relative degree of psychological and/or medical conditions associated with it. The biopsychosocial model views physical disorders such as pain as the result of a dynamic interaction among physiologic, psychologic and social factors, which perpetuates and may worsen the clinical presentation. Each individual experiences pain uniquely. A range of psychological and socioeconomic factors can interact with physical pathology to modulate patients' report of symptoms and subsequent disability.

Disease versus Illness

The biopsychosocial model just reviewed focuses on both disease and illness, with illness being viewed as a complex interaction of biological, psychological and social variables. As Turk and Monarch (2002) appropriately note, *disease* is defined as "an objective biological event" involving the disruption of specific body structures or organ systems caused by either anatomical, pathological or physiological changes. *Illness*, in contrast, is generally defined as a "subjective experience or self-attribution" that a disease is present. Therefore, illness refers to how a sick individual and members of his or her family live with, and respond to, symptoms and disability. This distinction between disease and illness is analogous to the distinction made between *pain* and *nociception*. Nociception involves the stimulation of nerves that convey information about tissue damage to the brain. Pain, on the other hand, is a more subjective perception that is the result of the transduction, transmission and modulation of sensory input. This input may be filtered through a person's genetic composition, prior learning history, current psychological status, and sociocultural influences. Loeser (1982) originally formulated a model outlining four dimensions associated with the concept of pain: the aforementioned dimensions of nociception and pain, as well as *suffering* (the emotional responses that are triggered by nociception or some other aversive event associated with it, such as fear or depression), and *pain behavior* (those things that individuals do when they are suffering or in pain, such as avoiding activities/exercise for fear of re-injury).

Subsequently, Waddell (1987) highlighted the fact that pain cannot be comprehensively assessed without a full understanding of the individual who is exposed to the nociception. He also made a comparison of Loeser's model of pain with an early biopsychosocial model of illness originally proposed by Engel (1977). Such a biopsychosocial model focuses primarily on *illness*. With this perspective, a diversity in pain or illness expression (including its severity, duration and psychosocial consequences) can be expected. The inter-relationships among biological changes, psychological status, and the sociocultural context all need to be considered in fully understanding the pain patient's perception and response to illness. Any model or treatment approach that focuses on only one of these core sets of factors will be incomplete.

The Importance of Biopsychosocial Interactions

Ray (2004) has provided an excellent overview of mind-body relationships, and how social and behavioral factors can act on the brain to influence health, illness, and even death. In our own biopsychosocial clinical research, we take such an interactive perspective, which recognizes the important afferent and efferent feedback between biological and psychological systems, as well as the effects of social mediators (see Gatchel, 2004). Pain is viewed as not purely a perceptual phenomenon, but the injury that has caused the pain also disrupts the body's homeostatic regulation systems which, in turn, produce stress and the initiation of complex programs to restore homeostasis. Melzack (1999) argues that recognizing the role of the stress system in pain syndromes substantially broadens the conceptualization of chronic pain and our ability to understand it. Chronic pain is a stressor that will "tax" the stress system. Prolonged activation of the stress-regulation systems will ultimately generate breakdowns of muscle, bone and neural tissue that, in turn, will cause more pain and produce a vicious cycle of pain-stress-reactivity. One important measure of the above pain-stress cycle is cortisol. As Melzack (1999) emphasizes, along with the activation of the sympathetic nervous system, "cortisol sets the stage for the stress response." He goes on to state that "...cortisol plays a central role because it is responsible for producing and maintaining high levels of glucose for the response. At the same time, cortisol is potentially a highly destructive substance because, to ensure a high level of glucose, it breaks down the protein in muscle and inhibits the ongoing replacement of calcium in bone." Indeed, cortisol is the main hormonal product of the hypothalamic-pituitary-adrenal (HPA) axis in humans (Miller & Tyrrell, 1995). Although increased cortisol secretion is considered an adaptive response of the organism when stressed (for purposes of energy mobilization), prolonged secretion can lead to negative effects such as muscle atrophy, impairment of growth and tissue repair, immune system suppression, etc. (Sapolsky, 1996) Melzack suggests that cortisol will serve as a good marker of the degree of stress that should closely parallel the development of chronic pain. McEwen (1998) also highlights the importance of evaluating cortisol pattern dysregulation under conditions of allostatic load increases due to stress. HPA axis underlying mechanisms may therefore help to explain individual differences in stress and pain, as well as other medical conditions such as fibromyalgia.

Melzack's neuromatrix theory of pain and stress provides an ideal theory-driven methodology for better understanding underlying biopsychosocial interactive processes. Fortunately, reliable measures of cortisol can be easily obtained in a non-invasive manner in human subjects. For example, Pruessner and colleagues (1997) reported three independent studies demonstrating that cortisol level after morning awakening, assessed by sampling saliva, is a reliable biological marker for adrenocortical activity. Extensive other research has shown that salivary cortisol provides an accurate index of free plasma cortisol. (Kirschbaum & Hellhammer, 1994) Studies with human subjects have also demonstrated a close relationship between stress and salivary cortisol levels (Smyth et al., 1997).

We are also starting to develop an even broader view of biopsychosocial mechanisms in pain by using new brain imaging technology. This technology has not yet been systematically applied to the investigation of psychopathology and pain. However, one of the most popular and powerful imaging techniques now available is functional Magnetic Resonance Imaging (fMRI), which uses high-powered and rapidly oscillating magnetic-field gradients in order to detect changes in brain functioning (e.g., Rosenzweig, Breedlove, & Leiman, 2002). It can create images of the brain which detect activities in its different parts, and it has advantages over earlier imaging techniques' spatial and temporal resolution, while not requiring patients to be injected with any substance such as radioactive material. This imaging currently can achieve fast temporal and 2-4mm spatial resolution in the human brain. A number of studies have demonstrated the effective use of fMRI in cortical regions and subcortical structures involved in pain processing (e.g., Bingel et al., 2002; Coghill, McHaffie, & Yen, 2003; Tuor et al., 2000). Recently, Gracely et al. (2002) used fMRI to demonstrate augmented pain processing in fibromyalgia patients. This was also found in low back pain patients (Gracely & Clauw, 2002) In addition, brain imaging studies have been used to investigate brain networks involved in placebo and opioid analgesia (Petrovic, Kalso, Peterson, & Ingvar, 2002), as well as the basic functional neuroanatomy of the placebo effect as related to psychopharmacological response in depressed patients (Mayberg et al., 2002). Thus, imaging may provide a powerful new technique to help document the impact of different therapies.

The Advent of Biopsychosocial, Interdisciplinary Treatment

The emergence of the biopsychosocial perspective has resulted in the development of the most promising treatment of chronic pain to date. It involves an interdisciplinary approach in which the mental health needs of patients require careful evaluation and treatment, along with the concurrent physical pain problem. The treatment effectiveness of a biopsychosocial, interdisciplinary approach to pain has consistently demonstrated the heuristic value of this model (Turk & Monarch, 2002). Patients with chronic pain are at increased risk for depression (Rush, Polatin, & Gatchel, 2000); suicide, identified by the Surgeon General as one of the top public health concerns in the U.S. (Fishbain, 1999; Parker, 1998); and sleep disorders (Hanscom & Jex, 2001). Ohayon and Schatzberg (2003) have also found that chronic pain conditions increase the duration of depressive mood disorders in the general population. As pain becomes more chronic, emotional factors play an increasingly dominant role in the maintenance of dysfunction and suffering. Affective disorders, anxiety disorders, and substance abuse disorders are the three major psychiatric concomitants of chronic pain (Dersh et al., 2002). The significance of psychopathology in pain comorbidity is further evidenced by the potentially common pathogenetic mechanisms involved in psychiatric disorders, such as depression and pain (Okasha et al., 1999; Polatin, 1991). Both nociceptive and affective pathways coincide anatomically. Furthermore, norepinephrine and serotonin, the two neurotransmitters most implicated in the pathophysiology of mood disorders, are also involved in the pain process. Finally, antidepressants have been found to have a mitigating effect upon chronic pain, even at doses considered to be sub-therapeutic for depression. Gallagher (2002) has documented the close neurochemical connection between pain and depression.

Treatment Effectiveness

There have been a number of reviews that have documented the clinical effectiveness of such interdisciplinary treatment of chronic pain patients (e.g., Deschner & Polatin, 2000; Gatchel, 1999; Okifuji, 2003; Wright & Gatchel, 2002). Such interdisciplinary programs are needed for chronic pain patients who have complex needs and requirements. One variant of interdisciplinary tertiary pain management programs—functional restoration—has been comprehensively described in detail in a number of publications (e.g., Gatchel & Mayer, 1989; Gatchel, Mayer, Hazard, Rainville, & Mooney, 1992; Kermond, Gatchel, & Mayer, 1991; Mayer & Gatchel, 1988, 1989; Mayer et al., 1989; Mayer & Polatin, 2000). Functional restoration has received increasing attention in recent years because of its documented clinical effectiveness. Research has shown that the functional restoration program, when fully implemented, is associated with substantive improvement in various important societal outcome measures (e.g., return to work and resolution of outstanding legal and medical issues) in chronically disabled patients with spinal disorders in both one-year follow-up studies (Bendix et al., 1996; Bendix & Bendix, 1994; Hazard et al., 1989; Hildebrandt, Pfingsten, Saur, & Jansen, 1997; Mayer et al., 1985; Mayer et al., 1986), as well as a 2-year follow-up study (Mayer et al., 1987). For example, in the 2-year follow-up study by Mayer et al., 87% of the functional restoration treatment group was actively working at 2 years post-treatment, as compared to only 41% of a non-treatment comparison group. Moreover, about twice as many of the comparison group of patients had both additional spine surgery and unsettled workers' compensation litigation relative to the treatment group. The comparison group continued with approximately a five-times higher rate of patient visits to health professionals and had higher rates of recurrence or re-injury. Thus, the results demonstrate the striking impact that a functional restoration program can have on these important outcome measures in a chronic group consisting primarily of workers' compensation cases (traditionally the most difficult cases to successfully treat).

Finally, it should be noted that the original functional restoration program was independently replicated by Hazard et al. (1989) in this country, as well as Bendix and Bendix (1994) and Bendix, Bendix, Vaegter et al. (1996) in Jousset, Fanello, Bontoux et al. (2004) in France, Hildebrandt et al. (1997) in Germany, and Corey, Koepfler, Etlin and Day (1996) in Canada. The fact that different clinical treatment teams, functioning in different states (Texas and Vermont) and different countries, with markedly different economic/social conditions and workers' compensation systems, produced comparable outcome results speaks highly for the robustness of the research findings and utility, as well as the fidelity, of this functional restoration approach. In addition, Burke, Harms-Constas, and Aden (1994) have demonstrated its efficacy in 11 different rehabilitation centers across 7 states. Hazard (1995) has also reviewed the overall effectiveness of functional restoration. Thus, the clinical effectiveness of functional restoration has been well documented. Moreover, Gatchel and Turk (1999) and Turk (2002) have reviewed both the therapeutic- and cost-effectiveness of interdisciplinary programs, such as functional restoration, for the wide range of chronic pain conditions.

Current Threats to Treatment Effectiveness

One of the major obstacles that pain management specialists now encounter is that insurance companies often contract the management of specific services, such as mental and behavioral services, to a separate mental health management company, often referred to as a mental health "carve out." This can also be true for physical therapy and occupational therapy services. Patients maintain maximum benefit coverage by using a professional who is on the "panel" of the preferred provider network (PPN), rather than paying higher out-of-pocket costs for an "out-of-network" professional. Unfortunately, this often prevents patients from being seen on a same-day basis by an interdisciplinary team of professionals.

Recent research has demonstrated that such "carve-out" policies can significantly compromise the effectiveness of pain management programs (Gatchel et al., 2001; Robbins et al., 2003). For example, in the Robbins et al. study, it was found that physical therapy "carve-out" practices had a negative impact on both the short-term and one-year follow-up outcome measures in patients undergoing an interdisciplinary pain management program. Thus, such insurance carrier policies of contracting treatment "carve outs" significantly compromise the effectiveness of an evidence- based, best standard medical care treatment such as interdisciplinary care for pain. This raises important medico-legal and ethical issues, as well as vocational implications, for patients' long-term improvement and independent financial security. This attempt to contain costs in the short term is also shortsighted, because chronic pain will continue to be a medical problem requiring additional future long-term treatment costs. With the new "Pain-Care Bill of Rights" issued by the American Pain Foundation, chronic pain patients are now in a position to begin demanding the best standard of care for their chronic pain (i.e., interdisciplinary pain management). Other clinical researchers have also demonstrated the negative impact on outcomes by not providing full integrated interdisciplinary care for pain patients when it is required (e.g., Keel et al., 1998).

Developmental Issues

The success of interdisciplinary therapies incorporating a cognitive-behavioral orientation in improving the clinical status of chronic pain patients (Gatchel & Turk, 1996; Morley, Eccleston, & Williams, 1999) further attests to the major role that mental health issues play in chronic pain. Important questions, though, still remain. How are mental disorders exacerbated by pain and, conversely, how does a predisposition toward a psychiatric disorder affect the experience of pain and the evolution of chronic disability? What are the underlying neuropathways? We now also need a strong mental health life-span research emphasis. Chronic physical and mental health problems have become significant for the elderly, and the prevalence of such conditions can be expected to increase with the aging population. Individuals 50 years of age and older are twice as likely to have been diagnosed with chronic pain. Epidemiologic projections suggest a chronic pain prevalence of at least 2% of the adult population (Verhaak, Kerssens, Dekker, Sorbi, & Bensing, 1998). Currently, there are approximately 35 million Americans age 65 years or older, accounting for 12.4% of the total population (U.S. Census Bureau, 2001). By the year 2030, it is projected that about 20% of the population will be 65 years or older (U.S. Census Bureau, 2000). Awareness of these population trends contributes to increased concern about health care issues among older adults, including mental health and pain problems. There has not yet been an organized focus on utilizing lifespan development approaches to the study of comorbid psychiatric and pain disorders.

Related to the above developmental issue, I have earlier presented a broad conceptual model of the transition from acute to chronic pain (Gatchel, 1991, 1996). This model has proven useful in developing pain management strategies. It proposes three stages that may be involved in the transition of acute low back pain into chronic low back pain disability and accompanying psychosocial distress. To summarize, it is proposed that *Stage 1* is associated with emotional reactions, such as fear, anxiety, etc., due to the perception of pain during the acute phase. Pain or hurt is usually associated with harm, and so there is a natural emotional reaction to the potential for physical harm. If the pain persists past a reasonable acute period of time (2 - 4 months), this leads to *Stage 2*, which is associated with a wider array of psychological reactions and problems, such as learned helplessness-depression, distress-anger, somatization, etc., that result from the now more chronic nature of pain. The form these problems take will depend upon the *premorbid* or pre-existing psychosocial characteristics of the individual, as well as current socioeconomic conditions. Thus, for a person with a premorbid problem with depression who is seriously affected economically by loss of a job due to pain, depressive symptoma- tology may be exacerbated during this stage. Similarly, a significant personality disorder may begin to severely hamper a person's ability to cope with the stress of chronic pain. This model does not propose that there is one primary preexisting "pain personality," but assumes a general non-specificity in terms of the relationship between personality-psychosocial problems and pain. This is in keeping with research that has not found any such consistent personality syndrome. Moreover, even though a relationship is usually found between pain and certain psychological problems such as depression (Romano & Turner, 1985), the nature of the relationship remains inconclusive. Some, but not all, patients develop depression secondary to chronic pain. Others show depression as the primary syndrome, of which pain is a symptom. Also, factors that mediate the relationship between depression and pain remain largely unknown (Turk & Rudy, 1988). Thus, it is assumed that certain predisposing psychosocial characteristics differ from one patient to the next, and may be exacerbated by the stress of attempting to cope with pain. Indeed, the relationship between stress and exacerbation of mental health problems has been documented (e.g., Barrett, Rose, & Klerman, 1979; Gatchel & Dersh, 2002).

The above conceptual model proposes that as the "layer" of behavioral/psychological problems persists, it progresses into Stage 3 which is viewed as the acceptance or adoption of a "sick role" during which patients are excused from their normal responsibilities and social obligations. This may become a potent reinforcer for not becoming "healthy." The medical and psychological "disabilities" or "abnormal illness behaviors" (Pilowsky, 1978) are consolidated during this phase. Research consistently demonstrates the important psychological changes that occur as a pain patient progresses from the acute to more chronic phases, such as the MMPI changes documented by Hendler (1982). This model also proposes that superimposed on these three stages is what is known as the physical "deconditioning syndrome" (Mayer & Gatchel, 1988). This refers to a significant decrease in physical capacity (strength, flexibility and endurance) due to disuse and the resultant atrophy of the injured area. There is usually a two-way pathway between the physical deconditioning and the above stages.

Some early indirect support for this model was provided by a study by Blanchard, Kirsch, Applebaum and Jaccard (1989) with one type of chronic pain—headache. These authors note that a prospective longitudinal study is needed to answer the question of whether psychosocial problems often seen in chronic headache are the consequences of years of living with chronic pain, or are predisposing factors in the initial development of the pain. However, in a series of statistical analyses of cross-sectional data on a large number of patients of various ages and at different points in their lifetime course of headaches, some modest support was found for the hypothesis that preexisting psychopathology may be a significant factor in "causing" chronic headache. Such results are quite intriguing and are partly in keeping with the above conceptual model. More recent data from my laboratory further supports the validity of this model (Gatchel & Dersh, 2002).

In summary, chronic pain is quite prevalent, consumes a high proportion of the health care dollar, and will increase with the "graying of America." It has a high comorbidity with mental health problems. Scientific research is just beginning to broaden our understanding of this diathesis. My ongoing research will continue to investigate the etiology, prevention and treatment of mental health problems in patients with chronic pain, and will focus on furthering our understanding of the development and nature of chronic pain when accompanied by psychiatric disorders, which will be discussed next.

Comorbid Psychopathology and Chronic Pain Disorders

In conducting clinical research, it became quite apparent that patients with chronic pain commonly exhibit increased levels of emotional distress and psychopathology that interfere with effective treatment. As a result, we started to conduct a series of studies to evaluate the prevalence of DSM Axis I and Axis II diagnoses of pain patients, derived from a structured interview format (the Structured Clinical Interview for DSM-IV; SCID). One of our initial studies evaluating the nature of the relationship between chronic pain and psychopathology assessed 200 chronic low back pain patients for current and lifetime psychiatric syndromes (Polatin, Kinney, Gatchel, Lillo, & Mayer, 1993). Even when the somewhat controversial category of somatoform pain disorder was excluded, 77% of patients met lifetime diagnostic criteria, and 59% demonstrated current symptoms, for at least one psychiatric diagnosis. The most common types were major depression, substance abuse, and anxiety disorders. In addition, 51% met criteria for at least one personality disorder. All of the prevalences were significantly greater than base rates for the general population. These are strikingly high rates of psychopathology in this chronic pain population, and are comparable to rates that have been reported in other studies (e.g., Fishbain, Goldberg, Meagher, Steele, & Rosomoff, 1986). We also found these rates to be higher than those in patients with acute low back pain (Kinney, Gatchel, Polatin, Fogarty, & Mayer, 1993). Subsequently, we found comparably high rates of psychopathology in other chronic pain disorders, such as temporomandibular disorder (TMD) (Gatchel, Garofalo, Ellis, & Holt, 1996; Kinney, Gatchel, Ellis, & Holt, 1992), as well as upper extremity disorders such as carpal tunnel syndrome (Burton, Polatin, & Gatchel, 1997; Mathis, Gatchel, Polatin, Boulas, & Kinney, 1994). Dersh, Polatin and Gatchel (2002) provide a more comprehensive review of such findings.

The Polatin et al. (1993) study also found that, of those patients with a positive lifetime history of psychiatric disorders, 54% of those with depression, 94% of those with substance abuse, and 95% of those with anxiety disorders had apparently experienced these syndromes *before* the onset of their back pain. These were the first results to suggest that certain psychiatric syndromes appear to precede chronic low back pain (substance abuse and anxiety disorders), whereas others (specifically, major depression) develop either before or after the onset of their low back pain. Depression was demonstrably high in chronic low back pain patients, and patients appeared to be divided equally between those who had depression before the onset of pain and those in whom depression developed after the onset of pain. This was one of the first studies to evaluate an important aspect of the "chicken and/or egg" question: what comes first, the pain or the psychopathology? We are continuing to evaluate the nature of the relationship between the two variables.

In another study, which led to the development of a prediction model to be used in our future studies, Gatchel, Polatin and Mayer (1995) found evidence of a "psychosocial disability factor" in low back pain patients. In this study, 421 patients presenting with acute low back pain complaints of less than six months were systematically evaluated with a comprehensive psychosocial assessment battery. Contact information was verified every three months by telephone for one year. Then, one year after the initial evaluation, all patients were contacted to participate in a structured telephone interview to document return-to-work status. The responses generated a logistic regression model which found that the following array of variables correctly classified 90.7% of the cases in terms of work status at one year: self-reported pain and disability scores, scores on Scale 3 of the MMPI, workers' compensation/personal injury insurance status, and gender. Thus, these results revealed the presence of a "psychosocial disability factor" associated with those injured workers most likely to develop chronic low back pain disability problems at one year. There were also no significant differences between the return-to-work and no-return-to-work groups in terms of physician-rated severity of the initial back injury or in the physical demands of the jobs to which the patients had to return. Such results again highlight the fact that chronic pain disability reflects not only the presence of some physical symptomatology, but that psychosocial characteristics make a significant contribution in determining which injured workers may develop chronic low back pain disability. In fact, some have argued that only a small amount of the total disability phenomenon in people complaining of low back pain can be attributed to physical impairment (Waddell, Main, & Morris, 1984). Indeed, most cases of low back pain are ill defined and physically unverifiable, and are often classified as "soft tissue injuries" that cannot be visualized or verified on physical examination. Even the correlation between radiographic-documented disc-space narrowing and disc rupture level including disc herniation is less than 50% (Pope, Frymoyer, & Anderson, 1984). Moreover, an MRI study by Jensen, Brandt-Zawadzki, Obuchowski, et al. (1994) found significant spinal abnormalities in patients *not* experiencing low back pain.

On the basis of the above study, we can now identify those acute low back pain patients who may require early intervention to prevent development of chronic disability. This has formed the basis for a subsequent early intervention translational research with "high-risk" patients (to be reviewed later in this Chapter). We are also simultaneously conducting similar research with temporomandibular disorder (TMD) patients. Based upon a series of studies (Epker, Gatchel, & Ellis, 1999; Garofalo, Gatchel, Wesley, & Ellis, 1998), we have developed a prediction model that accurately classifies 91% of acute TMD patients who go on to develop chronic problems.

Other Comorbidity Issues

Along with our research on psychopathology and chronic pain disorders, we are also involved in the development of treatment outcomes research of interdisciplinary approaches to other chronic comorbid mental health and pain disorders. As previously noted, interdisciplinary treatment emphasizes the importance of addressing the complex needs of chronic pain patients, including their psychosocial needs. As reviewed earlier, the first truly effective interdisciplinary approach to chronic low back pain patients—functional restoration—was developed by Mayer and Gatchel (1988), which subsequently generated numerous studies documenting its effectiveness. It has also been shown to be effective for cervical spine disorders (Wright, Mayer, & Gatchel, 1999), upper extremity disorders (Mayer, Gatchel, Polatin, & Evans, 1999), TMD (Gardea, Gatchel, & Mishra, 2001; Mishra, Gatchel, & Gardea,

2000), as well as heterogeneous pain disorders (Robbins et al., 2003). Gatchel and Turk (1999) provide a comprehensive review of the positive treatment- and cost-effectiveness of such an interdisciplinary approach.

In all of our studies, we have been interested in the management of the comorbid mental health problems experienced by patients undergoing treatment, and whether it would limit successful rehabilitation. In one such study, we used the SCID to assess the prevalence of current and lifetime DSM diagnoses in a sample of chronic low back pain patients beginning an intensive three-week interdisciplinary treatment program (Gatchel, Polatin, Mayer, & Garcy, 1994). These patients were then followed over time, with treatment outcome being defined as return-to-work status one year after program completion. Despite high rates of Axis I and Axis II psychiatric disorders in this sample, neither type nor degree of psychopathology was found to be predictive of a patient's ability to successfully return to work.

An equally interesting series of results showed that elevated rates of psychopathology significantly decreased following the interdisciplinary treatment of chronic low back pain patients (Owen-Salters, Gatchel, Polatin, & Mayer, 1996; Vittengl, Clark, Owen-Salters, & Gatchel, 1999). The Owen-Salters et al. study (1996) evaluated patients for current psychiatric disorders on admission to the interdisciplinary program, and again at six months following completion of the treatment program. The results documented significant decreases in the prevalence of psychiatric disorders, particularly somatoform pain disorder and major depressive disorder. In a methodologically similar study, Vittengl et al. (1999) found decreased prevalence of Axis II personality disorders six months after completion of the treatment program in chronic low back pain patients. These two studies from our clinical research group demonstrate that effective rehabilitation significantly decreases the high comorbid rates of psychiatric disorders often found in chronic low back pain patients. Thus, comorbid mental health and pain disorders can be effectively treated by interdisciplinary programs.

Patient Heterogeneity and Response to Treatment

Now that we have found interdisciplinary treatment programs to be effective in managing many chronic pain syndromes, we are beginning to evaluate variables that may predict which patients respond best to such programs (see Gatchel & Epker, 1999). As noted by Turk and Okifuji (1998), one must avoid the assumption of "pain-patient homogeneity" in terms of response to treatment. There may be many individual differences or heterogeneity in such responses. Individuals with the same medical diagnosis may vary greatly in their response to their symptoms. Turk and colleagues, for example, have revealed that patients with diseases and syndromes as varied as back pain, headache, and metastatic cancer may display comparable adaptation patterns, whereas patients with the same diagnosis may actually show great variability in their degree of disability (e.g., Turk & Gatchel, 1999; Turk, Okifuji, Sinclair, & Starz, 1998).

As Turk and Gatchel (1999) have indicated, the traditional approach of "lumping" patients with the same medical diagnosis or set of symptoms together (e.g., back pain, fibromyalgia, temporomandibular disorder), and then to treat them all the same way, is not appropriate. That is because many of these common diagnoses are relatively gross categories, and there may be unique individual biopsychosocial differences of patients who fall under these generic diagnoses. Thus, some patients may respond quite positively to a certain treatment, whereas others may actually show no improvement at all. Therefore, it is becoming more important to match a particular intervention to specific patient characteristics. As Turk and Rudy (1990) originally emphasized, the "pain patient homogeneity" myth must be debunked, and patient differences need to be taken into account in order to tailor the appropriate treatment program. Turk and Okifuji (2001) have provided a comprehensive review of the importance of the treatment-matching process and literature to support greater clinical efficacy of such a matching approach strategy.

A number of studies have already demonstrated that patients classified into different subgroups based on their behavioral and psychosocial characteristics responded differentially to identical treatments (Epker & Gatchel, 2000; Turk, 2002). This has been fairly consistently observed across different types of pain syndromes (e.g., cancer, fibromyalgia, headache, low back pain and TMD). The differences in the psychosocial profiles displayed by patients has led to attempts to categorize different subgroups of patients and then to evaluate differential response to a treatment. For example, several outcome studies have demonstrated the effective use of the Multidimensional Pain Inventory (MPI) as one way to categorize subgroups of patients (as adaptive copers, dysfunctional, or interpersonally distressed). Adaptive Coper patients report a high level of social support and relatively low level of pain and perceived interference with their lives. In addition, they usually report relatively high levels of activity despite their pain, and often respond well to pain management procedures. In contrast, dysfunctional profile patients tend to perceive the severity of their pain to be high and to report that pain interferes with much of their lives. They also report a high degree of psychological distress because of their pain and, as a result, usually report low levels of activity. Interpersonally distressed patients are similar to dysfunctional profile patients, but they also perceive that their significant others are not very understanding about their condition. They, therefore, think that they have no good social support to help them with their pain behavior problems.

Turk and Okifuji (1998) have reviewed additional research demonstrating the utility of the above MPI subgroups with other chronic pain conditions, including headache, TMD pain and fibromyalgia. Assessment of such MPI profiles will help to "tailor" the needs for treatment strategies to account for the different psychosocial characteristics of patients. For example, patients with an interpersonally distressed profile may need additional clinical attention addressing interpersonal skills to perform effectively in a group-oriented treatment program. Pain patients with dysfunctional and interpersonally distressed profiles display more indications of acute and chronic personality differences, relative to adaptive coper profile patients, and they would therefore require more clinical management (e.g., Etscheidt, Steiger, & Braverman, 1995). Such additional attention, however, would not necessarily be essential for adaptive coper profile patients.

Studies such as those above support the notion that, because patients' responses to treatment differ as a function of their psychosocial coping profiles, then specific treatment modalities are more likely to be better suited than others for each profile. An important issue for future clinical research is whether there are other types of biopsychosocial profiles that are more or less responsive to different treatment modalities. For example, variables that have been found to be predictors of pain-related disability outcomes, such as catastrophizing, fear of movement/re-injury, pain beliefs, anxiety and depression, etc., and their interactions with environmental factors, such as workplace variables, health care system variables, etc., need to be more closely evaluated (Turk & Monarch, 2002).

There are also a number of other inventories that are useful in helping to better tailor treatment to medical patients in general. These instruments are beneficial for treatment personnel who can use the results to identify the best treatment approach and to anticipate potential patient management problems. Two will be discussed here.

The Millon Behavioral Health Inventory (MBHI). Millon, Green and Meagher (1982) originally developed the MBHI, which is a 150-question true-false test based on 20 clinical scales that reflect medically related concerns, such as compliance with treatment regimens and reaction to treatment personnel. The MBHI's clinical scales include those that rate introversive style, cooperative style, social style, premorbid pessimism, pain treatment responsivity, and emotional vulnerability. Several of these scales are clinically meaningful in assessment of pain patients. For example, in our treatment programs for patients with chronic low back pain, we often find that people who score low on the cooperative style scale and high on the sensitive style demonstrate poor treatment outcome (Gatchel, Mayer, Capra, Diamond, & Barnett, 1986). These patients usually tend not to follow advice and can be unpredictable and moody. Obviously, such personality characteristics can be detrimental to any group-oriented treatment process. In marked contrast, patients scoring high on cooperative and sociable scales demonstrate excellent outcome. We have also found that patients who score high on the emotional vulnerability scale usually require additional psychosocial treatment in dealing with their pain and disability, as we found in treating chronic headache patients (Gatchel, Deckel, Weinberg, & Smith, 1985). The MBHI scales can be useful for helping treatment personnel to better understand important personality characteristics that are directly related to response to a medical treatment environment, such as an interdisciplinary pain management program.

The Millon Behavioral Medicine Diagnostic (MBMD). Millon and colleagues have recently developed the MBMD, which has some advantages over the MBHI. This was done because several important psychosocial characteristics were not evaluated by the MBHI (Bockian, Meager, & Millon, 2000). These include the following:

- Information concerning the presence of psychiatric indicators, such as anxiety and emotional stability, which could potentially influence patients' adjustment to their medical condition.
- Information on coping styles that reflect potential personality disorders.
- Information about other psychosocial variables related to cognitive appraisals (e.g., self-esteem, functional efficacy), resources (spiritual and religious), and contextual factors (functional abilities).
- Information about specific lifestyle behaviors (e.g., alcohol and substance abuse, smoking, exercise routine, eating patterns).
- Information about a patient's communication styles (e.g., tendencies toward disclosure, social desirability, preference for more or fewer details concerning medical information).

Such detailed information is useful for predicting patient compliance to a recommended treatment regimen, potential medication abuses, and emotional responses to stressful medical procedures (which, in turn, can be beneficial in health care management decision-making and the triage process for mental health treatment).

Early Intervention with High-Risk Acute Pain Patients

As reviewed earlier, our most recent research has focused on the use of the empirically developed "high-risk" acute patient profile associated with the development of chronic disability problems. Our first one-year prospective outcome study (Gatchel et al., 2003) clearly revealed that high-risk acute low back pain patients who received early intervention displayed significantly greater improvements in psychosocial functioning, pain levels, medication use, health care utilization and occupational outcomes. Greater cost savings were also found. We are currently conducting a similar study with acute TMD patients employing an abbreviated version of functional restoration, developed specifically for these research programs. Again, it involves an interdisciplinary team approach, and is based upon the assumption that almost all patients suffering from comorbid mental health and pain disability can be returned to a productive lifestyle through appropriate medical care/ physical reconditioning and psychosocial interventions such as coping skills training. This functional restoration is accomplished through an aggressive, individualized psychosocial and physical reconditioning program. Treatment is initially guided by quantified measurement of function, allowing the reconditioning to proceed safely, but providing quantifiable documentation of compliance, effort and eventual success. Psychosocial issues and return-to-work issues are simultaneously addressed. We have found that such issues can be effectively dealt with using psychosocial approaches (Turk & Gatchel, 2002). Table 1 provides the major components of functional restoration.

- Psychosocial and socioeconomic assessment to guide, individualize, and monitor cognitive-behavioral oriented interventions and outcomes
- Multimodal disability management program using cognitive-behavioral interventions
- Formal, repeated quantification of physical deficits to guide, individualize, and monitor physical training
- Physical reconditioning of the injured functional unit
- Generic work simulation and whole-body retraining
- Psychopharmacological interventions for detoxification and psychosocial management
- Interdisciplinary, medically directed team approach with formal staffings, frequent team conferences, and low staff-to-patient ratios
- Ongoing outcome evaluation, using standardized objective criteria

Table 1. Major Components of an Interdisciplinary Functional Restoration Program

Summary and Conclusions

We are entering an exciting period in psychopathology and chronic pain research, resulting from a major paradigm shift away from an outdated *biomedical reductionism* approach, to a more pragmatic and comprehensive *biopsychosocial model* which emphasizes the unique interactions among biological, psychological and social factors that need to be taken into account to better understand health and illness. Suls and Rothman (2004, p. 119) have recently reviewed the evolution of the biopsychosocial model, and noted how the reciprocal relationship of the biological, psychological and social processes has stimulated dramatic advances in health psychology over the past two decades. As they point out: "As a guiding framework, the biopsychosocial model has proven remarkably successful as it has enabled health psychologists to be at the forefront of efforts to forge a multilevel, multisystems approach to human functioning. However, considerable, perhaps even daunting challenges remain as models are needed that specify the processes that connect the biological, psychological, and social systems." Another major reason for the now increased embrace of the biopsychosocial model has been the heightened prevalence of chronic pain conditions in this country, which can be expected to continue to rise. Chronic pain most often is accompanied by comorbid psychopathology, thus necessitating the use of a biopsychosocial approach to assessment and intervention programs for such comorbid chronic illnesses. As reviewed in this Chapter, the biopsychosocial approach to one such prevalent comorbid medical problem—chronic pain—has been shown to be quite effective, and it will hopefully lead to further breakthroughs in the areas of etiology, assessment, treatment and prevention. Of course, the major paradigm shift to the biopsychosocial model is still in its infancy stage, and new developments can be expected in the future. Our major task will be to ensure that its continued evolution occurs in a scientifically rigorous manner, with consistent efforts toward the systematic translation of this new biopsychosocial approach to comorbid psychopathology and chronic pain into the clinical arena where it can be further validated.

References

Barrett, J. F., Rose, R. M., & Klerman, G. L. (Eds.). (1979). *Stress and mental disorder.* New York: Raven Press.

Bendix, A. E., Bendix, T., Vaegter, K., Lund, C., Frolund, L., & Holm, L. (1996). Multidisciplinary intensive treatment for chronic low back pain: A randomized, prospective study. *Cleveland Clinic Journal of Medicine, 63,* 62-69.

Bendix, T., & Bendix, A. (1994). *Different training programs for chronic low back pain— A randomized, blinded one-year follow-up study.* Paper presented at the International Society for the Study of the Lumbar Spine, Seattle.

Bingel, V., Quante, M., Knab, R., Bromm, B., Weiller, C., & Buchel, C. (2002). Subcortical structures involved in pain processing: Evidence from single trial MRI. *Pain, 99,* 313-321.

Blanchard, E. B., Kirsch, C. A., Applebaum, K. A., & Jaccard, J. (1989). Role of psychopathology in chronic headache: Cause or effect? *Headache, 29,* 295-301.

Bockian, N., Meager, S., & Millon, T. (2000). Assessing personality with The Millon Behavioral Health Inventory, The Millon Behavioral Medicine Diagnostic, and The Millon Clinical Multiaxial Inventory. In R. J. Gatchel & J. N. Weisberg (Eds.), *Personality characteristics of patients with pain.* Washington, DC: American Psychological Association Press.

Burke, S., Harms-Constas, C., & Aden, P. (1994). Return to work/work retention outcomes of a functional restoration program: A multi-center, prospective study with a comparison group. *Spine, 19,* 1880-1886.

Burton, K., Polatin, P. B., & Gatchel, R. J. (1997). Psychosocial factors and the rehabilitation of patients with chronic work-related upper extremity disorders. *Journal of Occupational Rehabilitation, 7,* 139-153.

Coghill, R. C., McHaffie, J. G., & Yen, Y. F. (2003). Neural correlates of interindividual differences in the subjective experience of pain. *PNAS, 100*(14), 8538-8542.

Corey, D. T., Koepfler, L. E., Etlin, D., & Day, H. I. (1996). A limited functional restoration program for injured workers: A randomized trial. *Journal of Occupational Rehabilitation, 6,* 239-249.

Dersh, J., Polatin, P., & Gatchel, R. (2002). Chronic pain and psychopathology: Research findings and theoretical considerations. *Psychosomatic Medicine, 64,* 773-786.

Deschner, M., & Polatin, P. B. (2000). Interdisciplinary programs: Chronic pain management. In T. G. Mayer, R. J. Gatchel & P. B. Polatin (Eds.), *Occupational musculoskeletal disorders: function, outcomes & evidence* (pp. 629-637). Philadelphia: Lippincott, Williams & Wilkins.

Engel, G. L. (1977). The need for a new medical model: A challenge for biomedicine. *Science, 196*(4286), 129-136.

Epker, J., & Gatchel, R. J. (2000). Coping profile differences in the biopsychosocial functioning of TMD patients. *Psychosomatic Medicine, 62*, 69-75.

Epker, J. T., Gatchel, R. J., & Ellis, E. (1999). An accurate model for predicting TMD chronicity: Practical applications in clinical settings. *Journal of the American Dental Association, 130*, 1470-1475.

Etscheidt, M. A., Steiger, H. G., & Braverman, B. (1995). Multidimensional pain inventory profile classifications and psychopathology. *Journal of Consulting & Clinical Psychology, 51*, 29-36.

Fishbain, D. (1999). The association of chronic pain and suicide. *Seminars in Clinical Neuropsychiatry, 4*, 221-227.

Fishbain, D. A., Goldberg, M., Meagher, B. R., Steele, R., & Rosomoff, H. (1986). Male and female chronic pain patients categorized by DSM-III psychiatric diagnostic criteria. *Pain, 26*, 181-197.

Frymoyer, J. W., & Durett, C. L. (1997). The economics of spinal disorders. In J. W. Frymoyer et al. (Eds.), *The adult spine* (2nd ed., Vol. 1, pp. 143-150). Philadelphia: Lippincott-Raven.

Gallagher, R. M. (2002). *The pain-depression conundrum: Bridging the body and mind.* Retrieved August 10, 2003, from http://www.medscape.com/viewprogram/2030

Gardea, M. A., Gatchel, R. J., & Mishra, K. D. (2001). Long-term efficacy of biobehavioral treatment of temporomandibular disorders. *Journal of Behavioral Medicine, 24*, 341-359.

Garofalo, J. P., Gatchel, R. J., Wesley, A. L., & Ellis, E. (1998). Predicting chronicity in acute temporomandibular disorders using the research diagnostic criteria. *Journal of the American Dental Association, 129*(4), 438-447.

Gatchel, R. J. (1991). Early development of physical and mental deconditioning in painful spinal disorders. In T. G. Mayer, V. Mooney & R. J. Gatchel (Eds.), *Contemporary conservative care for painful spinal disorders* (pp. 278-289). Philadelphia: Lea & Febiger.

Gatchel, R. J. (1996). Psychological disorders and chronic pain: Cause and effect relationships. In R. J. Gatchel & D. C. Turk (Eds.), *Psychological approaches to pain management: A practitioner's handbook* (pp. 33-52). New York: Guilford.

Gatchel, R. J. (1999). Perspectives on Pain: A Historical Overview. In R. J. Gatchel & D. C. Turk (Eds.), *Psychosocial factors in pain: critical perspectives* (pp. 3-17). New York: Guilford.

Gatchel, R. J. (2004). Comorbidity of chronic mental and physical health disorders: A biopsychosocial perspective. *American Psychologist, 59*, 792-805.

Gatchel, R. J., Deckel, A. W., Weinberg, N., & Smith, J. E. (1985). The utility of the Millon Behavioral Health Inventory in the study of chronic headache. *Headache, 25*, 49-54.

Gatchel, R. J., & Dersh, J. (2002). Psychological disorders and chronic pain: Are there cause and effect relationships? In D. C. Turk & R. J. Gatchel (Eds.), *Psychological approaches to pain management: A practitioner's handbook* (2nd ed., pp. 30-51). New York: Guilford.

Gatchel, R. J., & Epker, J. T. (1999). Psychosocial predictors of chronic pain and response to treatment. In R. J. Gatchel & D. C. Turk (Eds.), *Psychosocial factors in pain: critical perspectives* (pp. 412-434). New York: Guilford.

Gatchel, R. J., Garofalo, J. P., Ellis, E., & Holt, C. (1996). Major psychological disorders in acute and chronic TMD: An initial examination of the "chicken or egg" question. *Journal of the American Dental Association, 127*, 1365-1374.

Gatchel, R. J., & Mayer, T. G. (1989). Functional restoration for chronic low back pain, part II: Multimodal disability management. *Pain Management, 2*, 136-140.

Gatchel, R. J., & Mayer, T. G. (2000). Occupational musculoskeletal disorders: Introduction and overview of the problem. In T. G. Mayer, R. J. Gatchel & P. B. Polatin (Eds.), *Occupational musculoskeletal disorders: function, outcomes, and evidence* (pp. 3-8). Philadelphia: Lippincott Williams & Wilkins.

Gatchel, R. J., Mayer, T. G., Capra, P., Diamond, P., & Barnett, J. (1986). Quantification of lumbar function, Part VI: The use of psychological measures in guiding physical functional restoration. *Spine, 11*, 36-42.

Gatchel, R. J., Mayer, T. G., Hazard, R. G., Rainville, J., & Mooney, V. (1992). Functional restoration. Pitfalls in evaluating efficacy [editorial] [see comments]. *Spine, 17*(8), 988-995.

Gatchel, R. J., Noe, C., Gajraj, N. M., Vakharia, A. S., Polatin, P. B., Deschner, M., et al. (2001). Treatment carve-out practices: Their effect on managing pain at an interdisciplinary pain center. *The Journal of Workers Compensation, 10*(2), 50-63.

Gatchel, R. J., Polatin, P. B., & Mayer, T. G. (1995). The dominant role of psychosocial risk factors in the development of chronic low back pain disability. *Spine, 20*(24), 2702-2709.

Gatchel, R. J., Polatin, P. B., Mayer, T. G., & Garcy, P. D. (1994). Psychopathology and the rehabilitation of patients with chronic low back pain disability. *Archives of Physical Medicine and Rehabilitation, 75*, 666-670.

Gatchel, R. J., Polatin, P. B., Noe, C. E., Gardea, M. A., Pulliam, C., & Thompson, J. (2003). Treatment and cost-effectiveness of early intervention for acute low back pain patients: A one-year prospective study. *Journal of Occupational Rehabilitation, 13*, 1-9.

Gatchel, R. J., & Turk, D. C. (1996). *Psychological Approaches to Pain Management: A Practitioner's Handbook*. New York: Guilford.

Gatchel, R. J., & Turk, D. C. (1999). Interdisciplinary treatment of chronic pain patients. In R. J. Gatchel & D. C. Turk (Eds.), *Psychosocial Factors in Pain: Critical Perspectives* (pp. 435-444). New York: Guilford.

Goldberg, D., Privett, M., Ustun, B., Simon, G., & Linden, M. (1998). The effects of detection and treatment on the outcome of major depression in primary care:

a naturalistic study in 15 cities. *British Journal of General Practice, 48*(437), 1840-1844.

Gracely, R. H., & Clauw, D. J. (2002). *Functional magnetic resonance imaging evidence of abnormal pain-processing pathways in low back pain.* Paper presented at the Annual Meeting of the American College of Rheumatology, New Orleans, LA.

Gracely, R. H., Petzke, F., Wolf, J. M., & Clauw, D. J. (2002). Functional magnetic resonance imaging evidence of augmented pain processing in fibromyalgia. *Arthritis and Rheumatism, 46,* 1333-1343.

Gureje, O., Simon, G., & Von Korff, M. (2001). A cross-national study of the course of persistent pain in primary care. *PAIN, 92*(1-2), 195-200.

Hanscom, D., & Jex, R. (2001). Sleep disorders, depression and musculoskeletal pain. *SpineLine, 2*(5), 56-59.

Hazard, R. G. (1995). Spine update: Functional restoration. *Spine, 20,* 2345-2348.

Hazard, R. G., Fenwick, J. W., Kalisch, S. M., Redmond, J., Reeves, V., Reid, S., et al. (1989). Functional restoration with behavioral support: A one-year prospective study of patients with chronic low-back pain. *Spine, 14,* 157-161.

Hendler, N. H. (1982). The four stages of pain. In N. H. Hendler, D. M. Long, T. N. Wise, et al. (Eds.), *Diagnosis and treatment of chronic pain* (pp. 42-63). Littleton: PSG, Inc.

Hildebrandt, J., Pfingsten, M., Saur, P., & Jansen, J. (1997). Prediction of success from a multidisciplinary treatment program for chronic low back pain. *Spine, 22,* 990-1001.

Jensen, M. C., Brant-Zawadzki, M. N., Obuchowski, N., Modic, M. T., Malkasian, D., & Ross, J. S. (1994). Magnetic resonance imaging of the lumbar spine in people without back pain. *The New England Journal of Medicine, 331,* 69-73.

Joint Commission on Accreditation of Healthcare Organizations. (2000). *Pain Assessment and Management: An organizational approach.* Oakbrook, IL: Author.

Jousset, N., Fanello, S., Bontoux, L., Dubus, V., Billabert, C., Vielle, B., et al. (2004). Effects of functional restoration versus 3 hours per week physical therapy: A randomized controlled study. *Spine, 29*(5), 487-493.

Katon, W., Sullivan, M., & Walker, E. (2001). Medical symptoms without identified pathology: relationship to psychiatric disorders, childhood and adult trauma, and personality traits. *Annals of Internal Medicine, 134*(9 Pt. 2), 917-925.

Keel, P., Wittig, R., Deutschman, R., Diethelm, U., Knusel, O., Loschmann, C., et al. (1998). Effectiveness of in-patient rehabilitation for sub-chronic and chronic low back pain by a integrative group treatment program. *Scandinavian Journal of Rehabilitation Medicine, 30,* 211-219.

Kermond, W., Gatchel, R. J., & Mayer, T. G. (1991). Functional restoration for chronic spinal disorders or failed back surgery. In T. G. Mayer, V. Mooney & R. J. Gatchel (Eds.), *Contemporary conservative care for painful spinal disorders* (pp. 473-481). Philadelphia: Lea & Febiger.

Kinney, R. K., Gatchel, R. J., Ellis, E., & Holt, C. (1992). Major psychological disorders in chronic TMD patients: Management implications. *Journal of the American Dental Association, 123*, 49-54.

Kinney, R. K., Gatchel, R. J., Polatin, P. B., Fogarty, W. J., & Mayer, T. G. (1993). Prevalence of psychopathology in acute and chronic low back pain patients. *Journal of Occupational Rehabilitation, 3*(2), 95-103.

Kirschbaum, C., & Hellhammer, D. H. (1994). Salivary cortisol in psychoneuroendocrine research: Recent developments and applications. *Psychoneuroendocrinology, 19*, 313-333.

Kroenke, K., & Mangelsdorff, A. (1989). Common symptoms in ambulatory care: incidence, evaluation, therapy, and outcome. *Annual Journal of Medicine, 86*(3), 262-266.

Kroenke, K., Spitzer, R. L., & Williams, J. B. (1994). Physical symptoms in primary care. Predictors of psychiatric disorders and functional impairment. *Archives of Family Medicine, 3*(9), 774-779.

Loeser, J. D. (1982). Concepts of pain. In J. Stanton-Hicks & R. Boaz (Eds.), *Chronic low back pain* (pp. 121-155). New York: Raven Press.

Marketdata Enterprises. (1995). *Chronic pain management programs: A market analysis.* Valley Stream, NY: Author.

Marketdata Enterprises. (2001). *Chronic Pain Management Clinics. A Market Analysis.* Tampa, FL: Author.

Mathis, L. B., Gatchel, R. J., Polatin, P. B., Boulas, J., & Kinney, R. (1994). Prevalence of psychopathology in carpal tunnel syndrome patients. *Journal of Occupational Rehabilitation, 4*, 199-210.

Mayberg, H. S., Silva, J. A., Brannan, S. K., Tekell, J. L., Mahurin, R. K., McGinnis, B. S., et al. (2002). The functional neuroanatomy of the placebo effect. *American Journal of Psychiatry, 159*, 728-737.

Mayer, T., Gatchel, R., Polatin, P., & Evans, T. (1999). Outcomes comparison of treatment for chronic disabling work-related upper extremity disorders. *Journal of Occupational and Environmental Medicine, 41*, 761-770.

Mayer, T. G., & Gatchel, R. J. (1988). *Functional Restoration for Spinal Disorders: The Sports Medicine Approach.* Philadelphia: Lea & Febiger.

Mayer, T. G., & Gatchel, R. J. (1989). Functional restoration for chronic low back pain. Part I: quantifying physical function. *Pain Management, 2*, 67-75.

Mayer, T. G., Gatchel, R. J., Kishino, N., Keeley, J., Capra, P., Mayer, H., et al. (1985). Objective assessment of spine function following industrial injury: A prospective study with comparison group and one-year follow-up. *Spine, 10*, 482-493.

Mayer, T. G., Gatchel, R. J., Kishino, N., Keeley, J., Mayer, H., Capra, P., et al. (1986). A prospective short-term study of chronic low back pain patients utilizing novel objective functional measurement. *Pain, 25*(1), 53-68.

Mayer, T. G., Gatchel, R. J., Mayer, H., Kishino, N. D., Keeley, J., & Mooney, V. A. (1987). A prospective two-year study of functional restoration in industrial low back injury. An objective assessment procedure [published erratum appears in JAMA 1988 Jan 8;259(2):220]. *JAMA, 258*(13), 1763-1767.

Mayer, T. G., Mooney, V., Gatchel, R. J., Barnes, D., Terry, A., Smith, S., et al. (1989). Quantifying postoperative deficits of physical function following spinal surgery. *Clinical Orthopaedics & Related Research, 244*, 147-157.

Mayer, T. G., & Polatin, P. B. (2000). Tertiary nonoperative interdisciplinary programs: The functional restoration variant of the outpatient chronic pain management program. In T. G. Mayer, R. J. Gatchel & P. B. Polatin (Eds.), *Occupational musculoskeletal disorders: Function, outcomes & evidence* (pp. 639-649). Philadelphia: Lippincott, Williams & Wilkins.

McEwen, B. S. (1998). Protective and damaging effects of stress mediators. *New England Journal of Medicine, 338*, 171-179.

Melzack, R. (1999). Pain and stress: A new perspective. In R. J. Gatchel & D. C. Turk (Eds.), *Psychosocial factors in pain: Critical perspectives*. New York: Guilford.

Melzack, R., & Wall, P. D. (1965). Pain mechanisms: A new theory. *Science, 50*, 971-979.

Miller, W. L., & Tyrrell, J. P. (1995). The adrenal cortex. In P. Felig, J. P. Baxter & L. A. Frohman (Eds.), *Endocrinology and metabolism* (3rd ed.). New York: Guilford.

Millon, T., Green, C. J., & Meagher, R. B. (1982). *Millon Behavioral Health Inventory* (3rd ed.). Minneapolis: Interpretive Scoring System.

Mishra, K. D., Gatchel, R. J., & Gardea, M. A. (2000). The relative efficacy of three cognitive-behavioral treatment approaches to temporomandibular disorders. *Journal of Behavioral Medicine, 23*, 293-309.

Morley, S., Eccleston, C., & Williams, A. (1999). Systematic review and meta-analysis of randomized controlled trials of cognitive behavior therapy and behavior therapy for chronic pain in adults, excluding headache. *Pain, 80*, 1-13.

National Institute of Health Technology Assessment Panel. (1995, October). *Integration of behavioral and relaxation approaches into treatment of chronic pain and insomnia*. Paper presented at the National Institute of Health Technology Assessment Conference, Washington, D.C.

Ohayon, M. M., & Schatzberg, A. F. (2003). Using chronic pain to predict depressive morbidity in the general population. *Archives of General Psychiatry, 60*, 39-47.

Okasha, A., Ismail, M. K., Khalil, A. H., El Fiki, R., Soliman, A., & Okasha, T. (1999). A psychiatric study of nonorganic chronic headache patients. *Psychosomatic Medicine, 40*, 233-238.

Okifuji, A. (2003). Interdisciplinary pain management with pain patients: Evidence for its effectiveness. *Seminars in Pain Management, 1*, 110-119.

Owen-Salters, E., Gatchel, R. J., Polatin, P. B., & Mayer, T. G. (1996). Changes in psychopathology following functional restoration of chronic low back pain patients: A prospective study. *Journal of Occupational Rehabilitation, 6*, 215-223.

Parker, D. (1998). See suicide as preventable: A national strategy emerges. *Christian Science Monitor, 3*, pp. 8-9.

Petrovic, P., Kalso, E., Peterson, K. M., & Ingvar, M. (2002). Placebo and opioid analgesia—Imaging a shared neural network. *Science, 295,* 1787-1740.

Pilowsky, I. (1978). A general classification of abnormal illness behavior. *British Journal of Medical Psychiatry, 51*(2), 131-137.

Polatin, P. (1991). Predictors of low back pain. In A. White & R. Anderson (Eds.), *Conservative care of low back pain* (pp. 223-241). Baltimore: Williams & Wilkins.

Polatin, P. B., Kinney, R. K., Gatchel, R. J., Lillo, E., & Mayer, T. G. (1993). Psychiatric illness and chronic low-back pain. The mind and the spine—Which goes first? *Spine, 18*(1), 66-71.

Pope, M., Frymoyer, J., & Anderson, G. (1984). *Occupational low back pain.* New York: Praeger.

Pruessner, J. C., Wolf, O. T., Hellhammer, D. H., Buske-Kirschbaum, A., von Auer, K., Jobst, S., et al. (1997). Free cortisol levels after awakening: A reliable biological marker for the assessment of adrenocortical activity. *Life Sciences, 61*(26), 2539-2549.

Ray, Q. (2004). How the mind hurts and heals the body. *American Psychologist, 59,* 29-40.

Robbins, H., Gatchel, R. J., Noe, C., Gajraj, N., Polatin, P., Deschner, M., et al. (2003). A prospective one-year outcome study of interdisciplinary chronic pain management: Compromising its efficacy by managed care policies. *Anesthesia & Analgesia, 97,* 156-162.

Romano, J. M., & Turner, J. A. (1985). Chronic pain and depression: Does the evidence support a relationship? *Psychological Bulletin, 97,* 18-34.

Rosenzweig, M. R., Breedlove, S. M., & Leiman, A. L. (2002). *Biological Psychology.* Sunderland, MA: Sinauer Associates.

Rush, A., Polatin, P., & Gatchel, R. J. (2000). Depression and chronic low back pain: Establishing priorities in treatment. *SPINE, 25,* 2566-2571.

Sapolsky, R. M. (1996). Stress, glucocorticoids, and changes to the nervous system: The current state of confusion. *Stress, 1,* 1-19.

Smyth, J. M., Ockenfels, M. C., Gorin, A. A., Catley, D., Porter, L. S., Kirschbaum, C., et al. (1997). Individual differences in the diurnal cycle of cortisol. *Psychoneuroendocrinology, 22*(2), 89-105.

Suls, J., & Rothman, A. (2004). Evolution of the biopsychosocial model: Prospects and challenges for health psychology. *Health Psychology, 23,* 119-125.

Tuor, V. T., Malisza, K., Fonick, T., Papadimitropoulos, R., Jarmasz, M., Somorjai, R., et al. (2000). Functional magnetic resonance imaging in rats subjected to intensive electric and noxious chemical stimulation of the forepaw. *Pain, 65,* 123-167.

Turk, D., & Rudy, T. (1988). Toward an empirically derived taxonomy of chronic pain patients: Integration of psychological assessment data. *Journal of Consulting & Clinical Psychology, 56,* 233-238.

Turk, D. C. (2002). Clinical effectiveness and cost effectiveness of treatment for patients with chronic pain. *Clinical Journal of Pain, 18,* 355-365.

Turk, D. C., & Gatchel, R. J. (1999). Psychosocial factors and pain: Revolution and evolution. In R. J. Gatchel & D. C. Turk (Eds.), *Psychosocial factors in pain: Critical perspectives* (pp. 481-493). New York: Guilford.

Turk, D. C., & Gatchel, R. J. (Eds.). (2002). *Psychological approaches to pain management: A practitioner's handbook* (2nd ed.). New York: Guilford.

Turk, D. C., & Monarch, E. S. (2002). Biopsychosocial perspective on chronic pain. In D. C. Turk & R. J. Gatchel (Eds.), *Psychological approaches to pain management: A practitioner's handbook* (2nd ed., pp. 3-29). New York: Guilford.

Turk, D. C., & Okifuji, A. (1998). Treatment of chronic pain patients: Clinical outcomes, cost-effectiveness, and cost-benefits of multidisciplinary pain centers. *Critical Reviews in Physical and Rehabilitation Medicine, 10*(181-208).

Turk, D. C., & Okifuji, A. (2001). Matching treatment to assessment of patients with chronic pain. In D. C. Turk & R. Melzack (Eds.), *Handbook of pain assessment* (2nd ed., pp. 400-414). New York: Guilford.

Turk, D. C., Okifuji, A., Sinclair, J. D., & Starz, T. W. (1998). Interdisciplinary treatment for fibromyalgia syndrome: Clinical and statistical significance. *Arthritis Care & Research, 11*, 186-195.

Turk, D. C., & Rudy, T. E. (1990). Robustness of an empirically derived taxonomy of chronic pain patients. *Pain, 42*, 27-35.

U.S. Census Bureau. (2000). *Population projections of the United States by age, sex, race, Hispanic origin, and nativity: 1999 to 2100.* Washington, D.C.: U.S. Census Bureau.

U.S. Census Bureau. (2001). *The 65 years and over population: 2000.* Washington, D.C.: U.S. Census Bureau.

Verhaak, P. F. M., Kerssens, J. J., Dekker, J., Sorbi, M. J., & Bensing, J. M. (1998). Prevalence of chronic benign pain disorder among adults: A review of the literature. *Pain, 77*, 231-239.

Vittengl, J., Clark, L., Owen-Salters, E., & Gatchel, R. (1999). Diagnostic change and personality stability following functional restoration treatment in a chronic low back pain patient sample. *Assessment, 6*, 79-92.

Waddell, G. (1987). Clinical assessment of lumbar impairment. *Clinical Orthopedic Related Research, 221*, 110-120.

Waddell, G., Main, C. J., & Morris, E. W. (1984). Chronic low back pain, psychologic distress, and illness behavior. *Spine, 5*, 117-125.

Wright, A., Mayer, T. G., & Gatchel, R. J. (1999). Outcomes of disabling cervical spine disorders in compensation injuries. A prospective comparison to tertiary rehabilitation response for chronic lumbar spinal disorders. *Spine, 24*(2), 178-183.

Wright, A. R., & Gatchel, R. J. (2002). Occupational musculoskeletal pain and disability. In D. C. Turk & R. J. Gatchel (Eds.), *Psychological approaches to pain management: A practitioner's handbook* (2nd ed., pp. 349-364). New York: Guilford.

Chapter 9

Behavioral Prescriptions for Depression in Primary Care

David O. Antonuccio, Ph.D
University of Nevada School of Medicine
Elizabeth V. Naylor
University of Nevada, Reno

Depression is a prevalent and expensive condition. The primary care medical setting is where many if not most patients are seeking and receiving treatment for depression. Unfortunately, accurate assessment and effective treatment of depression remains limited in the primary care environment. Pharmaceutical interventions prevail as the predominant treatment delivered in primary care medical settings (Moore, 2004). While psychotropic medications can certainly help ameliorate mental and behavioral problems, all medical interventions carry with them certain risks and side effects (e.g., Antonuccio, Danton, DeNelsky, Greenberg, & Gordon, 1999). This chapter will briefly review the literature concerning the prevalence, costs, and treatment of depression, discuss how to effectively and efficiently diagnose depression in a time-limited primary care setting, and introduce behavioral prescriptions as a safe and practical alternative to the pharmaceutical treatment of depression in primary care.

Prevalence of Depression

The World Health Organization (2000) suggests that unipolar depression is currently the most prevalent psychiatric condition and predicts it will become the second most significant cause of global disease burden by 2020. It is estimated that major depression affects up to 24% of Americans at some time during their lives (Kessler et al., 2003). Furthermore, a variety of studies suggest that depression affects women twice as often as males (Antonuccio, Danton, & DeNelsky, 1995; Kessler et al., 1994; World Health Organization, 2000).

Depression in Primary Care

Up to one third of patients in waiting rooms of primary care settings may be experiencing clinically significant symptoms of depression (Robinson, 2003). Approximately 44% of depressed patients are receiving treatment for psychiatric problems in the medical setting (Greenberg, Stiglin, Finkelstein, & Berndt, 1993), an increase from 28% in 1990 (Greenberg et al., 1993). According to data collected from the 1987 and 1997 National Medical Expenditure Survey, the proportion of the population who received outpatient treatment for depression has increased 300% from .73 per 100 persons in 1987 to 2.33 per 100 persons in 1997; and, the proportion of depressed patients treated by primary care physicians increased significantly from 68.7% to 87.3% (Olfson et al., 2002). Despite the notable increase in both the prevalence and treatment of depression in primary care, a variety of studies suggest primary care physicians lack appropriate skills to accurately diagnose and effectively treat depression. For instance, primary care physicians missed the diagnosis of major depressive disorder in 66% of patients with the presenting symptomolgy (Schwenk, 1994); 32% of primary care patients with major depression remained undetected for up to one year (Rost et al., 1998); and, only 20% of primary care patients with major depression recovered in eight months as compared to 70% who recovered after receiving treatment from mental health practitioners (Schulberg et al., 1996).

A myriad of medical concerns often co-occur with depression. Depression has been associated with increased medical utilization, negative perceptions of health status, poor adherence to disease management regimes, and elevated risk of morbidity and mortality (Katon et al., 1992; Katon, et al., 1994; Wells et al., 1989). In addition, many who commit suicide visit a physician within months before killing themselves (Conwell, 1994; Pearson, Conwell & Lyness, 1997). All of these data strongly indicate that primary care physicians need to have available the best possible methods for recognizing and effectively treating depression as early as possible.

Costs Associated with Depression

Although the prevalence of depression has remained fairly stable at 18 million Americans (Greenberg et al., 2003), the costs associated with depression have increased at an alarming rate; from 44 billion dollars in 1990 (Greenberg et. al, 1993) to 83 billion dollars in 2000 (Greenberg et al., 2003). An estimated 60% of primary care office visits do not result in an official biological diagnosis (Cummings, Pallik, Dorken & Hinke, 2000); and, it's probable that many of these patients who are utilizing medical services are reporting somatic complaints, including sleep, appetite, and concentration problems that may be related to depression. Among individuals diagnosed with major depression, research has supported a link between the presence of chronic psychological conditions and emergency room visits; one of ten episodes of treatment involve an emergency room visit and can lead to a higher usage of inpatient services, costing at least $2500 per individual diagnosed with major depression (Cucciare & O'Donohue, 2003).

Symptoms/Recognition of Depression

Depression has a number of debilitating symptoms that are detailed below. Severe role impairment associated with depression has been documented in a variety of domains, including social and work roles (Kessler et al., 2003). The nine cardinal symptoms of depression are listed below (American Psychiatric Association, 2000):

1. Depressed mood. Patients with depression usually describe their mood as sad, discouraged, hopeless, helpless, "blue," or "down in the dumps" (or some other colloquial variant). Depressed mood of clinical depression differs from sadness and grief in that it persists for at least two weeks and is accompanied by undue pessimism about the future and diminished self esteem. Irritible mood may be present in adolescents and children.
2. Loss of interest or pleasure or, stated alternatively, decrease in the rate of engagement in activities, particularly pleasant activities.
3. Significant changes in weight or appetite
4. Sleep disturbance (insomnia or hyperinsomnia)
5. Psychomotor agitation or retardation
6. Fatigue, which may include feeling overwhelmed or burdened by financial problems, marital difficulties, and job responsibilities. Typically, the patient feels as if an insupportable weight is resting on her or his shoulders.
7. Feelings of worthlessness, self-reproach, or excessive or inappropriate guilt. Some depressed patients believe they are being punished for sins they have committed.
8. Decreased ability to concentrate
9. Recurrent thoughts of death or suicide

There are a variety of recognized diagnoses for depression (which are specified by the fourth revised addition of the Diagnostic and Statistical Manual of Mental Disorders; DSM-IV-TR; APA, 2000) that vary in presentation, duration, intensity, and severity. Diagnostic criteria for major depressive episode in adults require that five or more of the nine previously listed symptoms of depression, including depressed mood or loss of interest or pleasure, be present during the same two week period and present a change from previous functioning. In dysthymic disorder, symptoms are similar and persist off and on for at least two years; however, suicidal ideation is not present and the symptoms are not sufficiently severe to meet the criteria for major depressive episode. Adjustment disorder with depressed mood manifests with a similar pattern of symptoms that arise as a maladaptive response to an identifiable psychosocial stressor.

The behavioral prescriptions that will be described are proposed for use in treating adult outpatients with one of the following diagnoses: mild or moderate major depressive episode, dysthymic disorder (or depressive neurosis), adjustment disorder with depressed mood, or the "depressions of everyday living," such as grief reactions and affective reactions to illness, injury, or surgery. Hence, the behavioral prescriptions will be used for mild to moderate unipolar depression and *not* bipolar depression. Bipolar depression differs from unipolar depression in that is characterized by manic episodes, with or without depressive episodes (as detailed by the nine cardinal symptoms). A manic episode is characterized by a concentrated period of abnormally high affect or irritability and includes three or more of the following symptoms: increased self-esteem or gradiosity, diminished need for sleep, increased talking as compared to usual, distractibility, increase in goal-oriented activities or psychomotor agitation, and engaging in pleasurable activities that have likely negative results (APA, 2000).

Differential diagnosis can be complicated for three reasons: (1) Depression often produces the "vegetative" somatic symptoms listed previously, (2) Depression may also induce a variety of other somatic complaints, such as aches and pains, fatigue, disturbed sleep, and gastrointestinal complaints (Kroenke et al., 1994), and, (3) a significant percentage of cases of depression result from a medical disorder. In patients with concomitant cardiovascular disease, neurological disorders, cancer, diabetes, HIV disease, and several other physical disorders, there is a twofold greater risk of developing symptoms associated with a depressive disorder (Kroenke, 2003). Various medications have also been associated with depressive symptoms (Bardage & Isacson, 2000). Depression may resolve completely with successful treatment of the medical problem. Therefore, a thorough, careful medical evaluation should be done and developmental, psychosocial, and family histories taken for any patient with possible depression.

Assessment of Depression

The behavioral prescriptions to be proposed for use by primary care doctors should be limited to adult outpatients exhibiting mild to moderate degrees of nonsuicidal depression. Thus, accurate assessment of the severity of depression is essential. A thorough diagnostic interview should be undertaken in search of the DSM-IV-R criteria noted previously. Any indication of strong suicidal inclination, severe depression, psychosis, or previous manic episode (which warrants the diagnosis of bipolar affective disorder) should lead to referral of the patient to a mental health professional.

Further, two supplementary methods can be very useful in assessing the severity of depression. With the first, the patient rates current mood on a scale of 1 to 10, with 1 representing the most depressed and 10 representing the happiest he or she has ever felt. The physician can explore what was happening in the patient's life when mood was rated lowest or highest as a means of generating possible therapeutic approaches. Questions about what has worked to improve mood in the past may also prove helpful.

The second is a seven item questionnaire measure of depression designed for primary care settings known as the Beck Depression Inventory for Primary Care (BDI-PC; Beck, Guth, Steer, & Ball, 1997), which has demonstrated good reliability and validity (Steer, Cavalieri, Leonard, & Beck, 1999). This questionnaire requires 1-2 minutes of a patient's time and can be used as an excellent adjunct to a clinical interview. (This questionnaire can be purchased from The Psychological Corporation, 19500 Bulverde Road San Antonio, TX 78259 Telephone: 1-800-228-0752 Order Fax: 1-800-232-1223, Website: www.psychcorp.com.).

If depression, a potentially lethal condition, is suspected, the physician should spend at least 30 minutes with the patient, even if other patients are kept waiting. A depressed patient is likely to tell his or her history very slowly and be quite reluctant to reveal the depth of his or her feelings. The patient should be asked to describe mood, activity level, and interactions with others. Questions about personal current events (with emphasis on the degree of marital and job satisfaction and recent actual or perceived losses, such as death of a relative or friend or loss of job or status) and the patient's feelings about them are also important. Such special care and attention may not only reduce the risk of suicide but also improve the patient-physician relationship (Barrier, Li, & Jensen, 2003).

Treatment of Depression

Pharmaceutical interventions prevail as the predominant treatment delivered in primary care medical settings (Moore, 2004). Among adults 18-years-old and older, office visits where an antidepressant was mentioned in progress notes increased from 45.1 million in 1998 to 60 million in 2001. By 2001, antidepressants were mentioned in 7.1% of all office visits in outpatient settings (Moore, 2004). An analysis of the Medical Expenditure Survey in 1987 compared to 1997 found that the use of antidepressants as a treatment for depression increased from 37.3% to 74.5%, and the number of individuals receiving psychotherapy as a treatment for depression decreased from 71.2% to 60.2%, (Olfson et al., 2002). While psychotropic medications have been demonstrated as helpful in ameliorating mental and behavioral problems, all medical interventions carry with them certain risks and side effects (Antonuccio et al, 1999). As patients age and develop multiple health problems, the risks associated with combining medications also multiply. Consistent with the Hippocratic dictum, "first do no harm," the question arises about whether other nonpharmaceutical interventions can also be delivered in this setting to give physicians additional effective choices with fewer medical risks. This is especially important given that patients in a primary care setting often do not adhere to antidepressant medications due to side effects, lack of improvement in symptoms, or because they actually feel worse (Haslam, Brown, Atkinson, & Haslam, 2004).

Whether one subscribes to the Hippocratic dictum or takes a cost-benefit approach to treatment, it is impossible to ignore the fact that antidepressants are not medically benign treatments. The short-term side effects of the SSRIs are well established and commonly include agitation, sleep disruption, gastrointestinal problems, and sexual dysfunction (Antonuccio et al., 1999). Side effects and medical risks (including risk of dying) increase when SSRIs are combined with other medications (Dalfen & Stewart, 2001), as is often the case (Antonuccio et al., 1999). In addition, the withdrawal symptoms of SSRIs are substantial for many if not most patients (Coupland, Bell, & Potokar, 1996; Fava, 2002; Rosenbaum, Fava, Hood, Ashcroft, & Krebs, 1998). Though data are mixed and somewhat controversial, other potential risks that warrant further investigation include the association (though not established causal relationship) of SSRIs with breast cancer (e.g., Cotterchio, Kreiger, Darlington, & Steingart, 2000; Bahl, Cotterchio, & Kreiger, 2003; Halbreich, Shen, & Panaro, 1996; Moorman, Grubber, Millikan, & Newman, 2003; Sharpe, Collet, Belzile, Hanley, & Boivin, 2002), acts of deliberate self-harm (e.g., Donovan et al., 2000; Healy, 2002), manic episodes (e.g., Preda et al., 2001), and the possibility of irreversible biochemical changes predisposing some susceptible patients to chronic depression (e.g., Baldessarini, 1995; Fava, 1995; Fava, 2002).

The rationale behind the idea that behavioral prescriptions might be an effective alternative to drug prescriptions is that (1) psychotherapy (particularly cognitive therapy, behavioral activation, and interpersonal therapy) compares favorably with medications in the short term, even when the depression is severe (e.g., DeRubeis, Gelfand, Tang, & Simons, 1999), (2) psychotherapy appears superior to medications when long term follow-up is considered (Antonuccio, Danton, & DeNelsky, 1995; Hollon, Shelton, & Loosen, 1991), and (3) there are no apparent medical side effects. Several meta-analyses, reported in both psychiatry and psychology journals covering multiple studies with thousands of patients, are remarkably consistent in support of the perspective that psychotherapy is at least as effective as medication in the treatment of depression (e.g., Conte et al, 1986; DeRubeis et al., 1999; Dobson et al., 1989; Hollon et al, 1991; Robinson et al., 1990; Steinbrueck et al., 1983; Wexler & Ciccheti, 1992).

In the era of managed care, it is not enough to be effective; treatments must be cost-effective. Cost-benefit analysis demonstrates that cognitive-behavioral therapy (CBT) interventions are at least as cost-effective as antidepressant prescriptions. When medical cost-offset (Hunsley, 2003), relapse, and side effects are considered in a cost-benefit analysis, psychotherapy can be very cost-effective, particularly in a psychoeducational (e.g., therapist-assisted bibliotherapy) or group format (Antonuccio, Thomas, & Danton, 1997). A number of recent studies (Guthrie et al., 1999; Simon et al., 2001; McLeod, Budd, & McClelland, 1997) focus on the reduction of health care utilization cost via the development of psychosocial intervention programs including bibliotherapy for a variety of psychological conditions such as depression. More specifically, Antonuccio, Thomas, & Danton (1997) show that over a 2-year period, fluoxetine alone may result in 33% higher expected costs than individual CBT treatment for depression and the combination treatment may result in 23% higher costs than CBT alone. Integrating such psychological treatment into primary care settings results in a medical-cost offset or reduction in overall costs (Cummings et al., 2000).

The cognitive-behavioral model suggests that the quality of person-environment interactions can influence and be influenced by thoughts, behaviors, and feelings, and, that relationships among these factors are reciprocal. For example, separation from a spouse may lessen certain pleasant *behaviors*, which trigger *feelings* of depression, which lead to negative *thoughts* about the future, which result in more intense *feelings* of depression and even less energy for activities.

Cognitive-behavioral therapy is designed to intervene in one or more of these areas, to stop the downward spiral of depression, and to initiate an upward spiral. Typically, cognitive-behavioral interventions consist of "homework assignments" and other techniques aimed at helping the depressed patient change nonconstructive thoughts, increase pleasant activities, improve interpersonal skills, and learn relaxation techniques. They not only tend to alleviate the current episode of depression but also reduce the likelihood of future episodes by helping improve the patient's behavioral repertoire and coping ability.

It is impractical for physicians in a primary care setting to deliver effective psychotherapy for depression; however, it is reasonable to assume that they may be able to practically deliver components of empirically validated psychotherapies in the form of brief behavioral prescriptions. The homework assignments of cognitive-behavioral therapy can be translated into behavioral prescriptions, which fit the concept of treatment familiar to physicians. If medical problems and mental disorders other than depression have been ruled out, if suicide is not an acute risk, and if the diagnosis is mild or moderate depression, the physician can tell the patient that he or she appears to be experiencing an episode of depression. The fact that depression is very common should be made clear and the relationship between depression and physical symptoms explained. The patient should be assured that the duration of depression is usually limited and that taking some action is likely to speed recovery. The physician can then prescribe some safe, effective alternatives to pharmaceuticals. Behavioral prescriptions should direct the depressed patient to *do* something differently the very next day or at least before the next appointment. The physician can quickly learn to creatively match the behavioral prescriptions to the patient's life-style preferences. Figure 1 summarizes the diagnostic and therapeutic protocol described in this and the preceding section.

Essential Components of Behavioral Prescriptions

The keys to using behavioral prescriptions follow.

1. *Rapport.* A good patient-physician relationship can be a lifeline for the depressed individual. It can be established in a short time, even with a new patient through the use of open-ended questions and active listening (Barrier, Li, & Jensen, 2003).
2. *Confidence in methods.* No physician can exude total confidence in any clinical skill at first. Data supporting the effectiveness of these methods when used by primary care physicians are not yet available; however, research is currently underway to provide these data. Nonetheless, they are based on solid evidence of their effectiveness when used by mental health professionals.
3. *Step-by-step action.* On the basis of rapport with and knowledge of the patient, the physician can persuade the patient to take action in small steps. For example, the patient can be advised to reinstitute a recently ignored pleasant activity, curb self-destructive behavior, or confront an obsessive negative thought. Each of these actions is, at least in part, demonstrably under the patient's control.

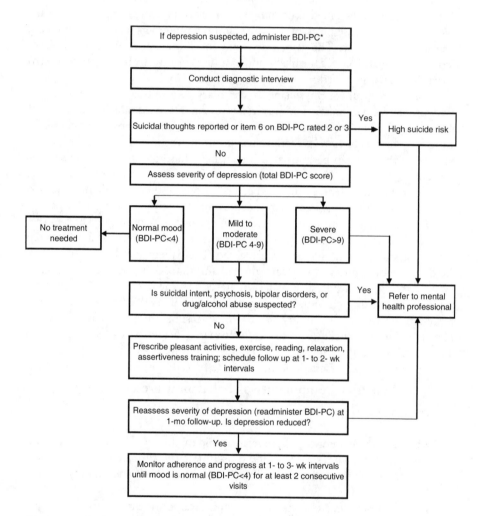

Figure 1. Protocol for diagnosis and behavioral prescription treatment of depression.
BDI-PC, Beck Depression Inventory-Primary Care

4. *Reversal of downward spiral of depression.* As noted previously, depression almost always entails a vicious spiral in which mood, thoughts, and behaviors facilitate one another's downward course. For instance, depressed mood may lead to negative thoughts (eg. I'll never find someone willing to marry me"), which lead to self-medication with alcohol, which leads to inactivity, which leads to an even more depressed mood and more negative thoughts. The result may be feelings of hopelessness, helplessness, and powerlessness. Behavioral prescriptions are potentially useful in reversing this spiral.

High Priority Prescriptions

The following general prescriptions need to be given high priority in a cognitive-behavioral approach to depression.

1. Prescribe an increase in positive or pleasant behavior. After asking the patient about enjoyable activities, prescribe one of them, e.g. a massage, skiing, dancing, listening to music, walking in the park, or calling a friend. The goal is to help the patient, over time, reestablish a regular pattern of positive behavior. Initially, the key is to persuade the patient to engage in at least one extra positive, pleasant activity, as often as from once a week to once a day.

2. Teach the patient how to substitute a realistic thought for an unduly pessimistic one. The extremely negative thoughts that plague depressed patients are often not provable and represent overgeneralization, catastrophizing, or perfectionism. For instance, "I will never find someone willing to marry me" is an extremely pessimistic statement about "forever" that cannot be shown to be true or false except over a lifetime. A more realistic thought may be, "The way I feel and act now makes me unattractive, so I want to work on changing my behavior." Consider prescribing that the patient read *Feeling Good* (Burns, 1999), a book devoted to strategies to enhance constructive thinking.

3. Evaluate the patient's use of such anxiety enhancing chemicals as caffeine and nicotine. Many depressed patients try to overcome their decrease in energy and activity level with coffee or cigarettes. The suggestion to cut back a little each day is appropriate. Also, consider prescribing relaxation exercises. Progressive muscle relaxation, imagery, meditation, and deep breathing are all examples of relaxation exercises. Relaxation audiotapes and CDs can be purchased online and at most bookstores. (One series is available through the Albert Ellis Institute, http://www.rebt.org/booksandtape/selfhelpaudiotapes.asp.).

4. Evaluate current use of alcohol and other drugs. Alcohol abuse or overuse in an attempt to self-medicate often exacerbates symptoms of depression. An explanation of the CNS effects of alcohol should be followed by the suggestion that no more than one or two alcoholic beverages be consumed in a 24-hour period. If the patient indicates that limiting drinking will be difficult, provide information on local treatment programs or prescribe attendance at Alcoholics Anonymous meetings.

5. Prescribe regular exercise. Many depressed patients, by the time they see a physician, have stopped exercising entirely, and some feel guilty about it. Physical exercise can not only improve the patient's overall health but also may, in and of itself, improve mood (Blumenthal et al., 1999; Babyak et al., 2000). Once you have convinced the patient that exercise can help, ask that the amount of weekly exercise (e.g. number of miles walked or jogged, minutes of aerobic exercise completed) be monitored. After a brief baseline period, prescribe an increase of 10%. Prescription of an exercise or aerobics class through a local YMCA, community education program, or college or university provides the opportunity for socializing as well as exercising.

6. If the patient seems to have problems with assertiveness or other social skills, prescribe an assertiveness training class. Keep a class schedule from the local community college handy.

7. Prescribe bibliotherapy. Three outstanding self-help books written for the layperson are *Feeling Good* (Burns, 1999), *Control your Depression* (Lewinsohn, Munoz, Youngren, et al., 1986), and *A Guide to Rational Living* (Ellis & Harper, 1975). Bibliotherapy as a treatment for depression has been empirically validated in a number of studies (Akerson, Scogin, McKendree-Smith & Lyman, 1998; Cuijpers, 1997; Jamison & Scogin, 1995; Gould & Clum, 1993; Pantalon, Lubetkin & Fishman, 1995; Scogin, Jamison & Davis, 1990; Scogin, Jamison, & Gochneaut, K., 1989; Smith, Floyd, Scogin, & Jamison, 1997). Cuipers' (1997) meta-analysis of bibliotherapy and depression examining six studies yielded an impressive mean effect size of 0.82 (with a 95% confidence interval of 0.50 –1.15). It is advised to have copies of each book in the office. Once the patient has selected one, prescribe reading at least one chapter a week and trying some of the homework assignments suggested. Also, suggest audiotapes designed to help the depressed patient change negative thinking patterns. (One series is available through the Albert Ellis Institute, http://www.rebt.org/booksandtape/selfhelpaudiotapes.asp.). Such prescriptions give the patient the sense that he or she can *do* something constructive about depression. Because the patient can attribute change to personal effort rather than to an external agent, more durable change is likely to result.

8. Be creative in writing cognitive-behavioral prescriptions. For example, some patients might benefit from being encouraged to obtain a companion animal. Research has demonstrated that a pet can help a patient to reduce loneliness, decrease depression, more effectively cope with stressful life events, improve activities of daily living, and increase social interactions (Geisler, 2004).

Follow-up and other considerations

As with medication prescriptions, the physician needs to tell the patient that adherence to behavioral prescriptions and progress will be carefully monitored. If the patient has not carried out some of the prescriptions, needling or criticism is counterproductive (the patient is already self-critical enough). Rather, constant encouragement is essential: the patient should be praised for what he or she has

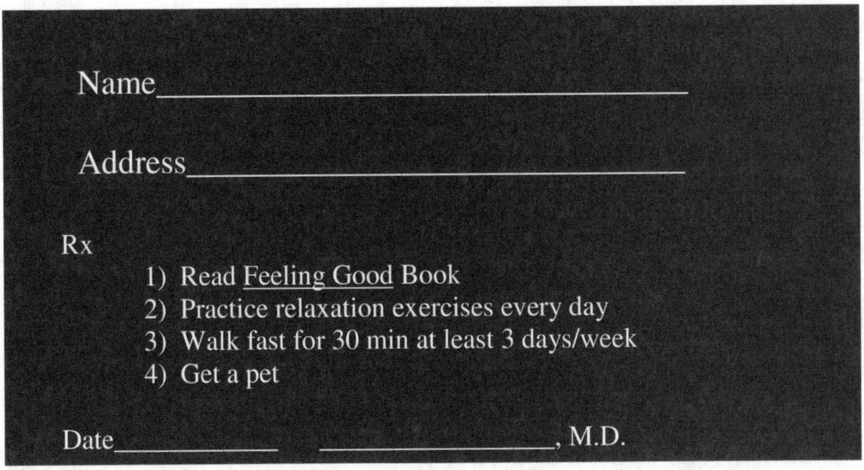

```
Name_____

Address_____

Rx
     1) Read Feeling Good Book
     2) Practice relaxation exercises every day
     3) Walk fast for 30 min at least 3 days/week
     4) Get a pet

Date_____      _____, M.D.
```

Figure 2. Sample behavioral prescription.

accomplished. In other words, it is important to focus on the part of the glass that is half full.

As with all treatment programs for depression, use of cognitive-behavioral interventions to treat a depressed patient calls for regular patient and provider contact which may be in a variety of forms, including face-to-face appointments or telephone and/or email communication (Simon, Ludman, Tutty, Operskalski, & Von Korff, 2004; Christensen, Griffiths, & Jorm, 2004). The patient and family must feel that they are important to the physician, who should convey empathy and hope. If no significant improvement occurs within six weeks, or if the physician is in doubt about progress, referral of the patient to a mental health professional is warranted. The physician should not operate outside her or his "comfort zone."

Cognitive-behavioral interventions have been demonstrated to benefit interpersonal and social functioning as well as ameliorate depressive symptoms, even with minimal patient-clinician contact (Simon et al., 2004; Christensen, Griffiths, & Jorm, 2004). Use of behavioral prescriptions is likely to help the physician be more effective in treating depressed patients and thereby increase the emotional and professional rewards of practice.

Conclusions

Depression is highly prevalent among adult outpatients, often goes unrecognized, and tends to frustrate the primary care physician. Components of cognitive-behavioral therapy delivered in short behavioral prescriptions offers the primary care physician an effective, safe means of treating mild or moderate depression. By writing behavioral prescriptions, the physician can encourage patients to engage in pleasant activities and exercise, change nonconstructive thinking patterns, and decrease use of anxiety-enhancing chemicals. This approach does not interfere with antidepressant or other treatment, entails minimal risks, can be carried out without extensive supplementary training, and is likely to be effective. Furthermore, it may reduce the physician's frustration and increase his or her sense of hope and confidence in dealing with depressed adult outpatients.

References

Ackerson, J., Scogin, F., McKendree-Smith, N., & Lyman, R. D. (1998). Cognitive bibliotherapy for mild and moderate adolescent depressive symptomology. *Journal of Consulting and Clinical Psychology, 66*, 685-690.

American Psychiatric Association. (2000). *Diagnostic and statistical manual of mental disorders, text revision* (4th ed.). Washington, DC: Author.

Antonuccio, D. O., Danton, W. G., & DeNelsky, G. (1995). Psychotherapy vs. medication for depression: Challenging the conventional wisdom with data. *Professional Psychology: Research and Practice, 26*, 574-585.

Antonuccio, D. O., Danton, W. G., DeNelsky, G. Y., Greenberg, R. P., & Gordon, J. S. (1999). *Raising questions about antidepressants. Psychotherapy and Psychosomatics, 68*, 3-14.

Antonuccio, D. O., Danton, W. G., & McClanahan. (2003). Psychology in the Prescription Era: Building a firewall between marketing and science. *American Psychologist, 58*, 1028-1043.

Antonuccio, D. O., Danton, W. G., & DeNelsky, G. (1995). Psychotherapy vs. medication for depression: Challenging the conventional wisdom with data. *Professional Psychology: Research and Practice, 26*, 574-585.

Antonuccio, D. O., Thomas, M., & Danton, W. G. (1997). A cost-effectiveness analysis of cognitive-behavior therapy and fluoxetine (Prozac) in the treatment of depression. *Behavior Therapy, 28*, 187-210.

Bahl, S., Cotterchio, M., & Kreiger, N. (2003). Use of antidepressant medications and the possible association with breast cancer risk. A review. *Psychotherapy and Psychosomatics, 72*, 185-194.

Baldessarini, R. J. (1995). Risks and implications of interrupting maintenance psychotropic drug therapy. *Psychotherapy and Psychosomatics, 63*, 137-141.

Bardage, C., & Isacson, D. G. (2000). Self reported side-effects of antihypertensive drugs: An epidemiological study on prevalence and impact on health-state utility. *Blood Pressure, 9*, 328-34.

Barrier, P. A, Li, T. J., & Jensen, N. M. (2003). Two words to improve physician-patient communication: What else? *Mayo Clinic Proceedings, 78*, 211-214.

Babyak, M., Blumenthal, J. A., Herman, S., Khatri, P., Doraiswamy, M., Moore, K., et al. (2000). Exercise treatment for major depression: Maintenance of therapeutic benefit at 10 months. *Psychosomatic Medicine, 62*, 633-638.

Beck, A. T., Guth, D., Steer, R. A, & Ball, R. (1997). Screening for major depression disorders in medical inpatients with the Beck Depression Inventory for Primary Care. *Behavior Research and Therapy, 35*, 785-791.

Blumenthal, J. A., Babyak, M. A., Moore, K. A., Craighead, W. E., Herman, S., Khatri, et al. (1999). Effects of exercise training on older patients with major depression. *Archives of Internal Medicine, 159*, 2349-2356.

Burns, D. (1999). *Feeling good: The new mood therapy.* New York, New York: Harper Collin Publishers.

Christensen, H., Griffiths, K. M., & Jorm, A. F. (2004). Delivering interventions for depression by using the internet: Randomized controlled trial. *British Medical Journal, 325*, Article doi:10.1136/bmj.37945.566632.EE. Retrieved November 7, 2004, from http://bmj.bmjjournals.com/cgi/reprint/328/7434/265.

Conte, H. R., Plutchik, R., Wild, K. V., & Karasu, T. B. (1986). Combined psychotherapy and pharmacotherapy for depression: A systematic analysis of the evidence. *Archives of General Psychiatry, 43*, 471–479.

Conwell, Y. (1994). Suicide in the elderly. In Schneider, L. S. Reynolds, C. F., Lebowitz, B. D., & Friedhoff, A. J. (Eds.), *Diagnosis and treatment of depression in late life: Results of the NIH consensus development conference* (pp. 397-418). Washington, DC: American Psychiatric Press.

Cotterchio, M., Kreiger, N., Darlington, G., & Steingart, A. (2000). Antidepressant medication use and breast cancer risk. *American Journal of Epidemiology, 151*, 951-957.

Coupland, N. J., Bell, C. J., & Potokar, J. P. (1996). Serotonin reuptake inhibitor withdrawal. *Journal of Clinical Psychopharmacology, 16*, 356-362.

Cucciare, M. A., & O'Donohue, W. (2003). Integrated care and the high utilizer: An explication of medical usage patterns and the role in the healthcare crisis. In N. A. Cummings, W. T. O'Donohue, & K. E. Ferguson (Eds.), *Behavioral health as primary care: Beyond efficacy to effectiveness* (pp. 95-110). Reno, NV: Context Press.

Cuijpers, P. (1997). Bibliotherapy in unipolar depression: A meta-analysis. *Journal of Behavior Therapy and Experimental Psychiatry, 28*, 139-147.

Cummings, N. A., Pallik, H., Dorken, M. S., & Henke, C. J. (2000). Medicaid, managed mental healthcare and medical cost offset. In J. L. Thomas & J. L. Cummings (Eds.), *The value of psychological treatment* (pp.324-335). Pheonix, AZ: Zeig, Tucker and Company Inc.

Dalfen, A. K., & Stewart, D. E. (2001). Who develops stable or fatal adverse drug reactions to selective serotonin reuptake inhibitors? *Canadian Journal of Psychiatry, 46*, 258-262.

DeRubeis, R. J., Gelfand, L. A., Tang, T. Z., & Simons, A. D. (1999). Medications versus cognitive behavior therapy for severely depressed outpatients: Meta-analysis of four randomized comparisons. *American Journal of Psychiatry, 156*, 1007-1013.

Dobson, K. S. (1989). A meta-analysis of the efficacy of cognitive therapy for depression. *Journal of Consulting and Clinical Psychology, 57*, 414–419.

Donovan, S., Madeley, R., Clayton, A., Beeharry, M., Jones, S., Kirk, C., et al. (2000). Deliberate self-harm and antidepressant drugs: Investigation of a possible link. *British Journal of Psychiatry, 177*, 551-556.

Ellis, A., & Harper, R. A. (1975). *A guide to rational living*. Englewood Cliffs, NJ: Prentice-Hall.

Fava, G. A. (1995). Holding on: Depression, sensitization by antidepressant drugs, and the prodigal experts. *Psychotherapy and Psychosomatics, 64,* 57-61.

Fava, G. A. (2002). Long-term treatment with antidepressant drugs: The spectacular achievements of propaganda. *Psychotherapy and Psychosomatics, 71,* 127-132.

Garber, J., & Flynn, C. (2001). Vulnerability to depression in childhood and adolescence. In R. E. Ingram & J. M. Price (Eds.), *Vulnerability to psychopathology: Risk across the lifespan* (pp. 175-225). New York: Guilford.

Geisler, A. M. (2004). Companion animals in palliative care: Stories from the bedside. *American Journal of Hospice and Palliative Care, 21,* 285-288.

Gould, R. A., & Clum G. A. (1993). A meta-analysis of self-help treatment approaches. *Clinical Psychology Review, 13,* 169-189.

Greenberg, P. E., Kessler, R. C., Birnbaum, H. G., Leong, S. A., Lowe, S. W., Berglund, P. A., et al. (2003). The economic burden of depression in the United States: How did it change between 1990 and 2000? *Journal of Clinical Psychiatry, 64,* 1465-1475.

Greenberg, P. E., Stiglin, L. E., Finkelstein, S. N., & Berndt, E. R. (1993). The economic burden of depression in 1990. *Journal of Clinical Psychiatry, 54,* 405-418.

Guthrie, E., Moorey, J., Margison, F. Barker, H., Palmer, S. McGrath, G., et al. (1999). Cost-effectiveness of brief psychodynamic-interpersonal therapy in high utilizers of psychiatric services. *Archives of General Psychiatry, 56,* 519-526.

Halbreich, U., Shen, J., & Panaro, V. (1996). Are chronic psychiatric patients at increased risk for developing breast cancer? *American Journal of Psychiatry, 153,* 559-560.

Healy, D. (2002). Conflicting interests in Toronto: Anatomy of a controversy at the interface of academia and industry. *Perspectives in Biology and Medicine, 45,* 250-263.

Hollon, S. D., Shelton, R. C., & Loosen, P. T. (1991). Cognitive therapy and pharmacotherapy for depression. *Journal of Consulting and Clinical Psychology, 59,* 88-99.

Hunsley, J. (2003). Cost-effectiveness and medical cost offset considerations in psychological service provision. *Canadian Psychology, 44*(1), 61-73.

Jamison, C., & Scogin, F. (1995). Outcome of cognitive bibliotherapy with depressed adults. *Journal of Consulting and Clinical Psychology, 63,* 644-650.

Katon, W., Von Korff, M., Lin, E., Bush, T., Lipscomb, P., & Russo, J. (1992). A randomized trial of psychiatric consultation with distressed high utilizers. *General Hospital Psychiatry, 14,* 86-98.

Katon, W., Von Korff, M., Lin, E., Walker, E., Simon, G., Bush, T., et al. (1995). Collaborative management to achieve treatment guidelines: Impact on depression in primary care. *Journal of the American Medical Association, 273,* 1026-1031.

Kessler, R. C., Berglund, P., Berglund, P., Demler, O. Jin, R., Koretz, D., et al. (2003). The epidemiology of major depressive disorder: Results from the national comorbidity survey replication (NCS-R). *Journal of the American Medical Association, 289*, 3095-3105.

Kessler, R. C., McGonagle, K. A., Shanyang, Z., Nelson, C. B., Hughes, M., Eshleman, S., et al. (1994). Lifetime and 12-month prevalence of DSM-II-R psychiatric disorders in the United States: Results from the National Comorbidity Survey. *Archives of General Psychiatry, 51*, 8-19.

Olfson, M., Marcus, S., Druss, B., Elinson, L., Tanielian, T., & Pincus, H. A. (2002). National trends in the outpatient treatment of depression. *Journal of the American Medical Association, 287*, 203-210.

Kroenke, K. (2003). Patients presenting with somatic complaints: Epidemiology, psychiatric co-morbidity and management. *International Journal of Methods in Psychiatric Research, 12*, 34-43.

Kroenke, K., Spitzer, R. L., Williams, J., Linzer, M., Hahn, S. R., deGruy, F. V., et al. (1994). Physical symptoms in primary care: Predictors of psychiatric disorders and functional impairment. *Archives of Family Medicine, 3*, 774-779.

Lewinsohn, P. M., Munoz, R. F., Youngren, M. A., & Zeiss, A. M. (1986). *Control your depression* (2nd ed.). Englewood Cliffs, NJ: Prentice-Hall.

McLeod, C. C., Budd, M. A., & McClelland, D. C. (1997). Treatment of somatization in primary care. *General Hospital Psychiatry, 19*, 251-258.

Moore, T. J. (2004). *Drug safety research: Special report. Medical use of antidepressant drugs in children and adults: 1998-2001*. Paper presented at the Feb. 2, 2004 FDA hearing on the use of antidepressants in children. Retrieved on March 2, 2004, from http://drugsafetyresearch.com/downloads/med_use_antidep.pdf

Moorman, P. G., Grubber, J. M., Millikan, R. C., & Newman, B. (2003). Antidepressant medications and their association with invasive breast cancer and carcinoma in situ of the breast. *Epidemiology, 14*, 307-314.

Pantalon, M.V., Lubetkin, B. S., & Fishman, S. T. (1995). Use and effectiveness of self-help books in the practice of cognitive and behavioral therapy. *Cognitive and Behavioral Practice, 2*, 213-228.

Pearson, J., Conwell, Y., & Lyness, J. (1997). Late-life suicide and depression in the primary care setting. *New Directions in Mental Health Service, 76*, 13-38.

Preda, A., MacLean, R. W., Mazure, C. M., & Bowers, M. B. (2001). Antidepressant-associated mania and psychosis resulting in psychiatric admissions. *Journal of Clinical Psychiatry, 62*, 30-33.

Robinson, P. (2003). Implementing a primary care depression primary care pathway. In N. A. Cummings, W. T. O'Donohue, & K. E. Ferguson (Eds.), *Behavioral health as primary care: Beyond efficacy to effectiveness* (pp 69-94). Reno, NV: Context Press.

Rosenbaum, J. F., Fava, M., Hood, S. L., Ashcroft, R. C., & Krebs, W. B. (1998). Selective serotonin reuptake inhibitor discontinuation syndrome: A randomized clinical trial. *Biological Psychiatry, 44*, 77-87.

Rost, K., Zhang, M., Fortney, J., Smith, J., Coyne, J., & Smith, G. R. (1998). Persistently poor outcomes of undetected major depression in primary care. *General Hospital Psychiatry, 20,* 12-20

Schulberg, H. C., Block, M. R., Madonia. M. J., Scott, C. P., Rodriquez, E., Imber, S. C., et al. (1996). Treating major depression in primary care practice. *Archives of General Psychiatry, 53,* 913-919.

Schwenk, T. L. (1994). Depression: Overcoming barriers to diagnosis. *Consultant, 34,* 1553-1559.

Scogin, F., Jamison, C., & Davis, N. (1990). A two-year follow-up of the effects of bibliotherapy for depressed older adults. *Journal of Consulting and Clinical Psychology, 58,* 665-667.

Scogin, F., Jamison, C., & Gochneaut, K. (1989). The comparative efficacy of cognitive and behavioral bilbliotherapy for mildly and moderately depressed older adults. *Journal of Consulting and Clinical Psychology, 57,* 403-407.

Sharpe, C. R., Collet, J. P., Belzile, E., Hanley, J. A., & Boivin, J. F. (2002). The effects of tricyclic antidepressants on breast cancer risk. *British Journal of Cancer, 85,* 92-97.

Simon, G. E., Ludman, E. J., Tutty, S., Operskalski, B., & Von Korff, M. (2004). Telephone psychotherapy and telephone care management for primary care patients starting antidepressant treatment. *Journal of the American Medical Association, 292,* 935-942.

Simon, G. E., Manning, W. G., Katzelnick, D. J., Pearson, S. D., Henk, H. J., & Helstad, C. P. (2001). Cost effectiveness of systematic depression treatment for high utilizers of general medical care. *Archives of General Psychiatry, 58,* 181-187.

Smith, N., Floyd, M., Jamison, C., & Scogin, F. (1997). Three-year follow-up of bibliotherapy for depression. *Journal of Consulting and Clinical Psychology, 65,* 324-327.

Steer, R. A., Cavalieri, T. A., Leonard, D. M., & Beck, A. T. (1999). Use of the Beck Depression Inventory for Primary Care to screen for major depression disorders. *General Hospital Psychiatry, 21,* 106-111.

Steinbrueck, S. M., Maxwell, S. E., & Howard, G. S. (1983). A meta-analysis of psychotherapy and drug therapy in the treatment of unipolar depression with adults. *Journal of Consulting and Clinical Psychology, 51,* 856–863.

World Heath Organization. (2000). *Women's mental health: An evidence based review.* Geneva: Author.

Wells, K., Steward, A., Hays, R., Burnam, M., Rogers, W., Daniels, M., et al. (1989). The functioning and well being of depressed patients: Results from the Medicaid Outcomes Study. *Journal of the American Medical Association, 262,* 914-919.

Wexler, B. E., & Cicchetti, D. V. (1992). The outpatient treatment of depression: Implications of outcome research for clinical practice. *Journal of Nervous and Mental Disease, 180,* 277–286.

Chapter 10

Examining Family-Based Treatments for Pediatric Obesity: A Detailed Review of the Last 10-Years

Brie A. Moore
University of Nevada, Reno
William T. O'Donohue
University of Nevada, Reno

Heightened awareness of the significant incidence of pediatric overweight and obesity and the resultant medical and psychological comorbidities give rise to questions regarding the short- and long-term effectiveness of treatments addressing weight management problems in children. This chapter presents a review of empirical studies of the treatment of pediatric overweight and obesity that meet minimal methodological criteria. The 14 studies reviewed are examined for information provided about the treatment of pediatric overweight and variables associated with successful long-term weight control. Given the limitations of the studies reviewed, guidelines for sample selection and description, research design, assessment and classification, and data analysis are provided. Recommendations for designing future multi-component, family-based, behavioral treatments are made.

As recently as a few decades ago, obesity in children was rare. In the 1960's, one in every twenty-four children ages 6- to 11-years-old was overweight (National Center for Health Statistics, 2002). With the exception of a few researchers (e.g., Bacon & Lowrey, 1967), the treatment of pediatric overweight also received little professional attention. Largely because of the increased availability of energy-dense foods and increasingly sedentary lifestyles, the prevalence of childhood overweight in the United States is rising at an alarming rate. The percentage of children who are overweight has increased two- to three-fold in the last 25 years (National Center for Health Statistics, 2002). Obesity now affects one in every five children in the United States and is the most prevalent nutritional disease of children in this country (Dietz, 1998). This increase is seen in both sexes and in children of all ages, with Mexican-American, African-American and Native-American children particularly at risk (Dietz, 2004). Childhood obesity has reached epidemic proportions.

These trends pose an unprecedented burden in terms of children's health and consequently, in future health care costs. Overweight children are commonly defined as those aged 2- to 20-years-old with body mass index (BMI) greater than the 95th percentile for age and gender. Although this definition is commonly accepted and widely used in research, it appears problematic as it implies 5% of all children would be considered overweight, regardless of their weight and the weight of others. Moreover, with the dramatic increase in the prevalence of overweight, it is unclear whether this definition is reflective of current normative data. Practitioners and researchers alike may find greater utility in the adoption of a more practical definition that is sensitive to the negative physiological sequelae of overweight. Such approaches include attention to cardiovascular risk factors including elevated blood pressure, total cholesterol, and serum lipoprotein ratios. Thorough assessment of overweight in children requires consideration of the child's age, height, weight, and growth patterns.

Overweight in children is associated with significant health problems and is an important early risk factor for both child and adult morbidity and mortality. Inactive and overweight children are more likely to have high blood pressure, abnormal insulin and cholesterol concentrations and more abnormal lipid profiles. In some populations, obese children now account for as much as 50% of Type 2 diabetes mellitus, a metabolic disorder related to obesity and sedentary lifestyles and historically rare in children (Fagot-Campagna et al., 2000). These changes increase the risk of early disability and death from heart disease, kidney disease, and other organ damage (Young-Hyman et al., 2001). Other important complications include asthma and sleep apnea, skeletal and joint problems, liver disease and gastrointestinal complications.

Often under acknowledged, yet highly prevalent, are the psychosocial comorbidities of pediatric obesity. The psychological stress of social stigmatization imposed on obese children may be as damaging as the medical morbidities. These commonly include poor self-esteem, body image disturbances, depression, social isolation, difficulty with peer relationships as well as poor academic achievement, and result in a great deal of suffering (Ebbeling et al., 2002). The American Academy of Pediatrics Committee on Nutrition (2003) has called for the development of effective treatment approaches for reducing body weight, increasing fitness, and determining long-term effects of weight loss on comorbidities of childhood obesity. Given its prevalence and resultant medical and psychological sequelae, decreasing the rates of obesity in children has been identified as a national health care priority (*Healthy People 2010*, 2004).

In the past decade, an increasing amount of professional attention has been given to the treatment of pediatric overweight (e.g., Epstein et al., 1995, 2001; Barlow & Dietz, 1998). Most efforts to reduce childhood obesity in children have used either family-based or school-based approaches. School-based interventions, despite their intensive, multi-site and sometimes multi-year designs, have not been successful in reducing the prevalence of childhood obesity (Ebbeling, 2002). Based on the literature, researchers have come to the conclusion that family-based behavioral interventions have become the standard of care for the evidence-based treatment of childhood obesity (Kazdin & Weisz, 1998). Despite these findings, providers who are concerned about childhood obesity may not believe that they have effective therapeutic strategies to help their patients control weight or the time to implement strategies that may be effective (Barlow & Dietz, 2002; Jelalian, Boergers, Alday & Frank, 2003).

In this review we address the question of the extent to which the research literature indicates that there are replicable treatments that reliably produce significant improvement in pediatric overweight. Towards bridging the gap between clinical research and pediatric obesity care, we have chosen to concentrate on family-based, behavioral obesity treatment programs targeting child weight loss, as this allows the review to be of a manageable size and because most extant treatment outcome studies have adopted this distinction.

We searched PsychInfo and MedLine databases for treatment outcome studies published in peer-reviewed journals from 1994 to the present. We chose this date to focus this review on the most current findings in the treatment of pediatric obesity and because epidemiological data document the highest prevalence of the epidemic since 1994 (National Center for Health Statistics, 2000). Additionally, excellent, comprehensive reviews of studies conducted prior to this date are provided by Epstein (1998), Haddock et al. (1994), and Jelalian and Saelens (1999). We also examine the reference sections of all articles and reviews obtained. Our basic criteria for inclusion were: (a) random assignment of subjects to conditions and (b) at least some comparison group (or a comparison condition in a single subject design). These criteria were judged to be the minimum necessary for some meaningful interpretation of data. Random assignment allows one to regard the groups as initially equivalent, and thus post-treatment differences cannot be attributed to initial differences. Comparison or control groups are necessary to provide a context for understanding the meaning of outcome data. The limitation of uncontrolled studies of treatment groups is that even if there are positive pre-post treatment changes, a no-treatment or placebo comparison group might reveal equal or even greater changes.

An overwhelming majority of the literature on pediatric obesity can be characterized as epidemiological or descriptive (e.g., correlational). In comparison, there is a dearth of controlled treatment outcome studies. Of the outcome studies located, those excluded from the review included single group pretest-posttest designs and those with comparison groups that did not employ random assignment to conditions. Fourteen total studies met the inclusion criteria for review.

Evaluation Criteria

The question motivating this review was: What evidence is there that there are replicable treatments that produce clinically significant and enduring improvement for pediatric overweight and obesity? For this question to be answered research needs to be designed with the following considerations:

Sample Selection and Description

The selection of the sample is a critical step because it determines the extent to which generalizations can be made to individuals not participating in the study. There are two groups of individuals to which generalization issues apply: clients and therapists. There are two broad strategies as to sample selection. One is to attempt to draw a representative sample of the larger pediatric population presenting as overweight and of therapists treating this population (Paul, 1967). However, representative sampling of clients is quite difficult to achieve, particularly when factors such as degree of overweight, comorbidities, ethnicity, family composition and socioeconomic status are considered. Thus, all studies reviewed utilized the second broad sampling strategy: convenience sampling of clients and therapists. Convenience samples are clearly unrepresentative of the larger population and may lead the reader to overestimate the social validity and replicability of a given treatment (Fisher, 1971). For example, Epstein et al. (2000) reported 461 families interested in participation, 171 families were screened and 90 families included in the study. Similarly, Golan and colleagues (1998) identified 160 children as being obese. One-hundred-forty of these met their inclusion criteria. Of these 140 children, only 60 families agreed to participate in the study. The inclusion of highly trained, specialized therapists may also severely limit the disseminability of a given treatment. Because pediatric obesity is a public health problem, the use of convenience samples may severely distort our understanding of the utility of presented treatments in addressing the magnitude of the problem. However, if samples are described thoroughly, then meaningful interpretation of the relevance of the results can still be achieved. Characteristics of the samples can be thoroughly described (regarding, for example, socioeconomic status, ethnicity, age, and degree of overweight) and thus their relationship to the larger population can be ascertained.

We found that samples in pediatric obesity research are biased toward higher socioeconomic status, moderately overweight, preadolescent and Caucasian children with few medical or psychological comorbidities. This is problematic as some researchers have found that results from middle class, Caucasian families have not generalized to families with diverse socioeconomic and ethnic backgrounds (e.g., Levine et al., 2001; Robinson et al., 2001). Similarly, therapists in the studies reviewed also appeared to be unrepresentative in that highly experienced therapists appear to be over sampled.

Moreover, it is useful if the client sample is sufficiently well-described to identify subgroups. This prevents drawing general conclusions that are not true of certain subtypes and provides prognostic information regarding the specific treatment. Samples must be thoroughly described in terms of the range and mean percentage overweight, the assessment criteria used to determine the degree of overweight (e.g., BMI, skinfold thickness, growth charts), medical and psychological comorbidities (e.g., blood pressure, cholesterol levels, externalizing or internalizing problems, Child Depression Inventory scores), motivation to engage in treatment, and how the child was initially identified as needing treatment (e.g., physician, parent, or school referral). Child age, percentage overweight, family composition, socioeconomic status, ethnicity, family and child history of weight control and obesity and treatment motivation, all appear to be important variables to include in a thorough description of the sample. Discipline, degree, age, gender, credentials, and experience should be variables that serve as a minimum description of therapists.

Study Design

In order for a treatment to be considered effective, it must be shown that it produces a better outcome than either no treatment or than the administration of a credible placebo. A no treatment control group is also essential for evaluating possible iatrogenic effects of treatment.

Moreover, a major problem plaguing the treatment of pediatric and adult overweight and obesity is the refractory nature of the problem, leading to a lack of generalization of treatment effects over time. Rapid increase in prevalence and resultant comorbidities has led to heightened awareness and a call for the development of interventions demonstrating long-term maintenance of treatment effects. Because of the refractory nature of pediatric obesity and the threat of relapse, study designs should include a number of follow-up periods to track durability of treatment effects. The studies of Epstein and colleagues (e.g., 1990, Epstein, Valoski, Wing, & McCurley, 1994) have served as exemplars of longitudinal research in this area.

Another concern is relevant to both valid causal inference and replicability. That is, it is critical that studies include an adequate description of treatment and fidelity checks to ensure professional or family adherence to the protocol. These steps allow one to have a clear understanding of exactly what treatment consisted of and that the treatment was consistently delivered across clients. Use of treatment manuals and fidelity checks is a highly desirable design feature, particularly because such use of treatment manuals enhances replicability of therapy for those practitioners who want to implement the therapy on the basis of its positive outcome data. In the reviewed studies, researchers were more likely to describe specific treatment components than to include manualized treatments or fidelity checks to ensure adherence. In fact, only one study reviewed included a treatment fidelity check. Moreover, upon further investigation, treatment manuals were not published or publicly accessible (sometimes despite contacting the authors), compromising treatment replicability and dissemination.

Another important design feature is blindness of subjects and therapists, particularly when therapists are also collecting data that were used as an outcome measure. Daily diet and activity behaviors are difficult to measure accurately and may be influenced by response biases due to demand characteristics.

Finally, another useful design characteristic is the measurement of process variables. For example, if a treatment involves nutrition education focused on training clients in the relative distribution of foods and servings in the FDA food guide pyramid and this treatment does not seem to result in significant improvement in the consumption of foods in accordance with the recommendations, two interpretations are plausible: (a) clients did not adequately learn the food pyramid, or (b) they learned the food pyramid but learning this did not significantly impact their eating behavior. A measurement of the extent to which knowledge changed in this case allows treatment process information that can be used to choose among these two plausible alternative explanations. Few studies we reviewed gathered any process data.

Behavior Change Assessment

Researchers must carefully choose what outcome measures they use. A problem plaguing obesity researchers is that gathering objective daily diet and activity behavior is often difficult. Thus, the heavy reliance on self-report. However, there are serious concerns about the validity of self-report regarding energy consumption of obese individuals (Bandidni, Scholler, Cyr, & Dietz, 1990). Additionally, when working with pediatric populations, self-report may be further compromised. These problems are further compounded when one considers the possibility of demand characteristics added in treatment studies. At a minimum, independent parent and child report should be gathered. Other studies have included assessment of weight change throughout treatment to increase confidence in self-report (e.g., Epstein, Valoski, et al., 1994). Although the criterion assessment for daily energy consumption may present a challenge, researchers have utilized instrumentation (e.g., accelerometers) to ascertain objective anthropometric, fitness and energy expenditure measures (e.g., Epstein, Valoski, Vara, McCurley, et al., 1995). Such instrumentation prevents the limitations associated with the sole reliance on self-report.

Another important measurement issue is the measurement of child psychological distress associated with obesity and its treatment. Historically, studies investigating this relationship have produced mixed results. For example, negative psychological effects such as low self-esteem and poor social adjustment have not been consistently found (e.g., Klesges et al., 1992). One suggested reason for this inconsistency in findings is methodological differences, including differences across studies in the definition and measurement of psychological distress (Epstein, Klein & Wisniewski, 1994).

If the psychological functioning of the obese child is conceptualized as a multi-determined phenomenon, factors other than level of obesity warrant our attention. For example, Epstein and colleagues (Epstein, Klein, et al.,1994) found that parental obesity and parental psychiatric symptoms showed a stronger relationship to psychological problems in moderately obese children than age, sex, or BMI. Similarly, in a later study, Epstein et al. (1998) observed significant improvements in child and maternal psychopathology as a result of undergoing a family-based behavioral weight control program. Future research should attempt to understand and measure those mechanisms (e.g., parenting practices, parent modeling, and/or family environmental factors) that could mediate the influence of parental problems on child psychological distress. This knowledge may give us better insight into the psychological treatment of the obese child and family.

Data Analysis

Due to methodological limitations, a number of concerns regarding data analyses and subsequent conclusions arise. With multiple comparison, the probability of Type I errors increase. Seldom are procedures used to compensate for the increase in family wise error rates. Second, between groups comparisons should be made whenever possible as these allow a context for ruling out major rival hypotheses such as placebo effects. However, some studies focus on within group comparisons of pre-post effects despite the inclusion of a comparison group. Third, attention should be given to the issue of adequate statistical power. Tests of insufficient power are likely to result in Type II errors, that is, there will be an unacceptably high probability of false conclusions that there are no group differences (no treatment effects) when actually there are simply two few cases in each cell. Sample sizes may be inadequate relative to the variance attributable to sources other than the treatment method to detect differences. In the studies reviewed, sample sizes varied considerably, with few researchers reporting power analyses.

Finally, treatment should be evaluated with respect to both clinical significance and social validity. Statistical analysis simply indicates that the groups are drawn from different populations; it says little about whether the magnitude of effects is sufficiently large to meet practical considerations. Jacobson and Truax (1991) have proposed a useful analysis for clinical significance. However, the large majority of studies reviewed failed to examine the clinical significance of the treatment of pediatric obesity. Social validity refers to the acceptability of the treatment to consumers (Wolf, 1978). Treatments that produce significant change may still be rejected by consumers or completed reluctantly with low levels of treatment satisfaction. This is a particularly important problem in pediatric studies as an important group of stakeholders are the children, who can be forced to participate in treatment by their parents. Additionally, due to time and reimbursement limitations, pediatricians are unlikely to implement costly, complicated or socially unacceptable treatments. Ideally, social validity measures should be gathered from parents, pediatricians (as key referral sources) and children.

It would have been advantageous to summarize results for studies reviewed using the statistical techniques of meta-analysis. However, combining the results of the studies reviewed here was inappropriate because: (a) the majority of studies included insufficient information about sample selection procedures; (b) the outcome measures differed across studies; (c) there were large differences in treatment procedures or the treatment procedures were inadequately described; and (d) the large variability across studies in length of follow-up periods. These factors made it difficult to determine the comparability of studies, which is a prerequisite for making the combination of their results meaningful.

Effectiveness of Treatment for Pediatric Overweight and Obesity

Review of Studies

Based on the review criteria mentioned above, all randomized, controlled outcome studies of pediatric obesity treatments are described in detail below. Previous research has documented that percentage overweight typically remains stable in the absence of intervention (e.g., Aragona, Cassady & Drabman, 1975; Kirschenbaum, Harris & Tomarken, 1984). Similarly, other studies have indicated that behavior modification of eating and physical activity behaviors is superior to education alone (Epstein, Wing, Steranchak, Dickson, & Michelson, 1980). Building on these findings, the second generation of literature reviewed here compares the relative efficacy of multiple active treatment components. The specific treatment components reviewed include: cognitive versus behavioral components, specific strategies for diet and physical activity modification, mastery criterion and reinforcement strategies, problem-solving strategies, and parent and child treatment focus.

Pediatric Diet and Weight Control

Cognitive vs. Behavioral Treatments. Across studies, considerable evidence exists for the efficacy of behavioral and cognitive treatment strategies for the psychosocial treatment of pediatric obesity. Although many empirically supported treatments have included cognitive components (e.g., problem-solving, cognitive restructuring), few have provided direct evidence for the relative contributions of behavioral and cognitive therapies. Herrera, Johnston, and Steele (2004) compared the relative efficacies of cognitive, behavioral and comparison group treatments for pediatric obesity. Fifty children recruited through a for-profit pediatric weight loss facility were included in the study. An additional 25 children who had received usual care at the facility were included in the comparison condition. Criteria for participation included: 1) child was at least 15% overweight for sex, age and height; 2) between 6- and 18-years of age; 3) at least one parent willing to participate in weekly sessions. The sample was 53% female, with an average age of 11.5-years-old, and 66.9% overweight. The attrition rate was 8%. Although ethnic identity information was not available for the comparison group, participants in the cognitive and behavioral conditions were predominately Caucasian (90%). The remainder of the sample described their ethnicity as Pacific Islander (4%), Hispanic (4%), or African American (2%). Socio-economic data for families were not presented, but families were described as middle-class. At pre-treatment, no significant differences across conditions were found for age, sex, or percentage over ideal BMI.

Families were randomly assigned to either the cognitive or behavioral obesity treatment condition. Across conditions, treatment was conducted with groups of 5 children and their parent(s) in 10 weekly, 120 minutes sessions. Treatment was provided by master's-level therapists supervised by doctorate-level licensed psychologists. Weekly multidisciplinary staff meetings were held to discuss treatment integrity. Anonymous archival data from 25 participants was randomly selected from a cohort of 75 children who had completed treatment at the weight loss facility. The comparison condition included nutritional education, exercise education and short- and long-term goal-setting instruction and evaluation. In addition to these components, the behavioral intervention included methods adapted from the Traffic Light Diet (described below; Epstein, Wing, Koeske, Andrasik, & Ossip, 1981), including self-monitoring of dietary intake and physical activity, parent and child praise of progress, parent and child modeling of appropriate health promotion behaviors, and contracting for contingent reinforcement of short-term goal attainment. In addition to the inclusion of common treatment components, the cognitive intervention condition also included parent and child monitoring of negative thoughts, restructuring/challenging negative thoughts, and self-reinforcement (use positive thoughts as motivation).

The primary dependent measure investigated in this study was change in percent overweight from week 1 (baseline) to week 10 (post-treatment). Treatment fidelity was also monitored throughout the course of the study. Two trained independent raters viewed a set of randomly selected videotapes comprising 25% of the treatment sessions and recorded the elements covered in each session. Kappa for the cognitive components was .69 ($p < .05$), while Kappa for behavioral variables was .59 ($p < .05$), indicating good and moderate levels of agreement, respectively (Cohen, 1960; Landis & Koch, 1977). Then, two trained graduate students, uninvolved in treatment classified sessions as either cognitive or behavioral. These ratings were compared to the treatment group's orientation with 100% accuracy, suggesting treatment fidelity was maintained for both conditions.

Results of this study indicated that overall, participants in each of the three conditions exhibited significant decreases in percentage over ideal BMI. Eighty-four percent of participants in the behavioral condition demonstrated significant improvement from pre- to post-treatment. Clinical significance was also addressed in this study using BMI classification categories from NHANES I. Categories included healthy ($< 85^{th}$ percentile), overweight (85th-95th percentile), obese (95th -97th percentile), and very obese ($> 97^{th}$ percentile). Forty-percent of participants in the behavioral condition demonstrated a reduction in BMI classification from either very obese to obese ($n=6$), obese to overweight ($n=3$) or from overweight to healthy ($n = 1$). Three participants (12%) in the cognitive condition changed BMI classifications from very obese to obese. In the comparison condition, six participants (24%) changed classification from very obese to obese ($n = 5$) or from obese to overweight ($n = 1$). No participant in any condition changed to a higher category. Analyses of changes in percent overweight revealed that the behavioral condition (-9.51%, $s.d. = 6.64$) was statistically superior to the comparison condition (-4.67%, $s.d. = 5.08$), but that the cognitive (-5.53%, $s.d. = 5.77$) and comparison conditions did not differ statistically in terms of change in percentage over ideal BMI.

This is the first study in the pediatric obesity literature to address the relative efficacy of cognitive and behavioral treatment components. Consistent with studies reviewed below (e.g., Epstein, Valoski, et al., 1994; 1998), these data provide additional support for the efficacy of family-based behavioral treatment for pediatric obesity. Although the small sample size, lack of a power analysis, and homogeneity of the sample may limit the generalizability of these findings, the inclusion of a valid control group and treatment fidelity ratings strengthen the conclusions which can be based on these data. This study contributes to the extant literature by investigating the effectiveness of behavioral treatment in the clinical realm. Additional strengths of this study include the addition of a discussion of clinical significance and the inclusion of a more diverse sample of participants than typically included in the literature. Children in this study represented a wide age-range and BMI classification. The reduction in degree of overweight experienced by the very obese (i.e., 60% over ideal BMI) children in this study suggests that behavioral interventions may be effective in preventing continued weight gain, improving BMI and possibly improving health status in very obese children. When viewed from a harm reduction model these results appear promising. However, given that only one participant experienced a clinically significant reduction in weight (i.e., from overweight to healthy), questions arise about the efficacy of this approach. Future studies investigating the relative long-term efficacy of these approaches should be pursued.

Traffic Light Diet. Over the past two decades, Epstein and colleagues (e.g., Epstein, 1990; Epstein & Wing, 1987) have provided support for both the short- and long-term efficacy of family-based behavioral treatments for obese children participating in clinical studies. The Traffic Light diet treatment includes a behaviorally oriented approach highlighting the role of parents as active participants in their children's habit change and weight loss (Epstein, Valoski, et al., 1994; Kazdin & Weisz, 1998). The "traffic light" diet entails clustering foods into three groups based on energy density. Foods containing high levels of saturated fats, refined sugar and overall high caloric values, such as candy, chips, and doughnuts are classified as "red" foods. "Yellow" foods, such as bagels, skim milk and fruits, are higher in calories, yet include the nutrients needed for a balanced diet. "Green" foods, including primarily vegetables, are very low in calories and rich with nutrients. The traffic light diet advises daily intake levels of food from each category. Although the specific parameters of the Traffic Light Diet differ across studies to some degree, typically, parents and children are instructed to consume between 1000 and 1200 calories per day and to limit red foods to no more than 15 per week.

Physical Activity. To address physical activity, participants receive parent and child specific manuals containing written information on the positive benefits of increased physical activity and the negative consequences of sedentary behavior. Participants are typically rewarded for engaging in either programmed exercise or lifestyle physical activity. Physical activity goals typically are set at first at 30 minutes per week and are then increased each time goals are met (e.g., by 30 minute increments with 180 minutes of moderate or high intensity exercise representing the highest goal).

Self-Monitoring. Participants are also instructed to use self-monitoring techniques, such as weighing themselves daily and graphing their weight. Participants also typically complete habit books noting physical activity, number of red foods consumed, and food and caloric intake.

Stimulus Control. When a behavior is more likely to occur in the presence of a discriminative stimulus, but not in its absence, the behavior is described as being under stimulus control. That is, a stimulus comes to control behavior when it predicts something about positive or negative reinforcement (Staddon, 2003). Typically, because of their flavor and the satiation they bring, high-fat and calorie-laden foods are inherently positively reinforcing, resulting in an increase in consumption. For many families and children, increased consumption of such foods (e.g., "comfort foods") may also be negatively reinforcing by facilitating avoidance of negative thoughts and emotions. To this end, behavioral weight control programs typically include a stimulus control component. Stimulus control strategies were also taught to increase cues for activity and decrease cues for sedentary behavior. For example, parents may be instructed to put the television in a room with uncomfortable chairs and to leave sports equipment visible to increase cues to engage in physical activity.

Reinforcement. Different types of reinforcement are used to increase the occurrence of program adherent heath promotion behaviors. For example, parents and children may be instructed to review habit books together each night and to use praise to increase desired behaviors. Parents and children may also jointly devise a point system to help attain behavioral goals. Points can be exchanged for mutually agreed upon reinforcers.

As dictated by the behavioral, family-based model, parents support child adherence to the program by actively modeling appropriate consumption, eliminating "red" foods from the home environment, and rewarding their children for compliance. The program also teaches skills to prevent noncompliance and promote adherence.

Using this approach to modifying diet and physical activity behaviors, investigations have vacillated between examining the relative efficacy of more operant-based approaches to specific habit change (e.g., Epstein et al., 1995; 2000; 2001) and evaluation of the efficacy of treatment components such as mastery criteria, contingency management (Epstein, McKenzie, Valoski, Klein, & Wing, 1994), and problem-solving (Epstein et al., 2000). Without an explicit rationale for successive investigations, the logic of this research program remains somewhat unclear. In the interest of advancing the treatment of pediatric obesity, future studies may benefit from the incorporation of a clearly explicated, logically coherent and continuous research program which builds upon and expands preceding findings. A number of studies incorporating this Traffic Light Diet are presented below.

In 2001, Epstein, Gordy, Raynor, Beddome and colleagues evaluated the effect of a parent-focused behavioral intervention on parent and child eating changes and percentage of overweight change in families at risk for childhood obesity. Thirty families with at least one obese parent and a 6- to 11-year-old non-obese child were recruited through physician referrals and by indicating interest by responding to media announcements. Families with children with a BMI less than the 85th percentile, at least one parent with a BMI greater than the 85th percentile, and one parent who was willing to attend treatment meetings were eligible for participation. Participants who had current psychiatric problems, diet or activity restrictions, or attended alternative weight control programs were excluded from treatment. In 28 of the 30 total families, the participating parent was obese. The average participating parent was 65.7% overweight, with a clustering of obesity-related risk factors in the family. Every family had at least one parent or grandparent with an obesity-related risk factor. Parents were confident they could lose weight, but less confident that they could make eating or activity changes or assist their children in making these changes.

Families were randomized to one of two groups in which targeted behaviors varied: a decreased intake of fat and sugar group or an increased intake of fruit and vegetable group. For all participants, weight-control treatment was provided to the parents for 8 weekly meetings, followed by four biweekly and two monthly meetings. Parents and children received workbooks which provided information on general weight control and prevention, the Traffic Light Diet (1,200-1500 calories per day with determinations for maintenance caloric intake levels post weight loss), developing a healthy eating and activity environment for children, behavior change techniques, and maintenance of behavior change. Children and parents cooperatively completed program-related activities in the workbook on a weekly basis. Participating parents met individually for 30-minutes each week with an individual therapist to review program-related parent-child activity and progress towards parent weight, diet and activity goals and attended a 30-minute group meeting. Non-overweight parents had no caloric restriction but were asked to meet their condition specific targeted dietary goal. Parents were also taught positive reinforcement strategies, including praise for target behaviors, stimulus control strategies, preplanning and problem-solving. Children were reinforced for completing program-related activities at home by having a sticker placed on a tracking sheet and, at the 6-month follow-up, with gift certificates contingent on the number of activities completed during the program. In the increase fruit and vegetable group, the goal was to incrementally increase intake of these foods to reach at least two servings of fruits and three servings of vegetables per day. Participants in the decrease fat and sugar group were provided incremental goals towards attainment of the goal to consume no more than 10 servings of high-fat/high sugar foods per week.

Primary dependent measures, collected at baseline, post-test (6-months) and 12-month follow-up, included anthropometric measures, food intake, and parental control over child eating. Percentage overweight was calculated by comparing the participant's BMI with the BMI at the 50th percentile for age and gender. Changes in eating habits over the past month were assessed using the Food Habits Questionnaire, while daily intake of fruits, vegetables and high-fat/high-sugar foods was assessed using the Food Intake Questionnaire, a measure validated for child and adult subjects against 24-hour dietary recalls with adequate reliability (Epstein et al., 2001). Parental control over child eating, concern about child overweight, and perception of parent overweight was assessed with the Child Feeding Question-naire-Short Version, a validated instrument (Birch et al., 1998). Socioeconomic status was assessed using Hollingshead's Four-Factor Index of Social Status. A particular strength of this study is the inclusion of a thorough medical history, which was assessed via interview regarding the prevalence of obesity and obesity related disorders in parents and grandparents, the perceived probability that the child would become obese, and confidence in parent's ability to change their and their children's eating and exercise habits. No significant differences existed between groups with the exception of more hypertension in families in the decrease fat and sugar group.

Results indicated that for both parents and children, differences in fruit and vegetable intake over time significantly differed by group, whereas high-fat/high-sugar intake significantly decreased across groups over time. Children also showed significant between-group differences in fruit and vegetable intake over time (+ 0.72 ± 1.11; -0.55 ± 1.31) and significant changes in high-fat/high-sugar food intake for both groups over time (- 4.5 ± 7.97; - 8.5 ± 7.58). Parents showed significant differences in percentage of overweight change by group, with parents in the increase fruit and vegetable group showing reductions of -12.01% overweight and parents in the decrease high-fat/high-sugar group showing reductions of -3.94% overweight. No changes in percentage overweight were observed over time for children in either group. The authors did not discuss the clinical significance of these findings. That is, it is unclear if adult participants achieved non overweight or non-obese status as a result of this intervention. Across groups, significant decreases were observed for the Food Habits Questionnaire, with decreases in the use of fat as a seasoning, using low-fat versions of high-fat foods, and increases in fruit consumption. Parents in the increase fruit and vegetable group showed significantly greater decreases in parent perception of being overweight on the Child Feeding Questionnaire as compared to parents in the decrease fat and sugar group. However, differences in parent control over eating were not significant.

The authors assert that the results of this study suggest that targeting fruit and vegetable intake in children increases intake of nutritionally dense healthy foods while simultaneously decreasing intake of low nutrient dense foods. The authors concluded that higher levels of dietary carbohydrate and fiber intake may enhance satiation, reducing caloric and fat intake and this target may also lead to heightened availability of such foods in the home. Furthermore, focusing on what may be eaten rather than prohibiting food may facilitate adherence to programs focusing on caloric restriction. However, it is unclear whether this intervention produced clinically significant behavior changes in both children and their parents. That is, children in the increased fruit and vegetable group, on average, increased their consumption of fruits and vegetables by less than one serving. However, both treatment approaches appeared to be more promising in reducing consumption of high-fat and high-sugar foods. This study presents empirical support for the Traffic Light Diet for treating obesity in parents. Future research is warranted to further elucidate the differential impact of promoting healthy diet behaviors versus targeting problematic dietary behaviors in the prevention and treatment of pediatric obesity.

Mastery Criteria and Contingent Reinforcement. Based on the assumption that the rate of change in diet and activity behaviors varies across children and families, Epstein, McKenzie, Valoski, Klein and Wing (1994a) compared a family-based treatment program that included mastery criteria and contingent reinforcement for eating, exercise and parent skills to a control condition yoked for presentations of behavioral skills, information and reinforcement. In this study, 40 families with obese 8- to 12-year-old children were recruited by referral from physicians, by response to public service announcements and from a database of previous participants. To be included, children must have met the following entrance criteria: a) 20-100% overweight for height; b) no parent greater than 100% overweight; c) no current psychiatric contact or counseling for parents or children; d) no history of an eating disorder and e) one parent willing to participate in treatment as the targeted parent. The average child in the study was 10.2-years-old, 59.6% over the 50th percentile for Body Mass Index (BMI), and 74% of the sample was female. The average participating parent was 39.4-years-old and 30.1% (s.d. = 20.9%) percent over the 50th percentile for BMI. Eighty-two percent of the parents were mothers and 54% of participating parents were obese. Families were on average middle class socioeconomic status. Ethnicities of the included families were not presented.

Families were randomized to one of two groups: an experimental or control condition. Treatment was provided over 26 weekly meetings and 6 monthly meetings. Weekly meetings were comprised of weight measurement and a didactic lecture focused on weight control or behavior change. All participants were presented with the Traffic Light Diet and exercise program (described above; Epstein, Wing & Valoksi, 1985). Daily caloric intake goals ranged from 900 to 1800 calories daily (early treatment) to 900 to 1200 calories (late treatment). Maintenance levels of caloric intake were determined individually. Participants engaged in a lifestyle activity program which allowed them to choose aerobic activities that they could incorporate into their daily routine, such as walking, swimming or bicycle riding. Adherence was evaluated via self-monitoring, with goals ranging from 50 calories expended daily, 7 days a week (early treatment) to 300 calories expended daily, 5 days a week (late treatment). Parenting manuals included information on behavioral principles for increasing and decreasing target behaviors. Presented concepts included, positive and negative reinforcement, modeling, stimulus control and contracting. Worksheets describing problem situations were discussed during weekly treatment meetings to promote understanding of the application of these procedures. Quizzes, contracting and parent lotteries were also used throughout treatment across groups.

In the experimental group, families progressed through 5 levels of treatment at their own rate based on mastery of information and behavioral skills. Progress was reinforced based on individual data. Advancement was also dependent on weight loss to increase assurance in the accuracy of self-reported behavior change. For parents, praise statements and stimulus control goals were also included. Staff members determined each week, via review of self-monitoring books, if participants could progress to the next level and whether or not reinforcers were delivered. The control group was designed to control for paced introduction of educational material by yoking progress in treatment and reinforcement to the progress of the experimental group. For families in the control condition, the same information was presented, but families were not required to demonstrate mastery of skills. Parents self-monitored their use of praise and stimulus control techniques, but were not praised by staff for their use of these skills. Reinforcers were provided via a lottery for attendance, rather than for changes in parenting skills. However, reinforcers were provided at the same frequency in both groups. Characteristics of the staff implementing the treatment, including credentials, experience, age, or skill were not presented.

Dependent variables included parent and child BMI, self-reported adherence to treatment, and knowledge of behavioral parenting skills. Data were gathered at baseline, 6-months, 12-months and 24-months. Adherence was measured for the first and last weeks of treatment. Parenting knowledge was measured via the knowledge of Behavioral Principles Questionnaire, which was administered at baseline and 1-year.

Results indicated that families in the experimental group showed significant reductions in BMI through 1-year as compared to families in the control group. At 1-year, children in the experimental group demonstrated a reduction in percentage overweight of 26.5%, whereas children in the control group showed significantly less weight reduction (-16.7% overweight). Children in the experimental group demonstrated a 59% greater improvement in percent overweight. However, differences between the experimental and control groups were not maintained at 24-months (-15.4 vs. -10.6, respectively). Similar trends were observed for overweight parents. In regard to program adherence, significant group differences were found in the number of "red" foods eaten each week (-35.8 $\pm$ 18.8 vs. 28.6 $\pm$ 15.7), days within calorie range (1.2 $\pm$ 3.8 vs. -1.0 $\pm$ 3.2), and days of complete reporting (1.3 $\pm$ 2.8 vs. -2.3 $\pm$ 3.0). No significant differences were found for meeting exercise goals or other adherence measures. Across groups, parents showed equivalent significant increases in knowledge of behavioral parenting skills throughout the course of treatment.

In this study, the authors skillfully applied behavioral principles in the service of augmenting treatment adherence and maximizing outcomes. Additionally, the inclusion of a credible placebo group strengthens the conclusions which can be drawn based on these data. By matching treatment to individual differences in knowledge acquisition and behavior change, participants can receive maximal benefits from a given treatment. However, due to the absence of a description of therapist skill, credentials and experience, it is unclear if this treatment could be generalizable to therapists in the community. Similarly, the intensive nature of this program raises concerns about its cost-effectiveness, further limiting its generalizability. Also, the present approach does not successfully address the long-term maintenance of treatment effects. Given the widespread prevalence and refractory nature of pediatric obesity, such concerns present important limitations to this treatment Readers are directed to Goldfield et al. (2001) for future studies addressing cost-effectiveness and to Epstein, Valoski, et al. (1994; discussed below) for long-term outcomes associated with this approach.

Long-term Outcomes. In 1994, Epstein, Valoski, et al. reported 10-year treatment outcomes for obese children in 4 randomized treatment studies. One hundred eighty-five families with a child of 6-12 years of age, who was 20%-100% overweight for age, sex, and height and one parent willing to participate in treatment, participated in one of four studies. With the exception of Study 3, where the authors directly investigated the role of parent obesity status additional entrance criteria entailed that at least one parent in each family was obese. Referral sources were not reported. Families that participated in Study 1 were intact. Family composition for the studies 2, 3, and 4 was not reported. Exclusionary criteria included: (a) current psychiatric diagnosis or treatment or (b) learning disability. Families were not excluded from treatment based on a history of psychiatric problems. Additional exclusionary criteria for Studies 2 and 4 included: (a) absence of a medical problem that limited exercise. Families were predominately middle-class. No additional data regarding the age, mean percentage overweight, family composition, or gender distribution of participants in each study were presented in this report. All families were presented with a treatment package consisting of weekly treatment meetings for 8- to12- weeks, with monthly meetings continuing for 6- to12-months from the beginning of the program. The Traffic Light Diet (900 – 1,200 kcal) was provided to all participants with the goal of reducing caloric intake and improving nutrient density. Participants recorded daily energy intake in food diaries, which were reviewed at weekly meetings. Once participants' weight was within 10% of their goal, daily caloric intake was increased by 100 kcal until weight gain was noted. Subsequent energy intake was adjusted to maintain growth. This level of precision in the diet represents a significant strength as energy intake was calibrated to the individual with developmental considerations in mind.

Of the 185 families originally randomized, an impressive 158 (85%) families were available at the 10-year follow-up. In Study 1, participants were randomized into three groups with varying targets: (1) Parent and child weight loss; (2) Child only weight loss or (3) A non-specific target control group. Additional detail on this study design was reported in Epstein, Valoski and colleagues (1990). Participants in Study 2 participated in a diet and lifestyle intervention, a diet only intervention or a wait-list, no treatment control (Epstein, Wing, et al., 1984). The inclusion of the no treatment control provides a useful contrast and interesting information regarding the effectiveness of these treatments. Exercise consisted of an energy expenditure of 2,800 kcal weekly or the equivalent of 4 miles per day for a 150 pound person. Participants in the diet only group also received information on low expenditure calisthenics and stretching, but were not reinforced for changes in activity. In Study 3, the effects of parental weight status and child self control on child weight loss were assessed. Families were comprised of either at least one obese parent or two non-obese parents. Participating families in Study 4 were randomized to one of three groups: (1) aerobic exercise; (2) lifestyle exercise or a (3) calisthenics control group (Epstein, Koeske, & Wing, 1984). The three groups were similar in time allocated to exercise, goal setting, and feedback. However, the calisthenics control group experienced considerably less calorie expenditure than the aerobic and lifestyle exercise experimental groups. In order to promote adherence, the weekly energy expenditure goal for the groups was equivalent to approximately 9 miles per week. Similar to study 1, contingencies were structured so that parents and children received reciprocal reinforcement and independent support for behavior change of each other. Unfortunately, relative differences in the diet only versus diet, lifestyle exercise, aerobic exercise and calisthenics groups cannot be directly compared (Study 1, 2, 4) due to variability across studies in parent or child weight change directed contingencies and differences in weekly energy expenditure goals across studies. The inclusion of no treatment or treatment as usual control groups, particularly in Studies 1 and 4, would also provide additional information regarding the effectiveness of these individual treatments. However, the impressive long-term data from the individual studies provide valuable empirical evidence regarding the short- and long-term effectiveness of family-based behavioral weight control programs.

Dependent measures across studies included height, weight, changes in percentage overweight and changes in percentage over BMI for age and sex. Epstein and colleagues strengthened the validity of these outcomes by acknowledging both the limitations of self-report data (adjustments were made for underreporting of obesity) and developmentally related changes in BMI (used age appropriate standards to compare changes in BMI over time to the 50th percentile for the child's age and sex). Additionally, these researchers considered clinical significance and the magnitude of changes by examining the percentage of children in each group who were not overweight (less than 20% overweight) at 10 years and the percentage of children who showed at least a 20% increase or decrease in weight over 10-years. The inclusion of measures of energy intake, caloric expenditure, activity perception, environmental support, also strengthens the conclusions drawn regarding the role of these variables in treatment outcome. Although psychometrics were not reported for the treatment adherence measure, this questionnaire serves as a fidelity check for participant adherence to treatment and has been associated with treatment outcome at 5-years (Epstein et al., 1992). In stark contrast to the heavy reliance on self-report data without reliability checks, the inclusion of these measures represents a considerable strength of the reported studies. In addition, to these measures, variables which may have significantly influenced participant weight status in the last 10-years, such as psychiatric and medical history, tobacco use, drug use, and participation in other weight control programs, were assessed via questionnaire and interviews.

Due to the combination of data across the four studies, sufficient power was achieved to detect treatment effects across groups and studies. Results indicated: (Study 1) participants in the treatment condition targeting both parent and child weight loss demonstrated significant improvements in percentage overweight at 5- and 10-year follow-up as compared to children in the non-specific control group (- 15.3% vs. + 7.6%, respectively); (Study 2) participants in the diet and lifestyle exercise group (-10.0%) and the diet only group (-8.4%) experienced long-term decreases in percentage overweight that were not significantly different between groups; (Study 3) although children with non-obese parents demonstrated greater decreases in percentage overweight (-11.1%) versus children with at least one obese parent (+3.1%), parent weight status does not significantly effect child weight loss outcomes and (Study 4) children reinforced for lifestyle activity (-19.7%) and aerobic activity (-10.9%) experienced significant reductions in percentage over- weight at 10-years as compared to children in the calisthenics control group (+12.2%). Forty-three percent of children who received the parent and child weight target intervention and 64% of children who received the lifestyle exercise intervention maintained decreases of 20%. Overall, combined results indicated that 30% of children participating in these family-based, behavioral pediatric weight loss studies were not obese after 10-years. These results persisted even when smoking, other weight control attempts and other potentially confounding factors were taken into account.

Although psychiatric functioning was included in the medical assessment as a possible confound and prevalence was described (11.6% sample experienced depression), inclusion of baseline measures of psychosocial functioning would have been a valuable addition to these data. Results indicated that children who developed psychiatric disorders were less obese and less successful in long-term weight control than children who did not, but the findings did not address changes in psychological functioning over time. A number of factors predicted 10-year changes. The most predictive was percentage overweight at 5-year follow-up. However, when 5-year results were removed from the regression equation, environ- mental factors, such as number of meals eaten at home, weight status and activity behaviors of persons with whom the child lives, daily self-monitoring of weight and support and encouragement of family and friends, accounted for a substantial portion of the variance (34%) in 10-year changes. These results are further strengthened by the inclusion of objective outcome measures, power analyses, and assessment and control of variables which could possibly compromise the accuracy of conclusions regarding the long-term effectiveness of these treatments.

Together, these outcome studies together provide valuable information about the effectiveness of family-based behavioral treatment for pediatric obesity and those specific strategies which are likely to maximize treatment outcomes. However, given the increasing prevalence of pediatric obesity, it is unclear how this approach can successfully address this problem at a public health level. Given the intensity of the treatment and the specialized skill and experience of multiple therapists involved in these studies, widespread dissemination of this approach appears to be a considerable challenge. Future studies should seek to streamline treatment to include those treatment components identified as most efficient and cost effective for a wide variety of children and families.

Activity and Weight Change. In 1995, Epstein, Valoski, Vara, McCurley, et al. investigated the role of decreasing sedentary behavior and increasing activity on weight change in obese children. Sixty-one families with 8- to 12-year-old children, who were recruited through media or referred by physicians and school nurses, participated in the study. Inclusion criteria included: (a) Child 20% to 100% overweight and (b) One parent willing to attend treatment meetings. Families were excluded from participation if either parent was greater than 100% overweight, if a family member was on an alternative weight control program, if the child or parent had current psychiatric problems or if there were medical conditions that would prevent exercise.

At baseline, body composition, fitness data and activity preference questionnaire data were collected for all participants. Percentage overweight was calculated for children and adults on the basis of height and weight data. Percent body fat was estimated using an electrical impedance monitor and waist-to-hip ratio was measured with a flexible measuring tape. Fitness was measured via physical work capacity (PWC_{150}), which was determined from the regression of heart rates onto a bicycle ergometry workload that produced a heart rate of 150 beats per minute. The sophistication of the included anthropometric and fitness assessments is a particular strength in that various physiological correlates of pediatric obesity and inactivity are measured. To assess activity preference, participants were asked to rate on a Likert-type scale (1 = never, 5 = every day) how often they engaged in each of 42 activities and their liking of these activities (1 = don't like, 5 = like). A computer-based laboratory choice paradigm (Epstein et al., 1991) was used to assess children's choices between sedentary and vigorous physical alternatives. Caloric intake and compliance data were collected during the last 2 weeks of treatment. Habit books containing self-monitoring data were used to estimate energy intake and compliance to treatment goals. Although families were provided weekly feedback on their monitoring, the heavy reliance on self-report and the known tendency for obese participants to underestimate their intake (Bandini, Scholler, Cyr, & Dietz, 1990) may limit the validity of these reports. Inclusion of a second reporter, for reliability purposes, could strengthen the quality of this dependent measure. Additionally, inclusion of psychosocial measures, such as depression, peer relationships, or self-esteem inventories would be a valuable addition to the assessment battery. Body composition, fitness data and questionnaire data were collected post-treatment and all but questionnaire data were gathered at 1-year follow-up.

The average child participant was 10.1 years of age, 51.8% overweight, with 33.2% body fat, a waist-to-hip ratio of .94, and physical work capacity (PWC_{150}) of 59.3 watts. The average mother was 29.8% overweight, with 34.5% body fat and a waist-to-hip ratio of .84; the average father was 33.4% overweight, with 26.3% body fat and a waist-to-hip ratio of .95. The sample was predominately Caucasian, middle-class, and female. No between group differences were observed at baseline on any child or adult measure. Data on family composition, non-exercise related medical comorbidities and psychosocial functioning were not reported.

Participants were randomized to one of three treatment conditions: sedentary, exercise, or combined. The groups differed in the activities that were reinforced. Parents and children attended treatment meetings (including a group and individual component) on a weekly basis for 4 months, followed by two monthly meetings and measurement at 1 year. During the meetings, parents and children were weighed and counseled together by a therapist and then attended separate group meetings for parents or children. No information regarding the qualifications or training of the therapists were provided. For both parents and children, individual meetings consisted of reviewing monitoring, providing feedback, and providing rewards. Parent meetings also included training in negotiating and contracting with the child.

All children, regardless of group assignment, received a comprehensive obesity treatment program consisting of both diet and activity components. The diet portion of the intervention consisted of the Traffic Light Diet (Epstein, Wing, & Valoski, 1985) with 7 or fewer instances of consumption of red foods per week, a total caloric intake to 1,000 to 1,200 calories per day, and use of the eating-right pyramid or the basic four food groups to maintain nutrient balance. Although calories were not restricted for non-overweight parents, they were asked to limit red foods to seven or fewer per week.

In the activity portion of the intervention, participants received information written manuals informing them about the benefits of increased activity and the negative effects of engaging in common sedentary behaviors like watching television, talking on the telephone and playing computer games. Participants in the exercise group were reinforced for increasing physical activity, while reinforcers were provided to children in the sedentary group for decreasing sedentary activity. Children and adults in the combined group were reinforced for decreasing sedentary activity and increasing physical activity. A five-level system of behavior change requirements was used to shape changes in the targeted behaviors. Parents and children moved through the levels independently, advancing one level at a time. Meeting these requirements resulted in a contract reward. Sedentary behavior goals involved a decrease from a goal of 35 hours or less per week of the targeted sedentary activities at Level 1 to 15 hours per week or less of sedentary behavior at Level 5, decreasing in 5-hour increments across the levels. Physical activity goals included increases from 30 to 150 activity points per week (30 point increments). Participants were instructed how to convert time spent in physical activity to activity points. If goals were met early in the program, maintenance of activity change behaviors throughout the remainder of treatment was required to receive the contract reward. In order to receive the contract reward, a weight goal was also added to Level 5 that required participants to either lose 3 lbs or maintain their weight for 3-week intervals, depending on whether the individual had reached his or her ideal weight.

In addition to diet and activity, treatment also incorporated a variety of behavioral principles. Epstein et al. (1995) incorporated a mastery approach to teaching families how to change eating and activity habits. This individualized program included parent and child manuals which contained practice situations, readings and quizzes. Participants also used self-monitoring to record their weight, food and caloric intake, number of red foods, and time spent in physical and sedentary activity. Monitoring of activity differed according to group assignment. Participants in the sedentary group recorded the time spent in targeted sedentary activities, whereas participants in the exercise group recorded the number of earned exercise points. The combined group participants recorded both time spent in sedentary behaviors and exercise points. Stimulus control was used to increase physical activity, limit access to red foods, and decrease cues for engaging in sedentary behaviors. Parental praise of child behavior and reciprocal contracting between parents and children were used to reinforce desired diet and activity behaviors.

Of the 61 participants, 55 completed both treatment and follow-up. Attrition occurred due to non-treatment related injury, death, and other unreported factors. No significant differences between groups were observed for any of the anthropometric variables at baseline. Significant between group differences in the rate of change were observed for percentage overweight and body fat. Results indicated that at post-treatment, children in the decrease sedentary behavior group achieved a greater reduction in percentage overweight than children in either the exercise or the combined group, with differences between the decrease sedentary behavior and exercise group significantly differing. At 12-months, children in the decrease sedentary behavior group showed significant differences in percentage overweight versus both other groups. A similar pattern of results was found for changes in body fat, with significant reductions for the decrease sedentary behavior group as compared to the exercise group at 12-months. For all groups, fitness and child waist-to-hip ratio improved over time. Post-treatment, children in the decrease sedentary behavior group showed a significant increase in preference for high-intensity activities as compared to children in the exercise group, who showed only a minimal increase in preference for such activities. Based on habit book data, no differences in compliance were observed across groups. Child caloric intake was significantly different across groups at post-treatment with children in the exercise group consuming more energy per day than children in the other two conditions. No differences in choice by treatment group or differential changes in activity choice over time were observed.

The results of this study provide empirical support for the assertion that physical activity is an integral component of treatment for pediatric obesity. Epstein and colleagues (1995) illuminate the differential impact of reinforcing reductions in sedentary behaviors versus reinforcing increases in physically active behaviors on reductions in percentage overweight and adiposity. The inclusion of the combined group appears to provide data to support that reinforcing physical activity reduces the effectiveness of reinforcing decreases in sedentary behavior. Thus, this commonsensical strategy for increasing activity appears to be incomplete. The authors conclude that providing children with a sense of choice and control may be reinforcing in itself and increase the reinforcing value of physical activities. Similarly, children in the exercise group may have attributed their behavior change to parental control, which may reduce the reinforcing value of engaging in physical activities and discourage long-term maintenance of active behavior. This assertion is consistent with the findings of Israel, Guile, Baker & Silverman (1994) suggestion that enhancing the child's active role in treatment may be associated with improved outcomes, but is at odds with other research highlighting the important role of parents as exclusive agents of change in the treatment of childhood obesity (Golan, Weizman, Apter & Fainaru, 1998). Further research manipulating levels of child and parent control are warranted. Although the authors claim that the exercise group provided a "powerful treatment comparison" for the decrease in the sedentary group and "further underscores the intervention received by the sedentary group" (p114), additional information regarding the effectiveness of this intervention could have been ascertained with the inclusion of either a no-treatment or treatment as usual control group. How these outcomes compare to monitoring effects is unclear. Additionally, blindness of raters and assessment of clinical significance were not discussed. Furthermore, the replicability and generalizability of this treatment approach is brought into question. Although, structuring treatment to include both group and individualized care increases the likelihood of maximizing outcomes (Epstein, Valoski, Wing, & McCurley, 1990), importantly, it does so at the expense of treatment efficiency. Thus, this structure presents a considerable obstacle to the effective and cost-effective treatment of pediatric obesity.

In a follow-up study, Epstein, Paluch, Gordy, and Dorn (2000) further investigated the effect of decreasing sedentary behaviors, in contrast to increasing physical activity, when included as a component of comprehensive obesity treatment program. Additionally, dose-response relationships between the amount of reduction in sedentary behaviors and weight loss and fitness outcomes were tested. Participants included 90, obese 8- to 12-year-old children and their parents, self-referred or referred by their physician. Children who were between 20% and 100% overweight, with one parent who was willing to participate in treatment, were included in the sample. Families subject to dietary or exercise restrictions, with current psychiatric problems, currently participating in other weight control programs, and whose parents were greater than 100% overweight were excluded from participation. Sixty-four percent of the participating parents were obese, with mothers, on average, 51.5% overweight and fathers, on average, 41.6% overweight.

Gender composition of the sample, average age, family composition, socioeconomic status and other sample descriptors were not reported.

Families were stratified by sex and randomly assigned to four groups: (1) decrease sedentary, low dose (reductions of sedentary activity of 10 hours per week); (2) decrease sedentary, high dose (reductions of sedentary activity of 20 hours per week); (3) increase activity, low dose (10 miles per week) or (4) increase activity, high dose (20 miles per week). The 6-month treatment included 16 weekly meetings, followed by 2 biweekly and 2 monthly meetings. One and 2-year follow-up assessments were held. Families received parent and child workbooks including information on self-monitoring, the Traffic Light Diet (limiting red foods to 10 per week), the assigned activity program, behavior change techniques and maintenance of behavior change. Additionally, families were provided additional nutritional information, including reading food labels, stimulus control strategies, and the use of preplanning as a problem-solving technique for difficult eating and activity situations. Parents and children were trained in positive reinforcement and reciprocal contracting. After anthropometric measures were collected, families met with individual therapists for 15- to 30-minutes to review weekly weight change and dietary behaviors, activity and the behavioral contract. Parents and children then attended separate 30-minute, individualized groups. Activity programs did not differ from Epstein et al. (1995).

Dependent measures were collected at baseline, post-treatment (6-months), and at 1- and 2-year follow-ups. Anthropometric measures included height, weight, BMI for age and sex, percentage overweight, body fat (via bioelectrical impedance), and fat free body mass data. Fitness was assessed via heart rate, Physical work capacity (PWC_{150}), maximal oxygen consumption and physical activity questionnaire (based on the Minnesota Leisure Time Activity Survey). Activity and sedentary analyses were based on complete data for 48 children. Socioeconomic data were also gathered. Assessments of psychosocial functioning were not utilized. Across groups, results indicated significant reductions in percent overweight from baseline to post-treatment (-25.5%) and through 2-year follow-up (additional -12.9%), representing a reduction of 38.4% from baseline. Physical work capacity also significantly improved across groups, with increases of 33% by 6-months and an increase of 55% by 24-months. No significant differences in the rate of change by group were observed for any anthropometric or fitness measures. For all participants, the intervention resulted in a significant increase in the percentage of time spent being active. Targeted sedentary behaviors significantly decreased, while nontargeted sedentary behaviors increased from baseline to post-treatment. Obese parents also demonstrated a significant decrease in weight throughout treatment. These findings were maintained at 2-year follow-up. Results of this study showed that these two approaches to promoting activity in obese children were associated with similar decreases in percentage overweight and increases in fitness through 2-year follow-up. Thus, the results of the previous study were not replicated.

However, it is difficult to fully understand the effect of treatment on changes in physical activity or fitness without the inclusion of a treatment as usual or no physical activity control group. For all anthropometric and fitness measures, results did not differ across groups. However, the marked increases in physical activity, as compared to previous research, may indeed be related to limited access to a variety of reinforcing physical activity options. Moreover, the lack of inclusion of habit books to record daily caloric expenditure poses a considerable problem for interpretation of results, as energy intake, as it interacts with sedentary and physical activity and plays an integral part in weight loss. This study provides further empirical support for targeting sedentary and physical activity in the treatment of pediatric obesity.

In 2001, Faith, Berman, Heo, Pietrobelli et al. investigated the effects of a contingent television intervention on physical activity, television viewing, and changes in body fat in obese children. Ten obese children, aged 8- to 12-years-old, indicated interest in the study by responding to newspaper advertisements targeting children who watch excessive amounts of television. Inclusion criteria included: (a) BMI above the 85th percentile for age and sex; (b) watched at least 2 hours of television per day; (c) did not engage in regular physical activity (d) went home directly after school most days of the week; (e) had no siblings within 7 years of age and (f) had sufficient physical space within the home to install the television cycle. Seven boys and 3 girls participated in the study. No demographic information or further participant description was provided. Of the 10 total participants, 2 withdrew before completion of the 12-week program due to cycle malfunction and non-treatment related factors. Children were randomized, using a computer pseudo-random number generator program, to the experimental TV cycle group or to a non-contingent cycle control group. Lifecycles ergometers were placed in homes of children in both conditions. A 2-week baseline period was followed by a 10-week intervention period in which the Lifecycle was activated for children in the experimental group to operate the television contingent on pedaling. Children in the experimental condition earned 2-minutes of television viewing for each minute of pedaling. Although they had free access to the Lifecycle, no reinforcement was provided for pedaling for children in the control group.

Primary dependent measures were pedaling and television viewing times, which were continuously recorded by the micro-computer of the television cycle. Screening measures included the Child Behavior Checklist (CBCL; Achenbach, 1991) and the Brief Symptom Inventory (BSI). However, no psychological measures were administered at conclusion of treatment. BMI and percent total body fat, as measured by either dual-energy x-ray absorptiometry or bioimpediance analysis were also assessed at baseline and post-treatment. These measures also provided data on arm and leg percent fat. Five children in the experimental condition and 4 control participants underwent anthropometric testing. Results indicated that children in the experimental condition, as compared to those in the control group, showed significantly greater reductions in percentage leg fat and percentage total body fat (-1.2% versus +.9%, respectively). However, the clinical significance of these changes in body composition was not discussed. Therefore, it appears unlikely that these minimal changes in body fat were significantly related to improvements in health status. Data on pedaling and television viewing time indicated that children in the treatment group pedaled 64.4 minutes per week on average during the 10-week treatment phase, whereas children in the control group pedaled 8.3 minutes per week on average. Although these increases are notable, these data still fall short of the 60-minute daily physical activity recommendation. Among the experimental group, pedaling time significantly increased from baseline to weeks 3 to 5, while television viewing time significantly decreased across the 12-week study. Across the 10-week treatment phase, the experimental group spent on average 1.6 hours each day watching television, whereas children in the control group watched an average of 21.0 hours of television per day. This study demonstrated marked decreases in television viewing with the introduction of the contingent cycle, as compared to children in the general population who view approximately 23 hours of television per week. Unfortunately, however, failure to include a number of outcome measures leaves many questions unanswered. How were children allocating their leisure time? Did children access other televisions? Were there any changes in energy consumption? Did increased physical activity generalize to other activities besides the television cycle? Further research is warranted. However, this study provides support for reinforcement of physical activity, stimulus control strategies and the powerful influence of structuring an environment to support and promote healthy diet and activity behaviors.

Problem Solving and Weight Control. Epstein, Paluch, Gordy, Saelens & Ernst (2000) examined the differential effectiveness of problem solving training in the treatment of childhood obesity. Families were self-referred or recruited from referrals from physicians or previous participants. Participants included 67 families with a child greater than 20% overweight, one parent willing to attend treatment meetings, and child reading at a third-grade level or higher. Families with a parent who was greater than 100% overweight or with a family member who was either involved in an alternative weight-control program, diagnosed with current psychiatric problems or with activity restrictions were excluded. The final sample consisted of 62 families. The sample of children was predominately Caucasian, with mean BMI values of 27.4 (SD = 3.2). Additional participant demographic data, including participant age, gender composition of groups, socioeconomic status, and family composition data, were not reported.

Families were stratified by gender and degree of child and parental obesity then randomized to three groups: (1) parent and child problem-solving; (2) child problem-solving or (3) standard family-based treatment. Treatment included 16 weekly meetings followed by two monthly meetings. Families were also seen at 1- and 2-years after randomization for treatment follow-up and data collection. During each weekly treatment meeting, participants were weighed, met with individual therapists for 15- to 30-minutes and attended individualized parent or child group meetings. Information regarding the credentials or experience of therapists was not reported. The treatment consisted of workbooks describing the traffic light diet, lifestyle physical activity, and behavior change techniques including self monitoring, positive reinforcement, stimulus control, and preplanning. Didactic training in problem-solving, based on research by D'Zurilla and Goldfried (1971) and Robin and Foster (1989), was provided in group formats. For families in the problem solving conditions, group leaders used problem-solving methods when questions were asked. Depending on treatment condition, problem solving methods or didactic responses were given when questions were asked in the group. Similar distinctions were made in worksheet and homework emphasis for both groups. Further description of the problem-solving training, its components, and how it was tailored towards the treatment of pediatric obesity was not provided. Height, weight, body mass index (BMI) z scores, child problem solving scores, measured by the Purdue Elementary Problem Solving Inventory (PEPSI; Fldhusen, Houtz, & Ringenbach, 1972), child psychological problems, assessed by the Child Behavior Checklist (CBCL: Achenbach, 1991), parent psychological problems, as measured by the Symptom Checklist – 90 (Derogatis, 1995) and adherence behaviors, assessed by the Adherence Questionnaire (a laboratory constructed questionnaire) served as the primary dependent measures for pretest, posttest, 1-year and 2-year follow-up. Psychometrics were not reported for the included assessment measures.

Results indicated no significant differences between groups at baseline or in adherence to treatment throughout the study. Parent problem-solving significantly improved over time for parents in the parent and child group, whereas parents in the standard group demonstrated no changes over time on this measure. Parent problem solving change was related to parent weight change and changes in parent distress, but changes in parent distress did not persist from posttest to 2-year follow-up. Comparisons of the rate of weight change between the parent and child group versus the standard group indicated that both groups demonstrated similar decreases in weight at post-test, but the standard group showed smaller increases in total weight from baseline to 2-year follow-up and posttest to 2-year follow-up. Children in the standard group had larger decreases in standard BMI from baseline to 3-year follow-up than demonstrated by children in the parent and child group. Overall, the child only (50%) and standard groups (47%) had a greater percentage of children with large BMI decreases than did the parent and child group (11%). Child problem-solving showed significant changes over time with increases from baseline through 1-year follow-up, while total behavior problems, internalizing behavior problems, and total competence significantly improved at post-test, 1-year and 2-year follow-up. Baseline total behavior problems (CBCL scores) and change in these scores over 2 years predicted changes in child BMI over 2 years. Changes in child problem-solving were not significantly related to changes in BMI, but were related to baseline problem-solving and changes in child competence.

Overall, the results of this study indicated no advantages for child or parent weight control when parent and/or child are provided problem-solving training. In fact, clinically relevant BMI changes suggest the combined parent and child training in problem solving may compromise the standard treatment by potentially distracting attention from child weight change behaviors and redirecting attention to parent problem-solving issues and weight control. A particular strength of this study is the inclusion of child and parent psychological assessments and discussions of clinical significance. Results indicated that children demonstrated statistically and clinically significant psychological changes for Total Behavior Problems and Internalizing Behavior Problems over 2 years. Additionally, results were discussed in terms of "smaller total increases in weight" (p. 718) overtime. This reporting strategy, compounded by inadequate description of participants, confuses the refractory nature of childhood obesity and the tendency for normal weight gain throughout development. No between group differences were observed over time in change in parent weight or parent treatment adherence. In contrast to previous research, problem-solving training does not significantly add to the standard treatment. The authors suggest that previous results may be attributable to elimination of characteristics of standard behavioral treatments, but do not extrapolate on this hypothesis.

Future research identifying effective and potentially iatrogenic components of behavioral pediatric obesity programs is needed. The present study did not address the contribution of parent versus child control in their discussion of the differential impact of the two problem-solving treatment modalities. Superiority of the child only problem solving group, as compared to the parent and child group, may be consistent with other research and add additional empirical support for the benefits of maximizing child control in the treatment of obesity (Israel, Guile, Baker & Silverman, 1994). This treatment also resulted in both short- and long-term improvements in psychological functioning; however, it was not addressed how these improvements related to changes in BMI throughout the study. For example, did treatment non-responders demonstrate improvements in internalizing and externalizing behavior problems despite no changes in weight status? Future research would benefit from incorporating an idiographic approach to data analysis, which distinguishing treatment responders and non-responders, in addition to the sole presentation of group data. The findings of the present study may be at odds with previous research due to methodological limitations. Because the sample size for each of the three groups was not reported, it is unclear whether there was sufficient statistical power to find significant differences if indeed they exited. This study provides additional empirical support for the effectiveness of the traffic light diet in the treatment of pediatric obesity and its psychological sequelae. However, the lack of a standardized treatment manual and treatment fidelity checks reduces the replicability of the findings and compromises the types of conclusions that can be drawn regarding the effectiveness of problem-solving in the treatment of weight control.

In a follow-up study, Epstein, Paluch, Saelens, Ernst et al. (2001) evaluated the effects of behavioral, family-based treatment on disordered eating, child behavior problems and weight control in obese 8- to 12-year-old children. Sixty-seven families participated in the study. In order to be eligible for participation participating families included a child between 8- and 12-years-old who was between 20% and 100% overweight and could read at the third-grade level and one parent willing to attend treatment meetings. Exclusionary criteria included: (1) either parent over 100% overweight; (2) any family member participating in an alternative weight control program; (3) parent or child with current psychiatric problems and (4) restrictions preventing exercise. Forty-seven families completed baseline and 2-years assessments, thus, 76% of the sample was used to evaluate percent overweight change. The sample was predominately Caucasian and middle-class, with boys significantly more overweight than girls and mothers representing the large majority of participating parents.

Families were randomly assigned to one of three groups: problem-solving skills taught to parent and child; problem solving-skills taught to child only; and no additional problem-solving skills control. The treatment program included 15 weekly meetings, followed by 2 biweekly meetings and 2 monthly meetings during the 6-month treatment, with follow-up 2 years after commencement of treatment. Family members met with an individual therapist for 15- to 30-minutes and then attended a parent- or child-specific, 30-minute group meetings. Problem-solving training differed across groups, while all participants received similar diet, activity and behavior change information. The Traffic Light Diet with an initial 1,000 to 1,200 calorie goal and consumption of 7 or fewer red foods each week was implemented. Parents and children were instructed to praise increases in targeted eating and lifestyle activity behaviors by using reciprocal contracts based on meeting the goal.

Dependent measures were collected at baseline and 2-years and included weight, BMI for age and sex, and Child Behavior Checklist competence and behavior problem scale scores (CBCL; Achenbach, 1991). Parents were also administered the Symptom Checklist -90 (SCL-90) to assess parent psychological functioning and the Binge Eating Scale to assess parental disordered eating or weight-related cognition with severe problems. Children were administered the Kids' Eating Disorder Survey to assess symptoms of disorder eating and possible eating disorders, a well-validated measure for children 10- to 13-years-old. Social support for eating and exercise habits was used to assess encouragement and participation of family and friends in implementing health-related eating and exercise behaviors.

Results indicated that problem solving did not enhance psychological changes, as addition of problem solving did not enhance weight control. A significant reduction in CBCL total behavior problem and internalizing behavior problem scores was exhibited by children across groups. Total problems reduced from 16.3% to 4.1% and for internalizing problems, the percentages went from 16.3% at baseline to 0% at 2-year follow-up. No significant overall change in child eating disorder scores were found, although girls' scores decreased substantially. Twelve children had elevated total eating disorder scores at baseline and 13 children had elevated scores at 2-years. Six of these data points represent maintenance, while 7 of these scores represent development of eating disordered behaviors. Six children who had elevated scores at baseline did not have elevated scores at the 2-year follow-up. Neither child age nor percent overweight was related to any of the symptoms of disordered eating or psychological measures. Parents showed significant reductions in weight, symptoms of binge eating, and decreases in parental distress. The percentage of parents who met clinical criteria for binge eating went from 4.2% at baseline to 0% at 2-years. Similar patterns were found for parental distress with reductions from 17.0% at baseline to 6.3% at 2-years. The degree to which families used incentives to support eating and exercise change and changes in child behavior problems were related to both changes in total child eating disorder scores and weight dissatisfaction. Changes in symptoms of disordered eating predicted total problems and externalizing problems, while decreases in parent distress predicted improvement in child competence, but not in child behavior problems.

Due to methodological limitations, conclusions from this study should be viewed cautiously. Without the inclusion of a no treatment control group, we have little understanding of how additional family variables impact the typical development of eating disorders in obese preadolescents. An increased attention and family support control group without a weight control emphasis may have provided interesting information. As the sample consisted of primarily pre-adolescent children, many disordered eating behaviors may have yet to develop. Similarly, age-appropriate measures are not available and a heavy reliance on child self-report further limits the sensitivity and validity of these data. Yet, addressing disordered eating habits at this young age may prove to be a valuable prevention strategy. The authors provided an important contribution to the literature by examining the potential iatrogenic effects of child and preadolescent weight control programs and the role psychological factors play in the development of eating disorders. While the inclusion of participants with behavior problems in the clinical range and attention to these sequelae of obesity represents a considerable strength of this research, like many studies in the treatment of pediatric obesity, sufficient attention to socioeconomic and ethnic diversity is lacking. With the heightened increase in risk of obesity for ethnically diverse children, future studies should address the behavioral and psychological functioning of obese children in these populations. This program was associated with significant changes in weight and improvements in psychological functioning in children and their parents, and limited changes in child self-reported disordered eating symptoms and weight dissatisfaction. Results suggest that child behavior problems and symptoms of eating disorders may interact in children who are participating in weight control programs. However, it is unclear whether reductions in child behavior problems leads to reductions in eating disordered behavior or if the reverse is true. Overall, this study provides support for the assertion that multi-component, behavioral weight control programs improve child behavior problems, competence and weight status.

Parent versus Child Control. Multi-component treatments for pediatric obesity have differed in their emphasis on parent versus child control. Several researchers have directly manipulated this factor. To investigate the efficacy of enhanced child self-regulation training in the treatment of childhood obesity, Israel, Guile, Baker and Silverman (1994) compared this experimental condition to a parent-focused treatment control condition. Thirty-four overweight children between the ages of 8- and 13-years-old were recruited to participate in the study via newspaper articles and letters to pediatricians and school nurses. Inclusion criteria included that children were at least 20% overweight for height, age and sex, received medical clearance from a physician, had at least one parent willing to attend sessions and an absence of any physical or psychological difficulty that would interfere with participation. Of the 34 families beginning treatment, 8 families failed to complete the full 26 week treatment. Six families were not available for follow-up at both 1 and 3 years post-treatment. The sample was not described in terms of ethnicity, socioeconomic status, percent overweight, family composition, or other demographic variables. At baseline, groups were not significantly different in terms of parental weight, child percent overweight, or child triceps skinfold.

Participants were randomized to a standard treatment or the Enhanced Child Involvement (ECI) intervention condition. Parents and children met in separate groups for 8 weekly, 90-minute sessions, followed by 9 biweekly sessions (total 26 weeks). Both groups received a multi-component intervention consisting of discussion and homework assignments regarding cue control, physical activity, food intake and rewards (CAIR). Families were asked to monitor the child's food intake, adherence to cue control rules and parents were asked to reward appropriate behaviors including staying under a prescribed calorie limit and meeting minimal physical activity recommendations. Parents also received parent training including techniques for identifying problem behaviors, planning a program to change behaviors, and program implementation. Parent training was supplemented with the text *Living with Children* (Patterson, 1976), which parents were required to read.

In the standard treatment condition, parent responsibility for completion of homework and child motivation was emphasized. In contrast, the ECI condition emphasized child management of weight loss efforts. Children were taught self-management skills throughout the treatment including instruction on goal setting, formulating and implementing behavior change plans, self-evaluation/progress monitoring, self-reward and problem-solving behaviors. Skills were taught didactically and homework exercises were provided. Parents in this condition were also to reward their children for engaging in self-management skills.

Children were evaluated at baseline, post-test (26-weeks), 1-year and 3-years post treatment on anthropometric measures, self-regulation and self-control measures. Percent overweight and percentage over tricep skinfolds norm were calculated via height, weight, and tricep skinfold thickness, respectively. Self-regulation and self-control was assessed via the Locus of Control Scale for Children (LOCSC; Nowicki & Strickland, 1973), the Self-Control Rating Scale (SCRS; Kendall & Wilcox, 1979), and The Eating and Activity Self-Control Scale (EASC; based on

Cohen, 1980). Measures of problem-solving included the Means End Problem-Solving Test (MEPS; Shure & Spivack, 1972), the Situational Competency Test for Overweight Children and the Parent's Situation Record (developed for this study). A Homework Questionnaire was also administered to assess parents' perceptions of the degree of responsibility their child took for homework completion. Psychometrics of the included instruments were not addressed.

Results indicated no differences between groups with respect to parental weight, child percent overweight or child triceps skinfold at post-treatment (26-weeks), 1 year or 3-year follow-up evaluation. Across conditions, children demonstrated, on average, a reduction of 13.1% overweight. The condition by time interaction, with percent overweight at baseline as a covariate, was not significant. However, these null findings may be due to insufficient power (post hoc power analyses for condition = .14 and for condition by time interaction = .19). Results for triceps skinfold data were similar. Across conditions, children demonstrated a mean reduction in percentage over triceps norm of 32.6%. The main effect for time was significant. During the follow up period, children in both groups tended to report a gain in percentage overweight and percentage over triceps skinfold norms. However, 44% of children in the experimental group remained below post-treatment percentage overweight at 3-year follow-up. In regards to self-regulation measures, analyses showed that groups were not significantly different on any measures post-treatment. Across groups, increases were observed in child perceptions of an internal locus of control, child self-control and parent control regarding weight behaviors. For children in the experimental condition, post-treatment locus of control scores significantly predicted changes in percent overweight with higher internal scores predicting smaller gains in percent overweight. Higher child self-control scores, but not parent control scores, were correlated with decreases in percent overweight during treatment. Although trends were in the predicted directions, these relationships did not persist at follow-up. Skills associated with refusals of temptations (Situational Record) were highly correlated with changes in percent overweight from post-treatment to 1-year follow-up. Most children did not achieve non-obese status.

Do to a lack of statistical power, the results of this study must be interpreted with caution. In general, these results provide additional data supporting the efficacy of multi-component behavioral treatments in reducing child overweight. However, the authors state that these results are "more modest than once might have been hoped for" and that success is "short lived" (p747). The authors interpret these findings, given their limitations, to suggest that enhanced self-regulation training and the increase involvement of children in treatment is promising. For example, control beliefs and behaviors post treatment were associated with more positive outcomes post-treatment. These findings may have implications for possibly beneficial skills to include in relapse prevention components of future programs. The inclusion of a no treatment control group may have also provided useful and interesting information. Dismantling studies and component analyses could contribute more knowledge to our understanding of the specific impact of self-regulation training on outcomes. Furthermore, the use of a convenience sample and the reported attrition rates bring into question the social validity of this treatment approach. Overall, the present findings do not allow a clear understanding of the construct of self-regulation or its relationship to child weight control. Future research investigating the efficacy of self-regulation training, with the inclusion of well-validated assessment measures, is warranted.

To test alternative intervention models, Golan, Weizman, Apter and Fainaru (1998) investigated the efficacy of a family-based approach in which the parents served as the exclusive agents of change as compared to that of a conventional approach, in which children serve as the agents of change. Sixty obese children aged 6- to 11-years-old, recruited from the public school system in central Israel, were included in the study. In order to be eligible for participation, children had to weigh greater than 20% above recommendations for age, height, and sex, have no history of psychiatric disorders and have both parents living at home. Parents had to agree to attend group sessions, complete questionnaires and undergo regular checkups. Children who refused blood sampling and parents who did not agree that their child needed obesity related treatment were excluded from participation. One-hundred-sixty children were identified as obese, 140 met inclusion criteria and 60 agreed to participate. The majority of the study was middle class, with at least one obese parent, and in 45% of the families, both parents were obese. Children were on average 8.9-years-old and 39.6% overweight as baseline. Gender distribution of the sample was not reported.

Children were randomized to an experimental group with parents as the sole agents of change or a control group with children as the sole agents of change. The groups were matched for sex and age and no difference in socioeconomic status was found between the groups. Parents in the experimental group attended 14, 1-hour long support and educational group sessions, led by a clinical dietitian. Sessions were held weekly for the first 4 weeks, biweekly for the next 4 weeks, and ever 6 weeks for the last 6 sessions. Parents were trained in eating behavior modification, nutrition education (including decreasing dietary fat), cognitive restructuring, parental modeling, problem solving, creating opportunities for physical activity, decreasing stimulus exposure, limits of responsibility and coping with resistance. Fifteen couples participated in each parent group. Five additional brief (15-minute) individual, whole family sessions were held during the last 7 months of the program to maintain contact with families and gather anthropometric data. Children in the control group were prescribed a reduced calorie diet and 30, 1-hour long group sessions led by a clinical dietitian, addressing physical activity, eating behavior modification, stimulus control, self-monitoring, nutrition education, problem solving and cognitive restructuring. Fifteen children participated in each group session. Individual sessions were provided in the event that a child missed a group, encountered difficulties in adherence, or requested a change in diet prescription. The first eight sessions were held on a weekly bases and the remainder biweekly for a total of 1 year. Because group size was limited to 15 participants and treatment was not reported as manualized, questions arise as to the standardization of treatment across participants within condition.

Primary dependent measures included anthropometric measurements (weight, height, percentage overweight), caloric intake and diet and activity behaviors, and were collected at baseline, post-treatment and 6-months after the end of the intervention. To assess caloric intake, food diaries were collected for 7 days and validated by a clinical dietitian using 24-hour recall. The Family Eating and Activity Habits Questionnaire, developed and validated by the authors, was used to assess changes in weight control behaviors post-treatment. Results indicated that attrition occurred at a significantly higher rate for children in the control group than for families in the experimental group. Whereas 29 families completed the experimental treatment, 21 families in the control group terminated participation prematurely. Parents and children in the control group reported heightened levels of stress, irritation, frustration and tension with weight control. Both groups of children demonstrated a decrease in percentage overweight during the study period, with significantly greater weight reduction observed for children in the experimental group. These differences emerged after the first 3-months of treatment, with 85% of these results maintained at follow-up. Children in the experimental group exhibited a 14.6% decrease in percentage overweight compared to an 8.1% decrease for children in the control group. Seventy-nine percent of children in the experimental group lost greater than 10% of their excess weight and 35% achieved nonobese status (less than 10% overweight). In comparison, 38% of children in the control group lost greater than 10% of their excess weight and 14% reached nonobese status. In contrast to other research, these authors divided children into three groups based on percentage overweight at baseline, but found no significant group by level of overweight interactions. Fathers in the experimental group experienced significant reductions in percentage overweight at posttest, whereas parents in both groups and mothers in the experimental group did not experience significant changes in weight status.

Superior outcomes by Epstein and colleagues (1990) may be attributable to the joint involvement of both parents and children as compared to the sole reliance on parents as agents of change in this study. Additionally, although the control group in this study was presented as "conventional," few other researchers assign children as the sole agent of change in behaviorally-based treatment of pediatric obesity, given the large role parents play in structuring the environment of the young child. Yet, the contrast in intensity of the two groups, with the parent only group receiving significantly fewer sessions, underscores the utility and cost-effectiveness of incorporating or exclusively targeting parents in treatment. Comparing outcomes of the parent only group to a parent-child control group would have provided interesting outcomes. Given the level of peer support likely in the child only groups, psychosocial functioning, including peer relationships, would have also been an interesting dependent measure. The authors also discuss a lowered resistance to change when children were not assigned an obvious "patient" status as an important contributor to the success of the parent only group. This assumption is in contrast to that presented in previous research, which highlights the importance of child control in successful behavior change (Epstein et al., 1995; Israel, Guile, Baker & Silverman, 1994). Also, given that reinforcers were not actively incorporated in the control group and there was no sustained incentive for healthy diet and activity behaviors, it is likely that such behaviors would likely not be maintained in their absence (Faith et al., 2001). Considerations of degree overweight and levels of parental involvement represented considerable strengths in this study. This research provides empirical support for the superiority in adherence and weight reduction of a family based approach that targets parents as the sole agents of change as compared to a child-centered approach to the treatment of pediatric obesity. Parent involvement appears to be a central feature in the effective and efficient treatment of pediatric obesity.

Noting the lack of impact of current research on the increasing prevalence of childhood obesity, presented additional data supporting the efficacy of their parent-centered approach to the treatment of childhood obesity. In a follow-up study, Golan, Fainaru & Weizman (1998) evaluated the efficacy of a family-based treatment approach in which parents were the exclusive agents of change in reducing child overweight and producing changes in eating-related behaviors. The authors utilized the sample, methodology and procedures presented in the previously described study. No additional sample descriptors were provided. In brief, 60 children, aged 6- to 11-years-old were randomized to an experimental group with parents as the exclusive agents of change, or a control group in which children were responsible for their own weight loss. Parent and child participants were evaluated on anthropometric variables both pre- and post-intervention. Parents also completed the Family Eating and Activity Habits Questionnaire, which was develop by the authors for this study to identify factors associated with obesity and weight loss in children including, activity level, stimulus exposure, eating related to hunger, eating style and food intake.

Results of this investigation replicated those of the previously described study (Golan et al., 1998). Whereas children in both groups demonstrated a significant decrease in percent overweight, children in the experimental group showed significantly greater weight reduction (-14.6%) than controls (-8.4%). Although neither group showed an increase in physical activity or a decrease in television viewing behaviors, after the intervention, parents in the experimental group reported significant reductions in overall food stimuli, with significant reductions specifically in the number of sweets, snacks, cakes and ice creams available in the home. In terms of eating behaviors, significant differences were observed between groups in the presence of parental questioning about hunger before meals and subsequent parent directives to eat regardless of level of reported hunger. Similarly, as compared to children in the control group who only demonstrated reductions in the frequency with which they ate between meals, children of parents in the intervention group reportedly ate less often while standing, in response to stress, while engaged in other activities, or between meals. Overall, regression analyses indicated that behavioral changes explained 27% of the variance in overweight reduction. Eliminations in eating between meals and while studying or watching television were identified as the main contributors.

This research provides additional empirical support to the assertion that parents play an integral role in the treatment of childhood overweight. More specifically, this study demonstrates that parent education in behavior modification strategies is an effective means of changing problematic eating styles and subsequently, for reducing child overweight. However, the lack of significant differences between groups in reductions in sedentary activity (i.e., television viewing) and physical activity (e.g., swimming, bicycle riding, etc.) may have been due to a lack of sensitivity or accuracy in the measurement of these behaviors or possibly due to insufficient statistical power to detect real differences. Although the implications of this study are promising, the study is limited by a strong reliance in retrospective, parent-report data. For example, parents may not always have insight into their child's psychological motivation for eating (e.g., stress-induced) or the amounts or types of food their child consumes throughout the day. Focusing on parents as the exclusive agents of change presents a viable alternative to traditional family-based treatments. However, this program also represents an intensive, "parent-demanding" (p1223) intervention model. Given its promise, future studies should examine more efficient versions of this model, with an emphasis on parent adherence, social validity and cost-effectiveness.

Family Risk. Research has provided evidence for the superiority of family-based treatment programs in controlling weight for both pediatric and adult populations. In 1999, Golan, Weizman, and Fainaru compared the impact of two behavioral approaches for the treatment of childhood obesity on parental weight, eating and activity habits, and cardiovascular risk factors. Sixty obese children, ages 6- to 11-years-old participated in a 1-year clinical intervention study. Eligible participants weighed at least 20% greater than the expected weight for age, height and sex and had both parents living at home. There were no statistically significant differences between groups in anthropometric or demographic variables. In the experimental group, 15 mothers and 21 fathers were obese and in the control group, 12 mothers and 17 fathers were obese. Children were randomly assigned to either an experimental intervention group targeting parents only (n =30) or a conventional intervention group targeting only children (n = 30) matched for age, sex, and percentage overweight. Both parents in the experimental group attended 14, 1-hour long group sessions, staggered over a 1-year period. During the groups, parents were instructed to alter the family sedentary lifestyle, reduce fat intake, decrease exposure to food stimuli, apply behavioral modifications and practice relevant parenting skills. In the control group, children attended 30 sessions conducted by a clinical dietitian, conducted weekly for the first 8 sessions and biweekly for the remainder of sessions. Individual counseling was offered when a child missed a group session or needed additional support. Children were instructed restrict their energy intake, reduce fat intake, and increase physical activity, problem solving, cognitive restructuring and to use social support.

Dependent measures included anthropometric measures, including height, weight, BMI and percentage overweight, blood pressure, blood samples, including total cholesterol, HDL, serum insulin, serum glucose and triglyceride concentrations, and weight loss for both children and parents. Family eating and activity habits questionnaires were completed at baseline and at 12-months. Reliability and validity of the questionnaire were evaluated and found to be adequate.

Results indicated that using parents as the sole agents of change for treating childhood obesity resulted in greater weight loss in both children and parents and greater improvement in the cardiovascular risk factors among children when compared to the intervention in which children were the main agents of change. Seven of 21 obese fathers lost more than 10% of their baseline weight, while no fathers in the control group obtained such results. Mothers overweight did not change in both groups. Degree of overweight at baseline was not significantly related to weight loss in either group. Post-treatment, fathers in the experimental groups demonstrated significant reduction in plasma glucose levels (-16%) and in triglyceride levels (-21%), indicating a statistically significant difference from changes in cardiovascular risk factors as compared to fathers in the control group. Mothers in the experimental group showed improvement in insulin (-15%) and triglyceride levels (-8%) compared to controls. Changes in eating and activity habits were not significantly different across groups. A significant reduction in overall presence of restricted household food was reported by the experimental intervention group. Parent attendance was found to be positively, significantly correlated with child weight loss. Mother's baseline weight negatively, significantly correlated with attendance in sessions and father's baseline weight, attendance, and risk of cardiovascular disease were negatively correlated as well. The contribution of weight loss and the change in behaviors to the improvement in blood parameters was similar in both groups. Child weight loss was significantly correlated with paternal total cholesterol and glucose level in the experimental intervention group. Overall, treatment of childhood obesity using a cognitive behavioral intervention is more effective when parents are the exclusive agents of change compared to focusing on child behavior change directly. This study provides additional empirical evidence for the positive benefits of family-based treatments for children and parents and the importance of the inclusion of a strong parenting component in future treatments.

Toward Cost Effective Treatments. Researchers are beginning to acknowledge the shortcomings of existing treatments in addressing the public health crisis of pediatric obesity. Current approaches have focused on individual attention to maximize outcomes, but have done so at the expense of efficiency. Individualized approaches have been criticized as requiring more staff and financial resources than many clinics can reasonably afford. As the prevalence of obesity continues to increase, a new trend in pediatric obesity research is the development and evaluation of more cost effective treatment approaches. To date, little scientific attention has been given to the development of cost-effective treatments.

Building on the established efficacy of Epstein and colleagues' treatment approach, Goldfield, Epstein, Kilanowski, Paluch and Kogut-Bossler (2001) evaluated the cost-effectiveness of mixed (group and individualized) treatment format as compared to group-only family-based treatment for pediatric obesity. Cost-effectiveness of treatment was defined as the magnitude of reduction in standardized BMI and percentage overweight per dollar spent for recruitment and treatment. Thirty-one families, recruited from newspaper advertisements and physician referrals, were included in the study. Eligible participants were between 20% and 100% overweight, with neither parent greater than 100% overweight, with at least one parent willing to participate in treatment, no family member participating in alternative weight control programs, no child or parent having current psychiatric problems and no dietary or exercise restrictions on the participating parent or child. The sample was 100% Caucasian, middle class and mild to moderately overweight. No significant differences between groups were observed at baseline for any parent or child demographic or anthropometric variable (except parent height).

Families were randomized to either the mixed or group only treatment condition. Families were seen at 6 and 12 months after treatment began for follow-up assessments. Participants in both conditions attended 13 sessions including 8 weekly meetings, 4 biweekly meetings and one monthly meeting. Parent and child groups were conducted separately and a mastery approach to teaching was utilized to teach families how to change eating and activity habits. Child and adult participants were given manuals including information on diet, activity, behavior change techniques, parenting and coping with psychosocial problems commonly experienced by obese children, such as teasing and body image concerns. The same therapists provided treatment for children in both conditions. Approximately half of the therapists were new and half were skilled and experienced in family-based treatment of pediatric obesity. The majority of therapists had master's degrees in psychology, nutrition, or exercise science. Therapists received a standardized training provided by the Childhood Weight Control Program.

All families received the Traffic Light Diet (Epstein, Wing & Valoski, 1985), to decrease energy intake and promote a balanced diet, as described earlier in this paper. In addition to calorie restriction, activity guidelines were set. Behavior modification principles, including stimulus control, reinforcement, and self-monitoring principles were utilized to reinforce program adherent behaviors and assist families in attaining behavioral goals. For children in the mixed treatment group, 40-minute group sessions were supplemented with 15- to 20-minute individual sessions. Individual treatment focused on identifying those behaviors that influence weight change, problem-solving around treatment barriers, determining the accuracy of the habit book, and evaluating and providing feedback on goal attainment and program progress. Participants in the group only condition received an additional 20- minute group session to equate the time spent in treatment across conditions. Children participated in the first 15- to 20-minutes of the parenting group to assist in the development of the point system.

Anthropometric (i.e., percentage overweight, BMI) were collected at baseline and at 6- and 12-months post-randomization. Total treatment costs were calculated by adding the cost of screening, recruitment and treatment for both treatment completers and non-completers. Treatment costs included the cost of materials, staffing, and travel expenses. Cost-effectiveness was calculated by dividing change in standardized BMI scores or percentage overweight by the total cost of treatment at the 12 month follow-up. This provided the researchers with a measure of improvement per dollar spent. To facilitate interpretation of the cost effectiveness data, the researchers presented changes as if $1000 was spent providing treatment for each family.

Results indicated a highly statistically significant change in percent overweight and standardized BMI over time. No main effects or interactions due to group or generation were found. Across groups, children demonstrated a reduction in percent overweight of 9.97% (s.d. = 8.74) from baseline to 6-months and a reduction of 8.04% (s.d. = 10.27) from baseline to 12 months. Over the same time periods, parents showed reductions of 6.67% (s.d. = 10.3) and 5.31% (s.d. = 14.13), respectively. Obese parents reduced percentages overweight by 7.03% (s.d. = 11.65) at 6-months and 5.70% (s.d. = 16.08) at 12-months. The cost of group treatment ($491.51) was significantly less expensive than the cost of the mixed group ($1390.70). In regards to cost effectiveness, the group treatment (0.005 percentage units overweight per dollar) was associated with larger decreases in percentage overweight per dollar spent at 12-months than the mixed group (0.014 percentage units overweight per dollar). In total, the mixed intervention was approximately 2.8 times more expensive per family than the group only intervention, given equivalent weight control results.

This study represents an important step towards conceptualizing and treating childhood obesity as a public health problem. Unlike other studies, the treatment delivery method, rather than the efficacy of the treatment was emphasized. Based on the sound empirical base for the family-based, behavioral treatment of pediatric obesity, future studies can now embark on developing and validating efficient treatment packages that are ready for and amenable to widespread dissemination. The authors hypothesize that although both treatment formats include similar components, the process by which they impact change may differ considerably. The group format, in particular, is highlighted as providing social support and problem solving. Moreover, individuals may become more independent in their weight loss efforts and less reliant on therapist influenced effects, as compared to participants in individual treatment. As both group and individual treatments produce comparable effects, the authors also note that future research discriminating those who would benefit from individual from those who would most benefit from group treatment would be valuable for enhancing outcomes.

A considerable strength of this study was the inclusion of more novice therapists and detailed descriptions of therapist skill levels and disciplines. This increases the generalizability of these findings to other therapist samples. However, the generalizability of these findings to the larger pediatric population may be severely limited. Due to the inclusion of a largely homogenous convenience sample future studies should investigate if these findings are replicable with more obese and more ethnically and socially diverse populations. Additionally information on family composition and its relation to anthropometric outcomes in family-based treatments may provide meaningful information about the generalizability and social validity of this program. Future studies would benefit greatly from following the lead of Goldfield and colleagues and investigate the active treatment components necessary for even more cost-effective, wider reaching treatment delivery methods equipped to address the public health problem of pediatric obesity.

Conclusions and Future Directions

Based on the current review of the literature, progress has been made in the psychosocial treatment of childhood obesity in the past decade. The most extensively studied and effective treatments are multi-component, family-based behavioral treatments. Research demonstrates that a number of treatment components are implicated in the effective treatment of pediatric obesity. These include: 1). *Diet and Nutrition Education*: Focusing on what to eat versus what not to eat may increase program adherence (e.g., Epstein, 2001). 2). *Parent Training*: Involving and educating parents augments treatment effects and promotes long-term maintenance of treatment gains (e.g., Epstein, Valoski, et al., 1994; Golan, 1998, 1999, 2004; Israel et al., 1994). 3). *Physical Activity and Contingency Management*: Reinforcing lifestyle activity or programmed activity, in addition to dietary modifications, may maximize short- and long-term weight loss outcomes (e.g., Epstein, Valoski, et al., 1994). Similarly, reinforcing decreases in sedentary activity, targeting behaviors such as television viewing, computer and game playing, may provide children with a sense of control and facilitate positive treatment outcomes (e.g., Epstein, 1995). 4). *Stimulus Control*: Structuring the environment to support and promote healthy diet and activity behaviors (e.g., maximizing cues of physical activity while minimizing cues of sedentary activity) may augment treatment adherence (e.g., Faith et al., 2001). 5). *Mastery Criteria*: Providing mastery criteria for behavior change and individually tailoring programs to address differential learning curves may improve treatment efficacy (e.g., Epstein, McKenzie, et al., 1994). Furthermore, cost-effective adaptations of these programs may result in comparable outcomes, demonstrate a greater capacity to address larger segments of the population, and require relatively fewer resources (Goldfield et al., 2001).

Based on the methodological limitations of these studies, as reasonably expected, average reduction in percentage overweight using these means cannot be clearly known. However, family-based behavioral treatments, ranging from 10-weeks to 26-weeks in duration, have produced post-test reductions in child percentage overweight of -9.51% (Herrera et al., 2004) to approximately -26.5% (Epstein et al., 1994a). Although long-term maintenance of these results varies considerably across studies, comparable reductions in overweight have been shown to persist at 1-year follow-up (-25.5%; Epstein et al., 2000). However, these findings were based on individuals who were selectively recruited based on motivation to change and likelihood of success. Moreover, when investigating long-term follow-up data, only a small portion of the sample maintained even modest results (Epstein et al., 1994b). These represent significant limitations given this is the most widely studied, efficacious program to date for the family-based treatment of pediatric obesity. Given these limitations, future studies are warranted.

Based on treatment outcome data, pediatric obesity specialists waiver on whether the treatment of pediatric obese children should be considered as an optimistic or an unrealistically optimistic endeavor (Israel, 1999; Israel et al., 1994). The "common-sense cure" for obesity – eating less and being more physically active – has proven exceedingly difficult to achieve (Ebbeling, Pawlak, & Ludwig, 2002). Disappointing results may be understood in several ways. First, it is possible that our existing technologies are not sufficiently efficacious to address the problem of pediatric obesity. In this case, efforts would be well spent investigating novel means of increasing the strength of existing approaches. However, given the scope of the epidemic of childhood overweight and obesity, the greatest limitation of existing research is the lack of the adoption of a public health perspective.

The rapid increase in the prevalence of overweight and obesity strongly indicate that behavioral and environmental factors have played a significant role in contributing to the current epidemic. Many underscore a "toxic environment" (Horgen & Brownell, 2002), characterized by the promotion and accessibility of energy dense foods and increasingly sedentary lifestyles, as the primary contributing factor. This "toxic environment" is increasingly present as fiscal pressures lead communities to choose development over open spaces, schools to eliminate physical education and provide vending machines and fast-food lunches, parents to adopt increasingly less healthy lifestyles for their families and providers to have little motivation to effectively treat pediatric obesity. These pervasive environmental factors likely undermine individual efforts to maintain a healthy bodyweight (Ebbeling et al., 2002).

Future studies need to look at the multiple layers of treatment possible rather than assuming the traditional individual model is the most effective approach to treatment. The field would benefit greatly from future research investigating the clinical effectiveness and social validity of low-cost, accessible and efficient, behaviorally-based pediatric obesity treatment programs. A few progressive researchers are already considering this notion (e.g., Tate, Wing & Winett, 2001; Saelens et al., 2002; Ebbeling et al., 2002; Harvey-Berino, Pintauro, Buzzell & Gold, 2004). Pediatric obesity researchers must begin to look beyond efficacy and consider the criticism that existing programs have not yet been translated to effective office care (Barlow et al., 2000). Treatment approaches that focus on increasing the magnitude of children that can be successfully treated in a cost-effective manner will surely be welcomed as viable means for addressing the current epidemic.

A public health model for the treatment of pediatric obesity is presented in Table 1. Although this model does not intend to be comprehensive, our purpose is to encourage researchers to identify novel avenues for intervention and to consider issues of scope and dissemination in designing future treatments. Moreover, this

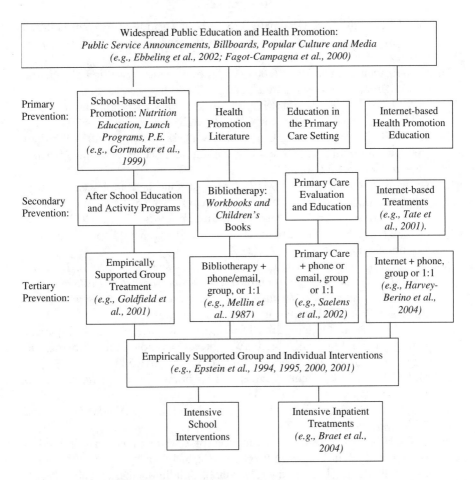

Table 1. Public Health Model for the Treatment of Pediatric Obesity. Note: Pharmacological interventions and bariatric surgery were not included as they are considered a last resort, only for children with complications (with careful consideration of risks), and beyond the scope of this review (Yanovski, 2001).

model is presented to encourage the collaboration of professionals, across disciplines, who have an impact on the behaviors and lifestyles of children who are overweight or at-risk for overweight. Together, families, schools, urban planners, and political leaders can take the fundamental measures needed to effectively detoxify the environment and create an atmosphere conducive to prevention and health promotion.

References

Aragona, J., Cassady, J., & Drabman, R. S. (1975). Treating overweight children through parental training and contingency contracting. *Journal of Applied Behavior Analysis, 8,* 269-278.

American Academy of Pediatrics. (2003). Policy Statement: Prevention of pediatric overweight and obesity. *Pediatrics, 112*(2), 424-430.

Bacon, G. E., & Lowrey, G. H. (1967). A clinical trial of fenfluramine in obese children. *Current Therapy Research Clinical and Experimental, 9,* 626-630.

Bandini, L. G., Schoeller, D. A., Cyr, H. N., & Dietz, W. H. (1990). Validity of reported energy intake in obese and nonobese adolescents. *American Journal of Clinical Nutrition, 52,* 421-425.

Barlow, S., & Dietz, W. (2002). Management of child and adolescent obesity: Summary and recommendations based on reports from pediatricians, pediatric nurse practitioners and registered dieticians. *Pediatrics, 110*(1), 236-238.

Barlow, S., & Dietz, W. (1998). Obesity evaluation and treatment: Expert committee recommendations. *Pediatrics, 102*(3), 29.

Birch, L. L., Johnson, S. L., Grimm-Thomas, K., & Fisher, J. O. (1998). *The Child Feeding Questionnaire (CFQ): An instrument for assessing parental child feeding attitudes and strategies. Operational definitions of factors, scoring and summing instructions.* University Park, PA: Pennsylvania State University.

Braet, C., Tanghe, A., Decaluwé, V., Moens, E., & Rosseel, Y. (2004). Inpatient treatment for children with obesity: Weight loss, psychological well-being, and eating behavior. *Journal of Pediatric Psychology, 22*(7), 519-529.

Cohen, J. (1960). A coefficient of agreement for nominal scales. *Educational and Psychological Measurement, 20,* 37-46.

Dietz, W. H. (2004). Overweight in childhood and adolescence. *New England Journal of Medicine, 350*(9), 855-857.

Dietz, W. H. (1998). Health consequences of obesity in youth: Childhood predictors of adult disease. *Pediatrics, 101*(3), 554-570.

Ebbeling, C. B., Pawlak, D., & Ludwig, D. (2002). Childhood obesity: Public-health crisis, common sense cure. *Lancet, 10*(360), 473-483.

Epstein, L. H., Gordy, C., Raynor, H., Beddome, M., Kilanowski, C., & Paluch, R. (2001). Increasing fruit and vegetable intake and decreasing fat and sugar intake in families at risk for childhood obesity. *Obesity Research, 9*(3), 171-178.

Epstein, L. H., Paluch, R. A., Saelens, B. E., Ernst, M. M., & Wilfley, D. E. (2001). Changes in eating disorder symptoms with pediatric obesity treatment. *Journal of Pediatrics, 139*(1), 58-65.

Epstein, L. H., Paluch, R. A., Gordy, C., Saelens, B. E., & Ernst, M. M. (2000). Problem solving in the treatment of childhood obesity. *Journal of Consulting and Clinical Psychology, 68*(4), 717-721.

Epstein, L. H., Paluch, R., Gordy, C., & Dorn, J. (2000). Decreasing sedentary behaviors in treating pediatric obesity. *Archives of Pediatric and Adolescent Medicine, 154,* 220-226.

Epstein, L. H., Kilanowski, C. K., Consalvi, A., & Paluch, R. (1999). Reinforcing value of physical activity as a determinant of child activity level. *Health Psychology, 18*(6), 599-603.

Epstein, L. H. (1999). Commentary: Future research directions in pediatric obesity research. *Journal of Pediatric Psychology, 24*(3), 251-252.

Epstein, L. H., Myers, M. D., Raynor, H. A., & Saelens, B. E. (1998). Treatment of pediatric obesity. *Pediatrics, 101*(3), 554-70.

Epstein, L. H., Myers, M. D., & Raynor, H. A.(1998). Predictors of child psychological changes during family-based treatment for obesity. *Archives of Pediatric and Adolescent Medicine, 152*(9), 855-861.

Epstein, L. H., Saelens, B. E., Myers, M. D., & Vito, D. (1997). Effects of decreasing sedentary behaviors on activity choice in obese children. *Health Psychology, 16*(2), 107-113.

Epstein, L. H., Valoski, A., Vara, L., McCurley, J., Wisniewski, L., Kalarchian, M., et al. (1995). Effects of decreasing sedentary behavior and increasing activity on weight change in obese children. *Health Psychology, 14*(2), 109-118.

Epstein, L. H., Klein, K. R., & Wisniewski, L. (1994). Child and parent factors that influence psychological problems in obese children. *International Journal of Eating Disorders, 15*(2), 151-158.

Epstein, L., McKenzie, S., Valoski, A., Klein, R., & Wing, R. (1994). Effects of mastery criteria and contingent reinforcement for family-based child weight control. *Addictive Behaviors, 19*(2), 135-145.

Epstein, L. H., Valoski, A., Wing, R. R., & McCurley, J. (1994). Ten-year outcomes of behavioral family-based treatment for childhood obesity. *Health Psychology, 13*(5), 373-383.

Epstein, L. H. (1992). Exercise and obesity in children. *Journal of Applied Sport Psychology, 4*(2), 120-133.

Epstein, L. H., McCurley, J., Wing, R., & Valoski, A. (1990). Five-year follow-up of family-based behavioral treatments for childhood obesity. *Journal of Consulting and Clinical Psychology, 58*(5), 661-664.

Epstein, L., & Wing, R. (1987). Behavioral treatment of childhood obesity. *Psychological Bulletin, 101*(3), 331-342.

Epstein, L. H., Wing, R. R., Koeske, R., & Valoski, A. (1987). Long-term effects of family-based treatment of childhood obesity. *Journal of Consulting and Clinical Psychology, 55*(1), 91-95.

Epstein, L. H., Nudelman, W., & Wing, R. (1987). Long-term effects of family-based treatment for obesity on nontreated family members. *Behavior Therapy, 18*(2), 147-152.

Epstein, L. H., Wing, R., Woodall, K., Penner, B., Kress, M., & Koeske, R. (1985). Effects of family based behavioral treatment on obese 5- to 8-year old children. *Behavior Therapy, 16*(2), 205-212.

Epstein, L. H., & Wing, R. (1983). Reanalysis of weight changes in behavior modification and nutrition education for childhood obesity. *Journal of Pediatric Psychology, 8*(1), 97-100.

Epstein, L. H., Wing, R. R., Steranchak, L., Dickson, B., & Michelson, J. (1980). Comparison of family-based behavior modification and nutrition education for childhood obesity. *Journal of Pediatric Psychology, 5*(1), 35-36.

Fagot-Campagna, A., Pettitt, D., Engelgan, M., Burrow, N., Geiss, L., Valdez, R., et al. (2000). Type 2 diabetes among North American children and adolescents: An epidemiologic review and a public health perspective. *Journal of Pediatrics, 136*(5), 664-672.

Faith, M., Berman, N., Moonsoeong, H., Pietrobelli, A. Gallagher, D., Epstein, L., et al. (2001). Effects of contingent television on physical activity and television viewing in obese children. *Pediatrics, 107*(5), 1043-1048.

Fisher, R. A. (1971). *The design of experiments* (9th ed.). New York: Hafner Publishing Company.

Golan, M., & Crow, S. (2004). Parents are key players in the prevention and treatment of weight-related problems. *Nutrition Reviews, 62*(1), 39-50.

Golan, M., Weizman, A., & Fainaru, M. (1999). Impact of treatment for childhood obesity on parental risk factors for cardiovascular disease. *Preventive Medicine: An International Journal Devoted to Practice & Theory, 29*(6), 519-526.

Golan, M., Weizman, A., Apter, A., & Fainaru, M. (1998). Parents as the exclusive agents of change in the treatment of childhood obesity. *American Journal of Clinical Nutrition, 67,* 1130-1135.

Golan, M., Fainaru, M., & Weizman, A. (1998). Role of behavior modification in the treatment of childhood obesity with the parents as the exclusive agents of change. *International Journal of Obesity Related Metabolic Disorders, 22*(12), 1217-1224.

Goldfield, G., Epstein, L., Kilanowski, C., Paluch, R., & Kogut-Bossler, B. (2001). Cost-effectiveness of group and mixed family-based treatment for childhood obesity. *International Journal of Obesity and Related Metabolic Disorders, 25*(12), 1843-1849.

Gortmaker, S. L., Peterson, K., Wieccha, J., Sobol, A., Dixit, S., Fox, M., et al. (1999). Reducing obesity via a school-based interdisciplinary intervention among youth. *Archives of Pediatric and Adolescent Medicine, 153,* 409-418.

Harvey-Berino, J., Pintauro, S., Buzzell, P., & Gold, E. (2004). Effect of internet support on the long-term maintenance of weight loss. *Obesity Research, 12,* 320-329.

Healthy People 2010.(2004). Chapter 19, Volume 2: Nutrition and Overweight. Retrieved on November 3, 2004 from, http://www.healthypeople.gov/Document/HTML/Volume2/19Nutrition.htm

Herrera, E. A., Johnston, C. A., & Steele, R. G. (2004). A comparison of cognitive and behavioral treatments for pediatric obesity. *Children's Health Care, 33*(2), 151-167.

Israel, A., Guile, C., Baker, J., & Silverman, W. (1994). An evaluation of enhanced self-regulation training in the treatment of childhood obesity. *Journal of Pediatric Psychology, 19*(6), 737-749.

Israel, A., Silverman, W., & Solotar, L. (1986). An investigation of family influences on initial weight status, attrition, and treatment outcome in a childhood obesity program. *Behavior Therapy, 17*(2), 131-143.

Jacobson, N., & Truax, P. (1991). Clinical significance: A statistical approach to defining meaningful change in psychotherapy research. *Journal of Consulting and Clinical Psychology, 59,* 12-19.

Jelalian, E., Boergers, J., Alday, S., & Frank, R. (2003). Survey of physician attitudes and practices related to pediatric obesity. *Clinical Pediatrics, 42*(3), 235-245.

Jelalian, E., & Saelens, B. (1999). Empirically supported treatments in pediatric psychology: Pediatric obesity. *Journal of Pediatric Psychology, 24*(3), 223-248.

Kazdin, A. E., & Weisz, J. R. (1998). Identifying and developing empirically supported child and adolescent treatments. *Journal of Consulting and Clinical Psychology, 66*(1), 19-36.

Kirschenbaum, D. S., Harris, E. S., & Tomarken, A. J. (1984). Effects of parental involvement in behavioral weight loss therapy for preadolescents. *Behavior Therapy, 15,* 485-500.

Klesges, R. C., Haddock, C. K., Stein, R. J., Klesges, L. M, Eck, L. H., & Hanson, C. L. (1992). Relationship between psychosocial functioning and body fat in preschool children: A longitudinal investigation. *Journal of Consulting and Clinical Psychology, 60,* 793-796.

Landis, J., & Koch, G. G. (1977). The measurement of observer agreement for categorical data. *Biometrics, 33,* 159-174.

Mellin, L., Slinkard, L., & Irwin, C. (1987). Adolescent obesity intervention: Validation of the SHAPEDOWN program. *Journal of the American Dietetic Association, 87*(3), 333-338.

National Center for Health Statistics (2002). Prevalence of Overweight Among Children and Adolescents: United States, 1999-2002. Retrieved on October 30, 2004 from, http://www.cdc.gov/nchs/nhanes.htm.

National School Boards Foundation. (2000). *Research and Guidelines for Children's Use of the Internet.* Available at: http://www.nsbf.org/safe-smart/full-report.htm

Saelens, B., Sallis, J., Wilfley, D., Patrick, K., Cella, J., & Buchta, R. (2002). Behavioral weight control for overweight adolescents initiated in primary care. *Obesity Research, 10,* 22-32.

Staddon, J. E. (1983). *Adaptive Behavior and Learning.* Cambridge: Cambridge University Press.

Tate, D., Wing, R., & Winett, R. (2001). Using Internet technology to deliver a behavioral weight loss program. *Journal of the American Medical Association, 285,* 1172-1177.

Wolf, M. (1978). Social validity: The case for subjective measurement, or how behavior analysis is finding its heart. *Journal of Applied Behavior Analysis, 11,* 203-214.

Yanovski, J. A. (2001). Intensive therapies for pediatric obesity. *Pediatric Clinics of North American, 48,* 1041-1053.

Young-Hyman, D., Schlundt, D. G., Herman, L., DeLuca, F., & Counts, D. (2001). Evaluation of the insulin resistance syndrome in 5- to 10-year old overweight/obese African-American children. *Diabetes Care, 24,* 1359-1364.